SURGICAL ANATOMY

SURGICAL ANATOMY
A Student's Manual

Sibani Mazumdar MBBS MS

Professor and Head
Department of Anatomy
Calcutta National Medical College
Kolkata, West Bengal, India

Ex-Professor
Department of Anatomy
Institute of Postgraduate
Medical Education and Research
West Bengal, India

Ex-Associate Professor
Department of Anatomy
North Bengal Medical College
Darjeeling, West Bengal, India
Calcutta Medical College
Kolkata, West Bengal, India
Nilratan Sircar Medical College
Kolkata, West Bengal, India

Foreword
Tulsibhai C Singel

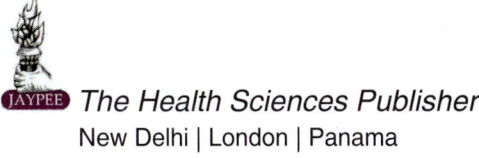

The Health Sciences Publisher
New Delhi | London | Panama

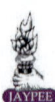

Jaypee Brothers Medical Publishers (P) Ltd

Headquarters

Jaypee Brothers Medical Publishers (P) Ltd
4838/24, Ansari Road, Daryaganj
New Delhi 110 002, India
Phone: +91-11-43574357
Fax: +91-11-43574314
Email: jaypee@jaypeebrothers.com

Overseas Offices

J.P. Medical Ltd
83 Victoria Street, London
SW1H 0HW (UK)
Phone: +44 20 3170 8910
Fax: +44 (0)20 3008 6180
Email: info@jpmedpub.com

Jaypee Brothers Medical Publishers (P) Ltd
17/1-B Babar Road, Block-B, Shaymali
Mohammadpur, Dhaka-1207
Bangladesh
Mobile: +08801912003485
Email: jaypeedhaka@gmail.com

Jaypee-Highlights Medical Publishers Inc.
City of Knowledge, Bld. 235, 2nd Floor, Clayton
Panama City, Panama
Phone: +1 507-301-0496
Fax: +1 507-301-0499
Email: cservice@jphmedical.com

Jaypee Brothers Medical Publishers (P) Ltd
Bhotahity, Kathmandu, Nepal
Phone: +977-9741283608
Email: kathmandu@jaypeebrothers.com

Website: www.jaypeebrothers.com
Website: www.jaypeedigital.com

© 2018, Jaypee Brothers Medical Publishers

The views and opinions expressed in this book are solely those of the original contributor(s)/author(s) and do not necessarily represent those of editor(s) of the book.

All rights reserved. No part of this publication may be reproduced, stored or transmitted in any form or by any means, electronic, mechanical, photocopying, recording or otherwise, without the prior permission in writing of the publishers.

All brand names and product names used in this book are trade names, service marks, trademarks or registered trademarks of their respective owners. The publisher is not associated with any product or vendor mentioned in this book.

Medical knowledge and practice change constantly. This book is designed to provide accurate, authoritative information about the subject matter in question. However, readers are advised to check the most current information available on procedures included and check information from the manufacturer of each product to be administered, to verify the recommended dose, formula, method and duration of administration, adverse effects and contraindications. It is the responsibility of the practitioner to take all appropriate safety precautions. Neither the publisher nor the author(s)/editor(s) assume any liability for any injury and/or damage to persons or property arising from or related to use of material in this book.

This book is sold on the understanding that the publisher is not engaged in providing professional medical services. If such advice or services are required, the services of a competent medical professional should be sought.

Every effort has been made where necessary to contact holders of copyright to obtain permission to reproduce copyright material. If any have been inadvertently overlooked, the publisher will be pleased to make the necessary arrangements at the first opportunity. The **CD/DVD-ROM** (if any) provided in the sealed envelope with this book is complimentary and free of cost. **Not meant for sale.**

Inquiries for bulk sales may be solicited at: jaypee@jaypeebrothers.com

Surgical Anatomy: A Student's Manual

First Edition: **2018**

ISBN: 978-93-5270-149-0

Printed at : Ajanta Offset & Packagings Ltd., Faridabad, Haryana.

Dedicated to

- *All categories of students (medical, dental, paramedical and nursing), whose respect for teachers and eagerness to know the subject inspired me always; and who find the romance in Anatomy*
- *My husband Dr Ardhendu Mazumdar—who is winner of many awards, always gives me inspiration*
- *My son Abishek and my daughter Juee, whose help in day-to-day life helps me to complete the book*
- *My parents Mrs Asha Rani Biswas and Late Ajit Kumar Biswas and My parents-in-law Late Mrs Urmila Mazumdar and Late Dr Aniruddha Mazumdar, whose blessings showered on me all the time*
- *Pupils all over the world and particularly to the generation next.*

Foreword

Dr Professor Sibani Mazumdar, author of two textbooks of anatomy with her husband (co-author), is an institute herself to the galaxy of anatomical world. She needs no further introduction, yet as senior dada (Bhaiya), I have the pleasure of introducing her since her book *Anatomy at a Glance: An Exam-oriented Text* has been translated into different languages of the world particularly in Chinese.

Her recent book (with guidance from Dr Ardhendu Mazumdar-Husband) is expressing its opening through M/s Jaypee Brother Medical Publishers (P) Ltd, New Delhi named as *Surgical Anatomy: A Student's Manual*:

- Students (Postgraduate and undergraduate) who know doctor comes from the Latin word *docere* which means "to teach", will have clinical acumen
- Short notes, surface anatomy, and radiology are represented by simple diagram
- Present NIIT, PG and UG, and DNB exam with explanatory notes is given
- She conducted the cultural and scientific program in NATCON 1996 where not only different delegates attended from India, but also from outside
- She is acting as Medical Council of India (MCI) inspector

- Her activity has been focused in media and press. Her husband Dr Ardhendu Mazumdar has been awarded as "Bharat Ratna" in 2016.
- In this year (2017) she has received Lifetime Achievement Award by Anatomical Society of India–West Bengal Chapter.

Tulsibhai C Singel

Professor
Department of Anatomy
Pacific Medical College and Hospital
Udaipur, Rajasthan

Ex-Professor and Head
BJ Medical College, Ahmedabad
MP Shah Government Medical College, Jamnagar
Government Medical College, Bhavnagar
Gujarat, India

Preface

On the occasion of publication of my present book, *Surgical Anatomy: A Student's Manual*, I express my gratitude to all my beloved students, colleagues, friends and teachers of the fraternity who have accepted and appreciated heartily my previous books, i.e. *Anatomy at a Glance: Exam-oriented Text* (which was also published in Chinese language) and *Dissection Manual, Living and Cross-sectional Anatomy* (the first dissection book by Indian author).

During my long association with teachers and students, I have always felt the need for a book of surgical anatomy as well as explanatory notes. I feel a good knowledge of anatomy will help surgeons to avoid some surgical complications during operations. So I wrote the book which is a brief compilation of short notes, explanatory notes, surface anatomy, radiology and points to remember, which will be very much helpful to all categories of students.

In this book I have marked PGE in some places which are the topics for postgraduate entrance examinations.

Sibani Mazumdar

Acknowledgments

- I express my deep gratitude to Shri Jitendar P Vij (Group Chairman) and Mr Ankit Vij (Group President) of M/s Jaypee Brothers Medical Publishers (P) Ltd, New Delhi along with Kolkata Branch for their constant encouragement in publishing this book.
- I would like to thank Dr Tulsibhai C Singel, Professor, Department of Anatomy, Pacific Medical College and Hospital, Udaipur, Rajasthan, who is my friend, philosopher and guide.
- I would like to thank all the teachers and postgraduate students of Department of Anatomy of Calcutta National Medical College, specially Dr Reshma Betal, Dr Sumita Dutta, Dr Abhijit Roy and Dr Biplab Goswami for their constant support.
- I express my deep gratitude to all the Heads of the Department of various medical colleges who gave me various suggestions during the preparation of the book.
- I also acknowledge some sincere students like Kunal Biswas, Kingshook Mukherjee and Raqueeb Mallik whose help in processing the book was outstanding.
- I am thankful to authors of various medical books who have enriched my knowledge through their valuable writing.
- I am indebted to *Late* Dr IB Singh and Dr Kakar for their permission to incorporate some pictures from their book.

Contents

1. General Anatomy — 1

Bones and Cartilages 2
Function of Bone *2*
Metaphysis (Short Notes) *3*
Characteristic Feature *4*
Law of Union of Epiphysis and the
Growing end of Long Bone *4*
Degeneration of Articular Cartilage
Results in Osteoarthritis *4*
Clinical Anatomy *4*

Joints 11
Definition *11*
Stabilizing Factor of Joint (Short Note) *12*
Certain Important Things about Joints *13*
Clinical Anatomy (Joints) *13*

Muscular System 16
Pennate Muscle (Short Notes) *19*
Clinical Anatomy *19*
Parallel Muscle (Short Notes) *20*

Nervous System 22
Autonomic Nervous System *24*

Arterial System 28

Terminology used in Description of Blood Vessels *31*

Veins 32

Lymphatic System 33

Clinical Anatomy *36*

2. Superior Extremity 38

Short Notes 39

Bones *39*
Muscles *40*
Nerves *44*
Arteries *58*
Spaces *62*
Others *70*

Explanatory Notes 73

Nerve Entrapment of the Upper Limb and Clinical Anatomy *82*

Surface Anatomy 83

Clinical Importance (Surface Anatomy) *83*

3. Inferior Extremity 94

Short Notes 95

Femoral Triangle *95*
Saphenous Opening *96*
Great Saphenous Vein *97*
Perforating Veins *100*
Iliotibial Tract *101*
Profunda Femoris Artery *102*
Interosseous Membrane (Lower Limb) *103*
Acetabular Labrum *104*
Popliteus Muscle *104*
Locking and Unlocking of the Knee Joint *105*
Superficial Peroneal Nerve *106*

Deep Peroneal Nerve *108*
Obturator Nerve *109*
Trendelenburg Test *111*
Factors that Increase the Stability of Hip Joint *111*
Extra-articular Ligament of Knee Joint *111*
Deltoid Ligament *112*
Spring Ligament *113*
Greater Sciatic Foramen *114*
Medial Longitudinal Arch of Foot *115*
Inguinal Lymph Nodes *115*

Explanatory Notes 116

Surface Anatomy of Lower Limb 123

4. Abdomen   126

Short Notes 127
Rectus Sheath *127*
Inguinal Canal *128*
Hesselbach's Triangle *130*
Gastric Triangle *131*
Stomach Bed *131*
Bare Area of Liver *132*
Common Bile Duct *133*
Calot's Triangle *134*
Extrahepatic Biliary Apparatus *134*
Portal Vein *135*
Peyer's Patches *136*
Esophageal Varices *137*
Second Part of Duodenum *138*
Renal Fascia *139*
Hepatorenal Pouch of Morison *140*
Porta Hepatis *141*
Epiploic Foramen *142*
Pelvic Mesocolon *143*
The Mesentery *144*

Lesser Omentum *145*
Coronal Section of Kidney *146*
Base of Urinary Bladder *147*
Membranous Urethra *148*
Ectopic Testis *148*
Ovarian Fossa of Lateral Pelvic Wall *149*
Celiac Trunk *150*
Pudendal Canal *151*
Ischioanal/Ischiorectal Fossa *152*
Fallopian Tube *153*
True Ligaments of Uterus *155*
Superficial Perineal Pouch *156*
Deep Perineal Pouch *157*
Pelvic Diaphragm *158*
Ileocecal Orifice *159*
Ligaments of Spleen *160*
Fascia of Colles *161*
Blood Supply of Vermiform Appendix *161*
Phimosis *162*
Bicornuate Uterus *162*
Cremasteric Reflex *163*

Explanatory Notes 163

Surface Anatomy of Abdomen which is Important to the Clinician and Surgeon 176
Planes *176*
Points *176*

5. Thorax 180

Short Notes 181
Sternal Angle *181*
Typical Intercostal Nerve *181*
Parietal Pleura *182*
Costodiaphragmatic Recess of Pleura *184*
Azygos Lobe of Lung *185*

Mediastinal Surface of the Lungs *185*
Root of the Lung *187*
Bronchopulmonary Segments *188*
Azygos Vein *190*
Accessory Hemiazygos Vein or Inferior Hemiazygos Vein *191*
Artery Supply to Heart (Coronary Circulation) *192*
Blood Supply of Interventricular Septum *193*
Superior Mediastinum *194*
Arch of Aorta *195*
Tetralogy of Fallot *196*
Pericardial Cavity *197*
Coronary Sinus *199*
Constrictions of Esophagus with Clinical Importance *200*
Thoracic Duct *201*

Explanatory Notes 202

Surface Anatomy of Thorax which is Helpful to Clinician and Surgeon 206

Clinical Anatomy (Heart and Pericardium) 208

6. Head, Neck and Brain — 211

Short Notes 212
Sutural Joint *212*
Scalp *213*
Lacrimal Apparatus *215*
Posterior Cricoarytenoid Muscle *216*
Palatine Tonsil *217*
Waldeyer's Ring *218*
Little's Area of Epistaxis *219*
Cornea *220*
Taste Buds *222*
Temporalis Muscle *223*
Hypoglossal Nerve *224*

Movement of Temporomandibular Joint *225*
Parotid Gland *226*
Thyroid Gland *228*
Orbital Fissure *230*
Nasal Cavity *231*

Brain and Eyeball 235

Filum Terminale *235*
Types of Sulci *236*
Neural Crest Cells *237*
Paracentral Lobule *237*
Blood–Brain Barrier *238*
Ciliary Body *238*
Iris *238*
Corpus Callosum *239*
Third Ventricle *242*
Aqueous Humor *243*
Arachnoid Granulations *244*
Rhomboid Fossa *244*
Circle of Willis *245*
Midbrain *247*

Explanatory Notes 249

Surface Anatomy of Head and Neck which is Helpful for Clinician 262

7. Histology 265

Short Notes 266

Transitional Epithelium P.G.E. *266*
Respiratory Epithelium *266*
Histology of Lung *266*
Histology of Duodenum *267*
Microanatomy of Appendix *268*
Histology of Ureter *269*
Histology of Parotid Gland *270*
Kupffer Cells *271*

Skin *271*
Classical Hepatic Lobule *273*
Histology of Esophagus *274*
Sructure of Lymph Node *275*
Suprarenal Gland *276*
White Pulp *277*
Histology of Fallopian Tube *278*
Histology of Spinal Cord (At T10 Segment) *280*
Dermatome *281*
Histology of Cerebellum *281*

Explanatory Note 282

Pimples or Acne is Common in Puberty *282*

8. Genetics   283

Definition *284*

Short Notes 284

Chromosome *284*
Karyotyping *285*
Classification of Chromosomes *285*
Codominant Genes *286*
Down's Syndrome (Mongolism) *287*
Nondisjunction *288*
Turner Syndrome *288*
Klinefelter Syndrome *290*
Barr Body (Sex Chromatin) or X Chromosome Inactivation *291*
Sex Chromosome *291*
Allelic Gene *292*
Translocation *293*
Philadelphia Chromosome *294*
Albinism *294*
Abnormalities Due to Alteration of Chromosomal Morphology *295*

Explanatory Note 296

Terms used in Genetics (Glossary) *297*

9. Embryology   300

Short Notes 301

Spermatogenesis *301*
Oogenesis *301*
Capacitation *303*
Morula *304*
Blastocyst *304*
Zona Pellucida *305*
Notochord *305*
Chorion *306*
Allantois or Allantoenteric Diverticulum *307*
Gastrulation *307*
Different Types of Placenta *308*
Placenta Previa *310*
Placental Barrier *310*
Umbilical Cord *311*
Amnion *311*
Meckel's Diverticulum *312*
Ectopic Pregnancy *313*
Somite *314*
Septum Transversum *316*
Physiological Umbilical Hernia *316*
Nonfusion of Müllerian Duct *317*
Abnormal form or Teratology *318*
Development of Certain Important Organs (Special Embryology) *319*
Nerves *332*

Explanatory Notes 347

10. Radiology: Imaging Technique   350

Conventional Radiography *351*
Standard Position used in Radiological Examination *352*

Other Methods of Imaging Technique *352*
Superior Extremity *354*
Anteroposterior view of Shoulder Joint *354*
Elbow Joint *355*
Posteroanterior view of Wrist Joint and Hand *357*
X-ray of Chest (PA view) *359*
Heart and Aorta *359*
Lungs *361*
Abdomen *362*
Contrast Radiography *362*
Pyelogram *365*
Hysterosalpingogram *367*
Head and Neck *367*
Cervical Spine *370*
Inferior Extremity *372*

11. Postgraduate Short Notes — 378

Mutagenic Agents *379*
Role of Y Chromosome *379*
Mucous Membrane of Small Intestine *379*
Palmar Arterial Arch *382*
Ethmoid Air Sinus *383*
Endochondral Ossification *383*
Blood Supply of Breast *385*
Point Mutation *386*
Duchenne Muscular Dystrophy *386*
Embalming Techniques *387*
Renshaw Cells *388*
Apoptosis *389*
Endocrine Cells of Gut *389*
Coronary Circulation *390*
Morphology and Maturation of T and B Lymphocyte *391*
Cervical Rib *393*
Immunohistochemistry *394*

Superior Colliculus and its Connections *395*
Retina and its Structure *396*
Submandibular Salivary Gland *397*
Frey Syndrome (Auriculotemporal
Syndrome or Gustatory Sweating) *399*
Pituitary *399*
Ossicles of Ear *402*
Movement of Ossicles *403*
Causes of Congenital Deafness *403*
Junctional Complexes *404*
Automatic Bladder *405*
Digital Synovial Sheath and Vinculae *405*
Role of Soft Palate in Swallowing and Phonation *406*
Acquired Immune Deficiency Syndrome *407*
Subphrenic Space *407*
Stem Cell *409*
Reticular Formation of Brainstem *410*
Blood Circulation of Brain *413*
Subclavian Steal Syndrome *414*
Cleidocranial Dysostosis *414*
Papez Circuit *415*
Embryological Types of ASD *415*
Sphincters of Gut *415*

Index *419*

CHAPTER 1

General Anatomy

CHAPTER OUTLINE

Bones and Cartilages
- Introduction
- Function of Bone
- Metaphysis (Short Notes)
- Characteristic Feature
- Law of Union of Epiphysis and the Growing End of Long Bone
- Degeneration of Articular Cartilage Results in Osteoarthritis
- Clinical Anatomy

Joints
- Definition
- Stabilizing Factor of Joint (Short Note)
- Certain Important Things about Joints
- Clinical Anatomy (Joints)

Muscular System
- Introduction
- Pennate Muscle (Short Notes)
- Clinical Anatomy
- Parallel Muscle (Short Notes)

Nervous System
- Introduction
- Autonomic Nervous System

Arterial System
- Introduction
  - Regions where pulsation is felt
- Terminology used in Description of Blood Vessels

Veins
- Introduction
  - Difference between artery and vein

Lymphatic System
- Introduction
  - Thoracic Duct
- Clinical Anatomy

Surgical Anatomy

BONES AND CARTILAGES

INTRODUCTION

Bones and cartilages are specialized connective tissue known as sclerous tissue; bones consist of bone cells (osteoblast—bone forming cells, osteocyte—mature cells, osteoclast—bone destroyer which helps in maintaining the shape of bone) and calcified matrix. As it has rich blood supply, bone can repair much more rapidly than cartilage. Lymphatics are absent in bone marrow.

FUNCTION OF BONE

- Provides mechanical support
- Gives attachment to the muscle
- Constitutes leverage action for augmentation of movement, and
- Is store house of bone marrow.

In case of adult, the site of bone marrow is withdrawn from the manubrium sterni and iliac crest.

Types of cartilages are shown in Table 1.1 and Figure 1.1.

Table 1.1: Cartilage (three types—depending upon the amount and type of protein fibers present in the matrix) (Short note)

Hyaline cartilage (e.g. articular, costal, respiratory) (Fig. 1.1) P.G.E	Elastic cartilage (e.g. epiglottis, pinna) (Fig. 1.1) P.G.E	Fibrocartilage (intervertebral disc) (Fig. 1.1) P.G.E
• Ground glass appearance of matrix	• More flexible than hyaline cartilage	• Resist stretch. Most compressible cartilage
• Collagen fibers present and they are very fine and evenly distributed	• Presence of abundant elastic fibers in matrix	• Abundant collagen fibers which are arranged in thick bundles
• In old age, segmental degeneration of cartilage and partially replace by bone	• No change in old age	• In old age, intervertebral disc becomes thin

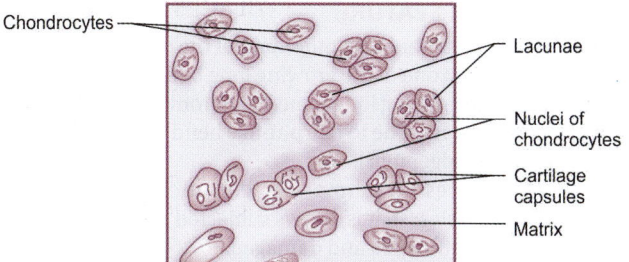
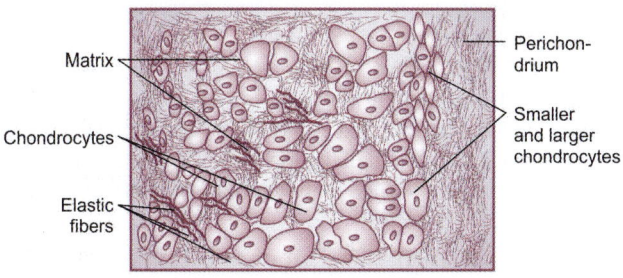
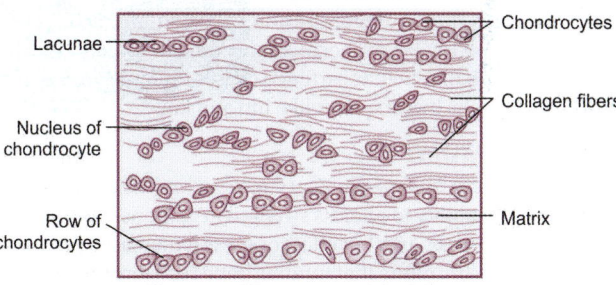

Fig. 1.1: Types of cartilages

METAPHYSIS (SHORT NOTES)

The epiphyseal end of diaphysis of growing bone is known as metaphysis. It is the most growing region of the bone.

Surgical Anatomy

CHARACTERISTIC FEATURE
- Its width is greater than any other part of the diaphysis.
- It is the vascular zone of the growing long bone.
- Infection of the growing long bone starts from here and gives rise to osteomyelitis. It is due to hairpin-like bend of the arteries (site of bacterial enlodgement).
- Metaphysis gives attachment to capsules, ligaments and sometimes muscles; so it is always subjected to stress and strain and hence become weak and damaged.
- Infection of metaphysis is common in children and known as osteomyelitis.

LAW OF UNION OF EPIPHYSIS AND THE GROWING END OF LONG BONE

The law states that the ends of long bone where ossification starts first unite last with the diaphysis and vice versa. So where the ossification starts first is the growing end of the long bone. The growing end lies opposite end of nutrient artery. In milking cow position the direction of artery is always downwards.

DEGENERATION OF ARTICULAR CARTILAGE RESULTS IN OSTEOARTHRITIS

Osteoarthritis is due to degeneration of articular cartilage. This cartilage lacks regeneration because it is devoid of pericondrium. The degeneration of articular cartilage causes difficulty in walking, if it affects the weight-bearing joint like hip and knee.

CLINICAL ANATOMY
- *Effect of exercise and mechanical stress on bone tissue*: Within limit bone has an ability to alter its strength in response to changes to mechanical stress. Another effect of stress is increased production of calcitonin-hormone that inhibits bone reabsorption. Removal of mechanical stress results in demineralization of bone. Main mechanical stresses are those that result from pull of skeletal muscle and pull of gravity. Athlete's bone is stronger and thicker than nonathlete.

- In whole span of life, male loses 15% of skeletal mass and female loses 30% of skeletal mass.
- *Vitamin D deficiency produces rickets in children. Vitamin D deficiency affects the mineralization of osteoids (Haversian system). There is poor absorption of calcium and in turn poor mineralization. There is bowing of legs and knocking of knees due to less strength of bone in children (Figs 1.2A and B).*
- *Osteoporosis*: Reduction of quality of bones both due to reduction of bony minerals and protein content (occurs in old age). It is more common in female in menopausal age group.

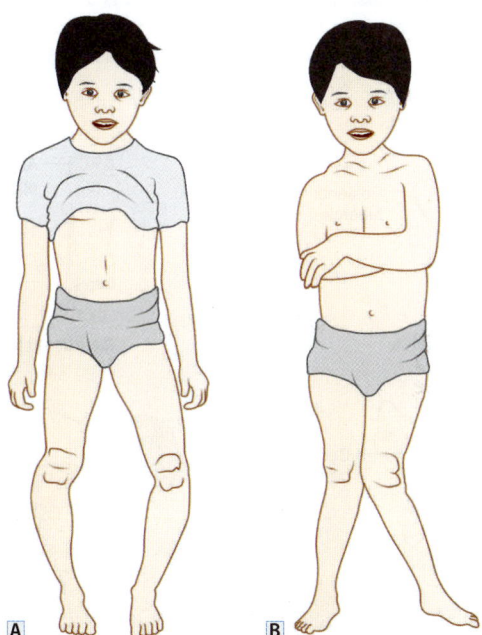

Figs 1.2A and B: Rickets in children: (A) Bilateral genu varum; (B) Bilateral genu valgum

- *Achondroplasia*: It is a congenital anomaly of skeletal system where limb bone is usually shorter but the development of trunk is normal size. This is due to defective endochondral ossification of epiphyseal plate of long bone.
- *Fracture of bone*: It may be partial or along the whole thickness.

Types of Epiphysis (Fig. 1.3, Short Note)

- *Pressure epiphysis*: It bears weight, e.g. head of femur, humerus. P.G.E.
- *Traction epiphysis*: It develops due to muscle pull, e.g. lesser tubercle of humerus is formed by pull of subscapularis. P.G.E.
- *Atavistic epiphysis*: Ancient history says it is a separate piece of bone but adheres to the host bone for nutrition, e.g. coracoid process of scapula, posterior tubercle of talus. P.G.E.

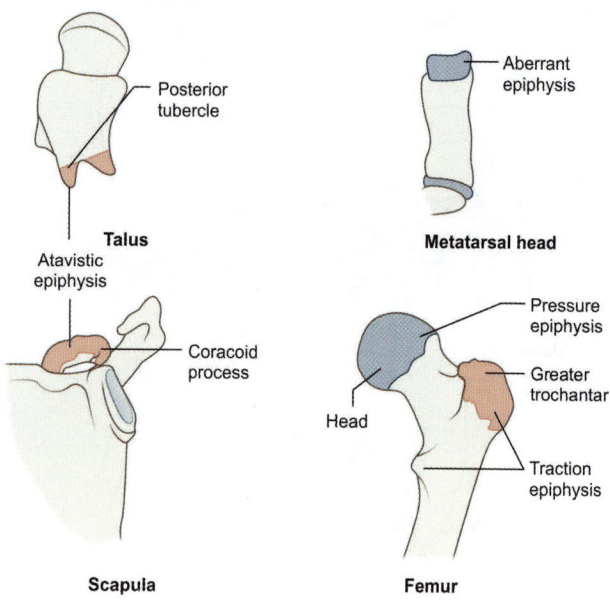

Fig. 1.3: Types of epiphysis

General Anatomy

- *Aberrant epiphysis*: Aberrant means extra. It is an extra epiphysis usually present at the head of first metacarpal. Normal epiphysis is present at the base. So, in spite of one epiphysis there are two.

Ossification (Fig. 1.4, Short Note)

The term ossification means bone formation. The bone formation starts in the embryonic period from a variety of preformed model. The model may be membranous, cartilaginous or membranocartilaginous. When ossification occurs in membranous model it is known as membranous ossification and when it occurs in cartilaginous model it is known as endochondral or cartilaginous ossification. In the developing bone, in the region of shaft, first there is proliferating zone, second zone is the zone of maturation. The third zone is the zone of

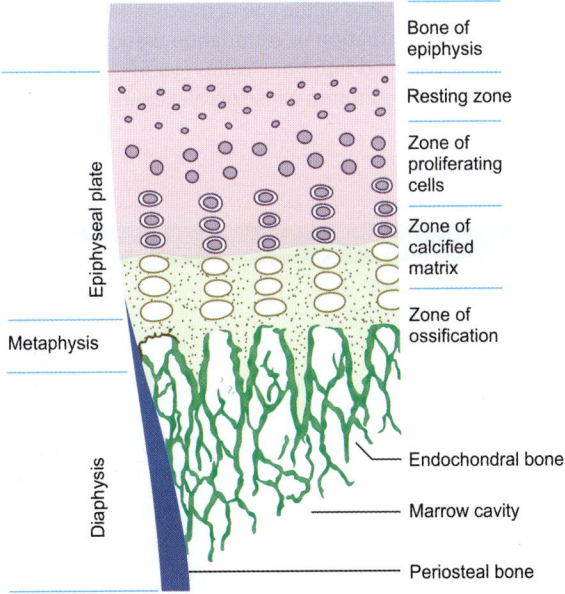

Fig. 1.4: Ossification

hypertrophy. The hypertrophic cartilage suffers from nutrition and death of cartilage occurs. This produces a gap known as primary areolae. This region is invaded by a blood vessel containing osteoblastic cells and osteoclasts. Thus, bone formation starts and it will gradually strengthen the broken model. The artery that enters into the primary areolae is known as nutrient artery. Osteoblasts deposit bone in a lamellar fashion. Osteoclasts is the bone destroyer, remodeled the shape of the bone.

Clinical Anatomy of Bones (in General)

- *Fracture:* Break in the normal outline of bone (Table 1.2 and Figs 1.5A to E).

Union of Fracture

During fracture there is bleeding at fracture site. It is organized as clot. The clot bridges end to end of the site of fracture. Fibroblasts invade the site and there is formation of granulation tissue (young vascular tissue). It will be changed into bony callus (young bone) and union takes place. The most common cause of thickening of bone is callus (Figs 1.6A to D).

Table 1.2: Types of fracture

Fracture type	Description	Comments
Simple	Bone breaks clearly or leanly but does not penetrate the skin	Sometimes called closed fracture
Compound	Broken end of bone protrudes through soft tissue and skin	More serious than simple fracture
Comminuted	Broken bone fragments into many pieces	Common in aged whose bones are more brittle
Greenstick	Bones break incompletely, much like green twigs break	Common in children whose bones are more flexible
Depressed	Broken bone portions are pressed inward	Typical in skull fracture

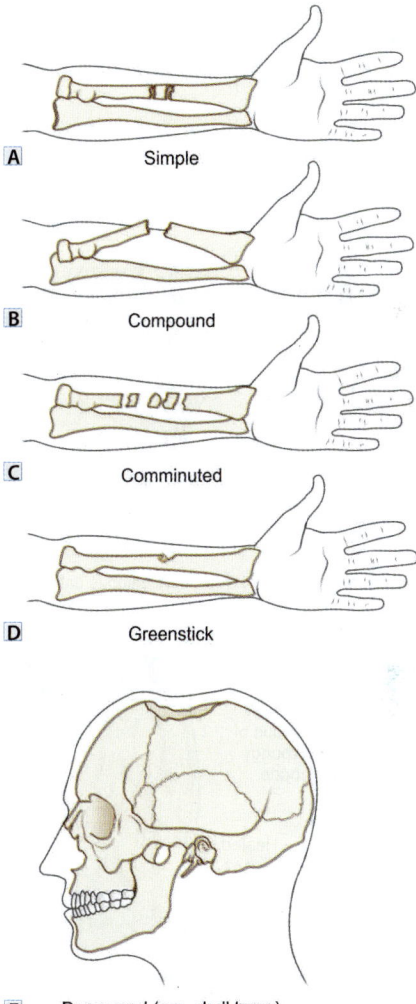

Figs 1.5A to E: Types of fracture

- Plaster or cast applied to heal fracture should not be removed before 6 weeks.
- Union of bone is rapid than cartilage. So, bone repair is rapid than cartilage.
- Greenstick fracture in children is common because of less deposition of inorganic material.

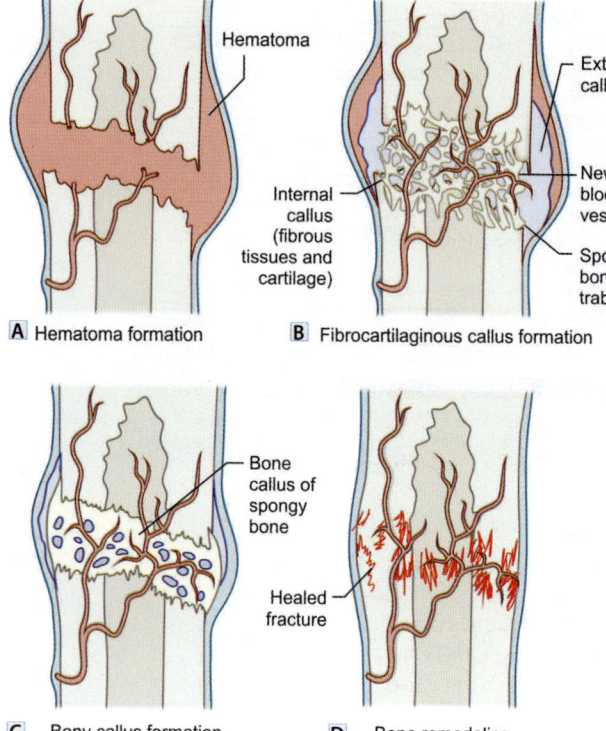

Figs 1.6A to D: Stages in union of fracture

General Anatomy

> **Points to Remember**
> - The area of prominence seen in the body are sacrum, ischial tuberosities, scapula, occiput, greater trochanter, heel, lateral and medial malleoli of ankle, olecranon and over tibial and femoral condyles (lateral and medial) where bedsores (pressure sores) can occur
> - X-ray features of a rickets are the following:
>   - *Epiphysis*: Delayed appearance
>   - *Metaphysis*: Cuping and spreading
>   - *Diaphysis*: Decrease bone density
>   - Bone deformities
> - In long bone metaphysis is the region where acute inflammation takes place known as osteomyelitis
> - Periosteum does not cover the sesamoid bones and three bony ossicles of middle ear
> - Malignant tumor of bone is known as osteosarcoma, usually affected the distal femur, proximal tibia or proximal humerus
> - Bone fractures are seen more often in person without adequate protein, calcium and vitamin D
> - Tuberculosis of short long bones are common (e.g. metacarpal and metatarsal)
> - Membrane bone are protective but not weight-bearing. They have very poor regenerative power
> - Long bone after growth is completed consists of solid structure without epiphyses, metaphyses or epiphyseal cartilage.

JOINTS

DEFINITION
Joints are defined as junction between two or more bones or bones and cartilage or between two cartilages.

Characteristics Features of Synovial Joints
- Wide range of movement is there.
- Bony surface is covered by hyaline cartilage.
- Presence of fibrous capsule which is lined by synovial membrane.
- Joint cavity is flushed by synovial fluid which is rich in hyaluronic acid and which nourishes the avascular articular cartilage.

Blood Supply of a Joint
Epiphyseal vessels enter the long bone at near the attachment of capsule and give anterior branch which ramify in plexus over synovial

membrane. It is seen application of temperature or pressure around a joint, reflexly after the blood flow. Hence, massage is important in case of child as well as in patient with disease.

Nerve Supply of a Joint

Segmental innervation of muscles regulate joint movement. Lasts formulation says four contiguous spinal segment regulate movement of particular joint. Upper two control flexion, adduction, medial rotation. Lower two control extension, abduction, lateral rotation.

Articular nerves contain sensory and autonomic fibers.
- *Hilton's law*: The law states that the nerve supply of a joint comes from nerve supply of nearby muscle and that nerve also supplies the skin over the joint. Therefore, in joint diseases irritation of nerve causes reflex spasm of muscles and referred pain to the skin overlying the muscles.

Physiology of Joint Motion
- *Depending on motion by synovial fluid*: The synovial fluid movement occurs by the compression of all articular cartilages and capsules.
- *Extensibility*: Joint mobility maintains the extensibility of articular tissue. If the joint is immobilized, the ligaments, tendons and cartilage loose its extensibility property and it leads to joint stiffness and hypomobility.

Factors that Limit the Range of Joint Motion

It depends not only on the bony configuration but also on muscle, ligaments and soft tissue envelop. These structures, lead to improper functioning of the joint in disease.

STABILIZING FACTOR OF JOINT (SHORT NOTE)
- Shape of articular surface of opposing bones
- Strength of capsular and intracapsular ligaments
- Strength of surrounding muscles of the joint
- Strength provided by rims of cartilage (glenoid labrum)
- Presence of fibrocartilaginous disc (menisci of knee joint).

CERTAIN IMPORTANT THINGS ABOUT JOINTS

- *0 position*: This is starting position of a joint. In case of shoulder, joint is arm located by the side of chest wall. Always start examination of joint from 0 position.
- Joint articular surfaces are avascular and it receives nutrition from synovial fluid.
- *Closed pack position*: In this position, the joint surfaces are congruent (fits with each other), the ligaments are tight. In this position, dislocation is rare. But damage of intra-articular structure is more common in closed pack position.
- *Loosed pack position*: Any position other than closed pack position is known as loose pack position of joint.

CLINICAL ANATOMY (JOINTS)

Common Joint Injuries

Sprain

It is a condition where the ligaments reinforcing a joint are stretched or torn. The lumbar region, the knee and ankle are common sites of sprain. RICE; R—for rest; I—for ice, C—for compression and E—for elevation, are the standard treatment for pulled muscle, stretched tendons or ligaments. Torn ligament do not heal well.

Cartilage Injuries (Figs 1.7A to C)

- It is common in knee joint, particularly in case of sportsman due to twisting force.
- The avascular cartilage (medial menisci) is unable to repair itself.

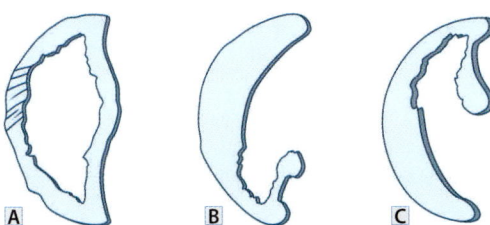

Figs 1.7A to C: Types of meniscal tear: (A) Bucket handle tear (most common); (B) Posterior horn tear; (c) Anterior horn tear

- The patient is unable to fully extend the knee and there is true locking.

Dislocation (Fig. 1.8)
- It involves displacement of articular surfaces of bones.
- It is usually accompanied by sprains, inflammation, and joint immobilization, like fracture, dislocation must be reduced (go back to original position). Shoulder joints, finger joints, thumb, patella and temporomandibular joint are commonly dislocated.
- *Subluxation* is the partial dislocation of a joint. Shoulder joint is commonly subluxated due to loose capsule on inferomedial aspect.
- *Temporomandibular joint* is also dislocated due to loose capsule; even a large yawning produces dislocation. Anterior dislocation of this joint is common. Acromioclavicular joint is also commonly dislocated.

Epiphyseal Injury
Epiphyseal injury occurs in growing long bone. The injuries occur through the weakest area of epiphysis (i.e. through the zone of hypertrophic cartilage). Epiphyseal injury may often be missed as fracture. To clear the doubt (in children), both sided X-ray must be taken for comparison.

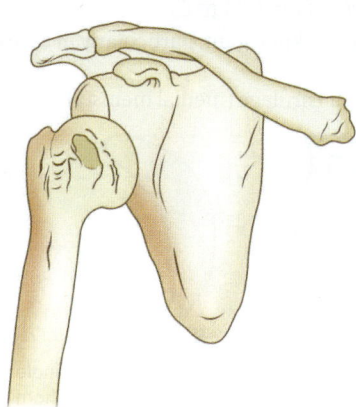

Fig. 1.8: Dislocation of shoulder

Inflammation and degenerative disease of joint includes bursitis, tendinitis and various forms of arthritis.

- *Osteoarthritis:*
  - Most common degenerative joint disease accompanied by stiffness, pain and discomfort.
  - Most common in aged (above 40 years) particularly in women. It is due to wear and tear of articular cartilage and bone demineralization.
  - Weight-bearing joints are mostly affected, e.g. knee joint.
- *Rheumatoid arthritis:*
  - Occurs in any age group (three times more in female).
  - It is most crippling arthritis (due to autoimmune disease) involving severe inflammation of joints.
  - Small joint like, joint of finger, wrist, ankle and feet are affected in the same time (both sides are involved).
- *Joint replacement:* It is a procedure of total or partial replacement of diseased joint by prosthesis (artificial aid). It is most commonly done in knee, hip and shoulder joints. Lifespan of prosthesis is 10–15 years (Fig. 1.9).

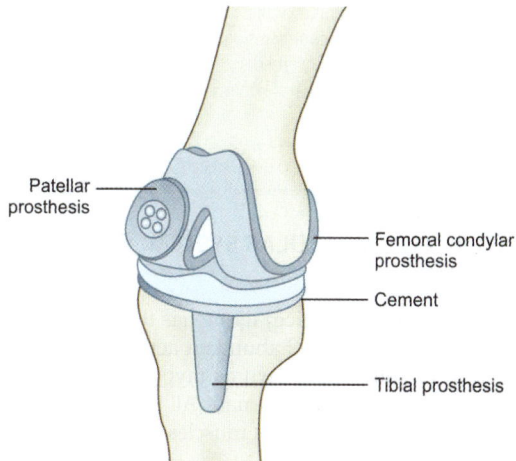

Fig. 1.9: Total knee replacement

- *Arthroscopy:* It is an imaging technique by which a doctor can examine the internal structure of a joint through a small puncture, without the use of extensive surgery.

Q. Greenstick fracture of bone in children? Explain.

Ans. In children, bone cells and collagen fibers are more and minerals and calcium are less. So, bones in case of children are more elastic and the fracture is not involving the full thickness of bone and is known as greenstick fracture.

Must Know Factor of Joint

- Joints are of three varietiess: (1) fibrous, (2) cartilaginous, and (3) synovial.
- All synovial joints possess (1) a cavity enclosed by (2) a fibrous capsule, which is lined inside by (3) synovial membrane.
- Factors maintaining the stability of the joints are: (1) bony configuration, (2) ligaments, and (3) muscles surrounding the joints (e.g. shoulder joint).

> **Points to Remember**
> - Joints are classified as fibrous, cartilaginous and synovial
> - There are more number of joints in a child than in adults. The primary cartilaginous joints at the ends of long bones after fusion disappear in adults
> - Joints are essential for better movements
> - Joints help in increasing the length of bones, increasing the size of cranial, thoracic and pelvic cavities
> - Joints in ear ossicles of middle ear are synovial joints
> - Joints in the laryngeal cartilage help us in speech.

MUSCULAR SYSTEM

INTRODUCTION

Muscle (mouse-like appearance) tissue has the special property of contractility due to presence of abundant actin and myosin protein filament. Muscle cells are known as myocytes. In men, muscle tissue constitutes 40–50% of body mass. All the muscles of body are developed from mesoderm except muscles of hair follicle (arrector pili), muscles of iris which developed from ectoderm. It is important to know that blood flow in skeletal muscle is extremely changeable and varies with muscle activity. Muscles and nerve can tolerate 6 hours of ischemia (lack of blood supply), after that muscle is replaced by connective tissue which reduces the power of muscle. There are three types of muscles (Table 1.3).

Table 1.3: Types of muscles *(Short Notes)*

Features	Skeletal (Fig. 1.10)	Smooth (Fig. 1.11)	Cardiac (Fig. 1.12)
Shape of fibers	• The fibers are cylindrical	Fibers are fusiform or spindle-shaped	Fibers are cylindrical and branched (intercalated disc present at the junction) P.G.E.
Position of nuclei	• Peripherally situated multiple nuclei P.G.E.	Single central nucleus P.G.E.	Single central nucleus P.G.E.
Cross striations	• Numerous prominent cross striation showing light and dark band P.G.E.	No such features	Cross striation may or may not be present (when present, it is faintly stained)
Situation	• They are usually attached to body skeleton	Muscle of organs like gastrointestinal tract, urinary tract, etc.	Present in heart musculature P.G.E.
Function	• Voluntary in function	Involuntary in function	Involuntary in function
Regeneration	• Limited	Limited	No
Contraction	• Quick, forceful	Slow, sustained contraction (peristaltic contraction)	Continuous rhythmic contraction
Nerve supply	• Somatic	Autonomic	Autonomic

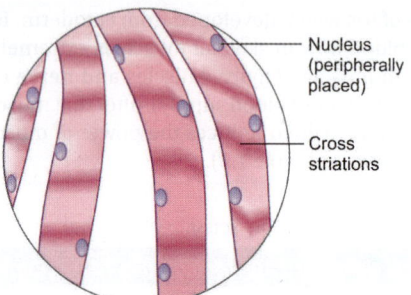

Fig. 1.10: Skeletal muscle

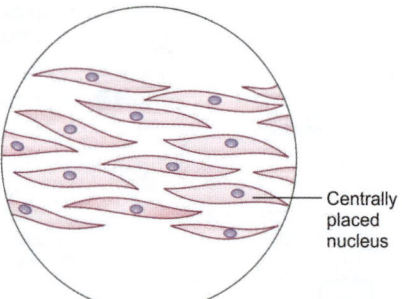

Fig. 1.11: Smooth muscle

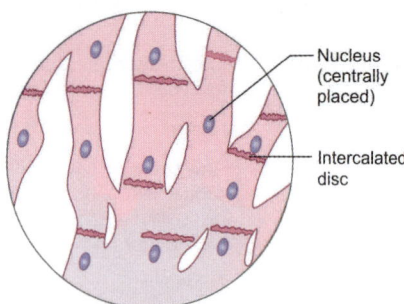

Fig. 1.12: Cardiac muscle

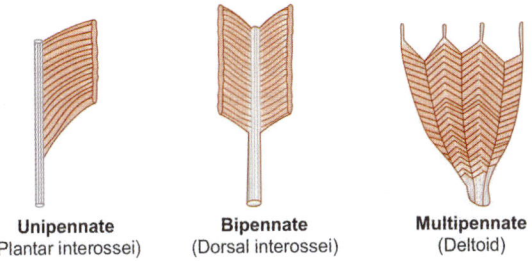

Fig. 1.13: Types of pennate muscles

PENNATE MUSCLE (SHORT NOTES)

Muscle tissue has got the property of contractility. According to orientation of muscle fibers, there are different varieties of muscles. Pennate muscle is one of them. The orientation of its fibers resemble that of a feather, hence the name. Here the muscle fibers are so arranged that their pull is oblique. They are attached to the sides of a tendon. There are different types of pennate muscles (Fig. 1.13):

- *Unipennate*: The muscle fibers are oblique and attached to one side of the tendon, e.g. flexor pollicis longus.
- *Bipennate*: The oblique muscle fibers are attached on both sides of the tendon giving a feathery appearance, e.g. interosseous muscle.
- *Multipennate*: More than one bipennate muscle fibers lie side by side, e.g. deltoid.
- *Circumpennate*: The muscle fibers originate from periphery and converge obliquely on central tendon, e.g. tibialis anterior.

CLINICAL ANATOMY

- *Effect of exercise on muscles*:
    - Regular aerobic exercise results in increased efficiency endurance (tolerance), strength, and resistant to fatigue of skeletal muscles.
    - Resistance exercise causes skeletal muscle hypertrophy (increase in size) and gains in skeletal muscle strength.
- *Muscle tone*: It is the partial state of contraction of muscle. Muscle tone increases at rest and diminishes during activity. Less muscle

tone is known as hypotonia. Excessive tone is known as hypertonia (rigidity and spasticity). Both conditions are seen in diseased state.
- *Cramp*: Sustained spasm of an entire muscle (lasts for a few seconds to several hours) causing the muscle to become tough and painful; common in calf, thigh and hip muscle.
- *Spasm*: A sudden involuntary muscle twitch (range from mere irritation to very painful) due to chemical imbalance; common in eyelid, facial muscle.
- *Muscle strain*: Excessive stretching and forcible tearing (due to overuse and abuse)—the injured muscle is painful and inflamed. Quadriceps and hamstring muscle strain are very common in athletes.
- *Muscle injury*: Very common; formation of hematoma (blood accumulated swelling) within the muscle, e.g. hamstring, gastrocnemius hematoma.
- *Wasting*: Wasting due to disuse and confinement in bed due to peripheral nerve injury.
- *Muscle atrophy*: When the motor nerve supply of a muscle is destroyed, the muscle undergoes atrophic and degenerative changes.

Common patterns of muscle fascicle arrangement are strap, quadrilateral, fusiform, triangular, pennate, spiral, etc. Muscles with parallel fibers shorten most. Pennate muscles shorten less.

Classification of voluntary muscle (according to shape and direction of muscle fibers) has been shown in Figure 1.14.

PARALLEL MUSCLE (SHORT NOTES)

The muscles fibers are parallel to the line of the pull. The fibers are long but their numbers are relatively few.

Types

Parallel muscles are divided into following subtypes (Fig. 1.15):
- Quadrilateral, e.g. quadratus lumborum
- Strap muscle, e.g. sartorius
- Strap with tendinous intersections, e.g. rectus abdominis
- Fusiform muscle, e.g. biceps brachii.

General Anatomy

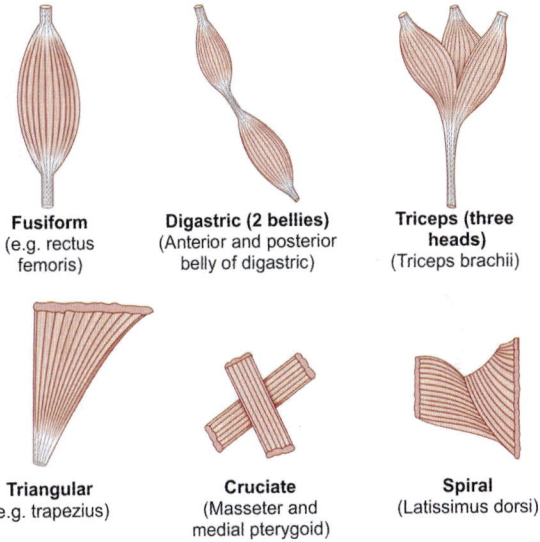

Fig. 1.14: Classification of voluntary muscle (according to shape and direction of muscle fibers)

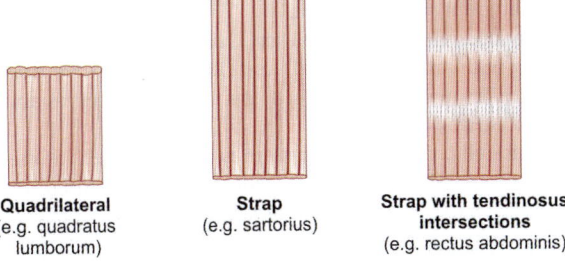

Fig. 1.15: Types of parallel muscles

Functions

- Range of movement is more due to the mere length of fibers
- Force of contraction is less due to less number of muscle fibers.

> **Points to Remember**
>
> - Heat rigor occurs above 43°C where the muscle protein gets denatured
> - Smooth muscle has got most good regenerative capacity than skeletal and cardiac muscle
> - Smooth muscle fiber does not contain myofibrils
> - Fibrillation is abnormal contraction of cardiac muscle
> - *Myasthenia gravis*: In this disease, there is defective synthesis of acetylcholine at motor end plate of the muscle. It produces fatigue of muscle contraction. Young female and old male are mostly affected. There is fatigue of ocular muscle, facial muscles. There is difficulty in chewing, whistling, speech and swallowing. Neck muscles are weakend and do not have normal posture. Respiratory difficulty may result. This is an immune disorder
> - *Myopathy*: A disease of muscles where there are pathological, electrical, biochemical changes of muscle. It may be congenital, endocrine, inflammatory or metabolic disorder.

NERVOUS SYSTEM

INTRODUCTION

The nervous system is controlling and communicating system of our body. Its main functions are to monitor, integrate, and response to information on the environment.

It is divided into two major parts: (1) *central nervous system* (CNS) (including brain and spinal cord) and (2) *peripheral nervous system* (PNS) (12 pairs of cranial nerves, 31 pairs of spinal nerves and their associated ganglia).

Functionally, the nervous system is again divided into *somatic nervous system* (which controls *voluntary* function) and *autonomic nervous system* (ANS) (control *involuntary* function).

Histology of Nervous Tissue

The structural and functional unit of nervous system is neuron (Fig. 1.16). They have a cell body and cytoplasmic processes called axon and dendrites. All neurons have one axon with few exceptions.

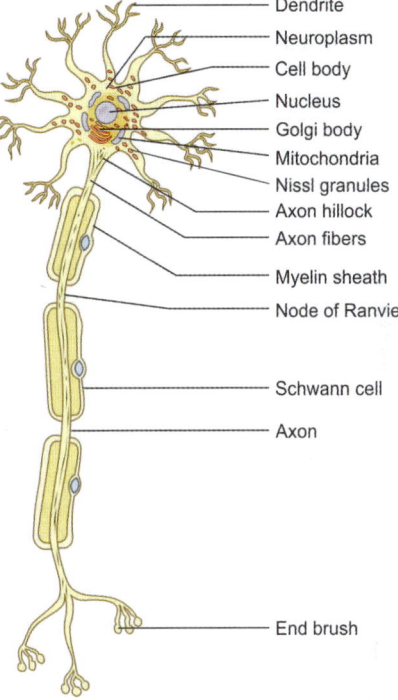

Fig. 1.16: Structure of a neuron

Axon transmits impulse away from nerve cell. The axon hillock is the most excitable part of the axon. The axon ends in enlarged terminals which secretes neurotransmitter. The large axons (nerve fibers) are myelinated. Myelination is done by Schwann cell in PNS and oligodendrocyte in CNS. In some places, the myelin sheath is absent known as nodes of Ranvier. The purpose of myelination is propagation of wave of excitation rapidly and also insulation. Myelinated nerve fibers are seen in muscles where reaction speed is needed; whereas unmyelinated fibers occur in transmission of visceral pain.

Neuroglia

These are the supporting cells of CNS. There are different types of neuroglial cells:
- *Astrocytes*: They are concerned with the nutrition of the nervous tissue. They are of two types:
  1. Protoplasmic astrocyte
  2. Fibrous astrocyte.
- *Oligodendrocytes* are like Schwann cells. They myelinate the CNS.
- *Microglia*: Their action is that of macrophages.
- *Ependymal cells*: They are short columnar cells lining the cavities of CNS.

Clinical Anatomy
- Proliferation of glial cells is called "gliosis". A CNS lesion is healed by gliosis.
- Tumor of the glial cells is the most common tumor of CNS.

Spinal Nerves

Spinal nerves are united ventral and dorsal roots, attached in a series, to the side of the spinal cords. They are 31 pairs: 8 cervical, 12 thoracic, 5 lumbar, 5 sacral, and 1 coccygeal. These emerge through intervertebral foramina. Except T_2-T_{12}, all ventral rami join one another forming nerve plexuses. This plexuses occur in the cervical, brachial, lumbar and sacral regions.

AUTONOMIC NERVOUS SYSTEM

It is the part of nervous system that controls automatic activity of our body (i.e. involuntary activity) like heart, smooth muscles and gland. It is divided into two parts—sympathetic and parasympathetic and both parts have afferent and efferent nerve fibers.

Sympathetic Trunk (Fig. 1.17)

They lie on either side of vertebral column; extends from base of the skull to the coccyx. It looks like a knotted thread. There are three cervical ganglia: (1) superior cervical ganglia (largest, formed by the fusion of upper four cervical ganglia), (2) middle cervical ganglia (smallest of the three, formed by the fusion of fifth and sixth cervical ganglia) and (3) inferior cervical ganglia (intermediate in size, formed

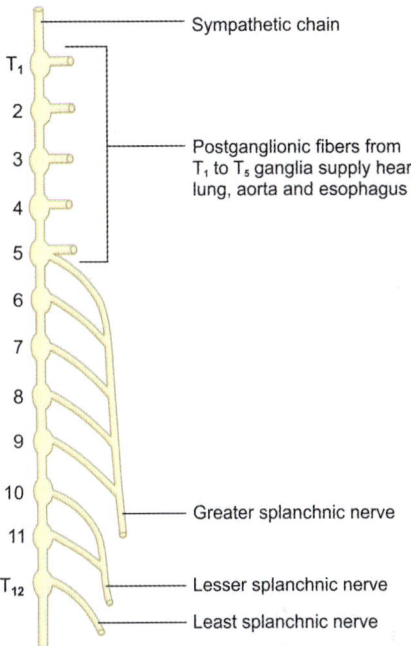

Fig. 1.17: The thoracic part of the sympathetic trunk and its splanchnic branches (schematic)

by the fusion of seventh and eighth cervical ganglia. This ganglia lies between carotid sheath and prevertebral fascia, eleven thoracic, four lumbar, four sacral ganglia. The sympathetic ganglions are structures where synapse (white rami) between pre- and postganglionic fiber takes place. The right and left trunk coverage medially and form ganglion impar (unpaired) in front of coccyx. Most preganglionic fibers reach the sympathetic trunk; they have three types of termination:

- They may terminate in the ganglion they have entered. These postganglionic nerve fibers (known as rami), now pass through the thoracic spinal nerve and supply the smooth muscle of blood vessels and sweat glands.

Surgical Anatomy

- The fibers may ascend high up and terminate in cervical ganglia or lower fiber may descend down in lower lumbar and sacral ganglia.
- Some of the preganglionic fibers may pass through the ganglia on thoracic part of sympathetic trunk without synapsing. These fibers form *three splanchnic nerves*.
    - *Greater splanchnic nerve*: Arise from fifth to ninth thoracic ganglia pierces the diaphragm and synapses (neuroneuronal junction) with celiac plexus.
    - *Lesser splanchnic nerve*: Arise from tenth and eleventh thoracic ganglia, pierces diaphragm and synapses with lower part of plexus.
- *Least splanchnic nerve*: Spinal nerves correspond to the same segment of spinal cord, but the sympathetic pathways do not correspond with the segment of spinal cord.
    - T_1 segment—passes up and goes to head region
    - T_2 segment—goes to neck
    - T_3-T_6 segment—into thorax
    - T_7-T_{11} segment—for abdomen
    - T_{12}-L_2 segment—for leg

According to some author, the parasympathetic system is represented as D division [i.e. digestion, defecation, diuresis (urination)]. The sympathetic system is represented as E division (i.e. excitement, exercise, embarrassment and emergency). Autonomic function is controlled at different levels: (1) reflexes are controlled at spinal cord and brainstem level, (2) hypothalamus controls the integration with autonomic, somatic and endocrine response, and (3) frontal lobe of cerebral cortex controls ANS at subconscious level via limbic connections. The efficiency of ANS decreases in old age.

Preganglionic fibers are cholinergic in both sympathetic and parasympathetic; postganglionic sympathetic fiber is adrenergic except for sweat gland and arrector pili muscle. Postganglionic neuron of parasympathetic is cholinergic. Parasympathetic is essential for life.

Clinical Anatomy

Autonomic nervous system is involved in every important process that goes in our body. Most autonomic disorders reflect, excess, or deficient controls of smooth muscle activity. Unlike CNS, the ANS can be easily and effectively controlled by drugs.

- *Hypertension (high blood pressure)*: It may result from excessive sympathetic activity. It is known as stress-induced hypertension.
- *Vaso-occlusive disease*: They are Raynaud's disease affecting the upper limb, Buerger's disease affecting the lower limb. It is characterized by gradual cyanosis (bluish coloration); pain in the affected region in severe cases gangrene (tissue death) may result. To treat severe cases, sympathectomy (cutting of sympathetic trunk in a particular segment) is done. The involved vessels dilate, re-establishing adequate blood supply to the affected region.
- *Congenital megacolon (Hirschsprung's disease)*: In this condition, parasympathetic innervation of the distal part of colon fails to develop. As a result, distal colon is immobile and dilated. The condition is corrected surgically.
- *Achalasia (not relaxed)*: A condition where esophagus is unable to propel food in the lower part due to parasympathetic neuron deficiency. The distal esophagus becomes dilated and vomiting is common.
- *Horner's syndrome*: It results from an interruption of the sympathetic nerve supply to head and neck. The affected person exhibits constriction of pupil (myosis), slight drooping of eyelid (ptosis), vasodilatation of skin arterioles (flashing of face) and loss of sweating (anhidrosis). Common sites of lesion are brainstem, cervical part of spinal cord or stellate ganglion.

Points to Remember

- Neuropathy is a disease of nerve which may affect sensation, movement, gland or organ function depending upon which nerve is involved.
- *Neuropraxia*: It is temporary interruption or physiological block of conduction without loss of action continuity.
- Axonotmesis is the loss of relative continuity of axon and its myelin but connective tissue framework is preserved.
- Neurotmesis is total destruction of entire nerve fiber.
- Myelin sheath of PNS is formed by Schwann cells and that of CNS is formed by oligodendrocytes.

ARTERIAL SYSTEM

INTRODUCTION

All animals and human being require a mechanism to distribute oxygen and nutrition throughout the tissues of body and to collect waste product and carbon dioxide from the tissues. So, there is requirement of blood—vascular system. It requires a muscular pump—the heart. Various types of blood vessels like (1) arteries, (2) arterioles (3) capillaries, (4) sinusoids, (5) venules, and (6) veins are present within the body.

- Arteries: Arteries are of three types:
    1. *Elastic or large size arteries*: Here tunica media (middle coat) contains more elastic tissue, e.g. aorta, carotid, subclavian, axillary, and common iliac arteries.
    2. *Muscular or medium size arteries*: Most widely distributed. Tunica media consists of predominantly muscle fiber, e.g. brachial, radial, femoral, gastric, superior mesenteric arteries.
    3. *Arteriole*: It is the smallest arteries having a diameter of 100 micron. They act as resistant vessel to maintain peripheral blood pressure.
- Capillaries: Primary exchange vessel. Carry blood from arteriole to venule. Arteriole, capillaries and venules together constitutes microcirculation.
- Sinusoids: Large lumen and tortuous course. Absent or incomplete basement membrane. Very porous (Table 1.4).

Angiogram: Visualization of arterial tree by radiopaque dye is known as angiogram. At the upper limb brachial artery (just above the cubital

Table 1.4: Differences between sinusoids and capillaries (Fig. 1.18)

Sinusoids	Capillaries
• Wider, irregular spaces	• Narrow regular space
• Lined by endothelial, reticuloendothelial cells, which may be interrupted, fenestrated	• Lined by continuous endothelial cells
• Basal lamina is not continuous	• Basal lamina is continuous

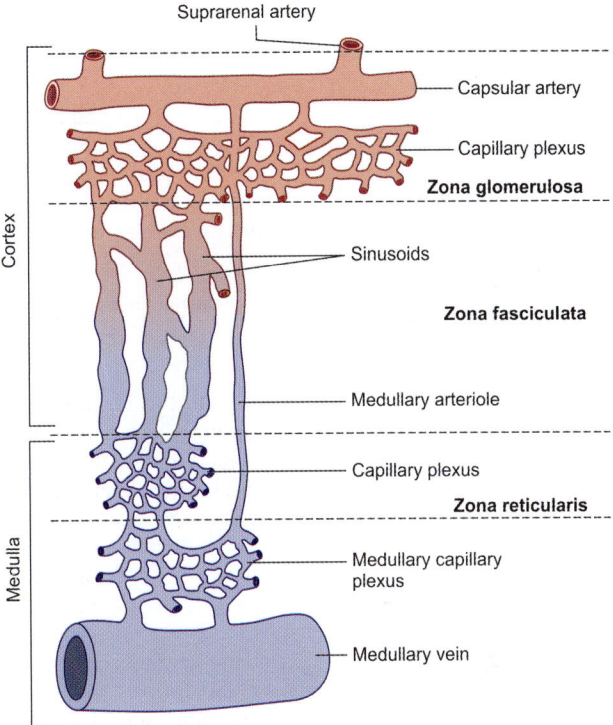

Fig. 1.18: Comparison between capillary and sinusoids (seen within suprarenal gland)

fossa) and radial artery (region where radial pulse is felt) are the common site, common carotid artery in neck (near its bifurcation) and femoral artery in lower limb (just below the inguinal ligament) in the site of choice for angiography (Fig. 1.19 and Table 1.5). Various regions in the body where arterial pulsations can be felt are shown in Figure 1.19.

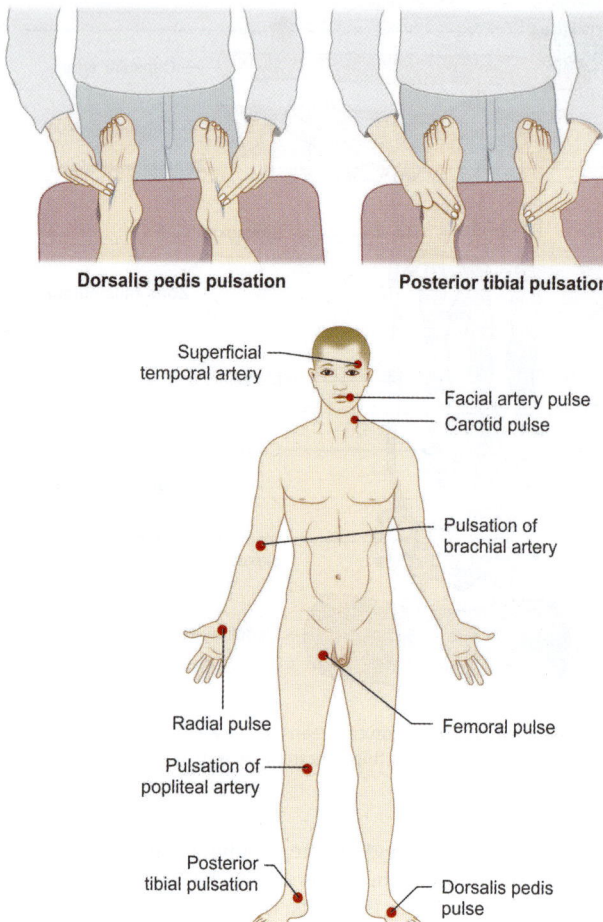

Fig. 1.19: Regions where arterial pulsation is felt (peripheral arterial pulse)

Table 1.5: Body regios where pulsation in felt

Pulse	Location	Condition required for feeling the pulse
Temporal	In front of auricle at the root of the zygomatic arch	Easily felt in children and in adult easily accessible site by anesthetist
Facial	At the anterior-inferior angle of master	Easily accessible site by anesthetist
Carotid	Along the anterior border of sternocleidomastoid in neck of the upper border of thyroid cartilage	It is the accessible site during cardiac arrest
Brachial	Medial to the tendon of biceps brachii in the cubital fossa	This pulse is required to measure the blood pressure
Radial	At wrist in front of forearm on radial side	Clinician used to access the rate and character of the pulse
Femoral	Below the inguinal ligament midway between anterior superior iliac spine and symphysis pubis	Used during cardiac arrest
Dorsalis pedis	Over dorsum of foot between extensor retinaculum of great and other toe	Used to access the circulation of lower limb in case vaso-occlusive disease

TERMINOLOGY USED IN DESCRIPTION OF BLOOD VESSELS

- Angina pectoris: Chest pain
- Artery: Carries more oxygenated blood away from the heart
- Embolous: Plug
- Infarction: Virtually blood less area
- Ischemia: Lacking adequate blood supply
- Stenosis: Narrowing
- Vein: Carries poorly oxygenated blood towards the heart
- End artery: The artery which have no precapillary anastomosis
- Vasa vasorum: A vessel supplying a vessel is known as vasa vasorum. It is present in tunica adventitia coat of large vessels. E.g. coronary arteries.

> **Points to Remember**
> - In old age, the arteries become stiff and prominent. This phenomenon is known as arteriosclerosis.
> - In arteriosclerosis usually large- and medium-sized arteries are affected.

VEINS

INTRODUCTION

Veins are the channels that carry blood toward the heart. Poorly oxygenated blood is carried by all veins in the body except pulmonary veins which carries oxygenated blood. It possess thin muscle wall and numerous than the arteries. Veins are elliptical in collapsed state and circular in filling state. Venous valves are numerous in distal part of lower extremity and the number of valves decreases proximally. There is no valve in superior and inferior vena cava. It is formed from capillary tissue fluid (micromolecular in nature). Blood vessels are arranged in following pattern. Arteries have supply function, capillary (terminal vascular bed) have exchange function and veins have reservoir function. In human body four types of venous system are present: (1) caval system, (2) portal venous system, (3) azygos venous system, and (4) paravertebral veins.

Must know:

Differences between artery and vein have been given in Table 1.6.

Table 1.6: Difference between artery and vein

Artery	Vein
• Takes more oxygenated blood away from the heart (except pulmonary artery)	• Carries deoxygenated blood toward the heart (except pulmonary vein)
• Valves absent	• Valves present
• The wall is thick, muscular and elastic	• The wall is thin, less muscular and nonelastic
• The lumen is smaller	• The lumen is bigger
• Are not collapsible	• Are collapsible
• Contain blood under high pressure	• Contain blood under low pressure
• Blood flows fast	• Blood flows slow
• Blood flows by jerks caused by beating of heart	• Blood flows evenly without any jerks

Points to Remember

- Venous insufficiency is the most common disorder of the venous system, and is usually manifested as varicose vein.
- Deep vein thrombosis is a condition in which a blood clot forms in a deep vein, which leads to pulmonary embolism and chronic venous insufficiency.
- Emissary vein (medium size vein) present in head and neck are valveless.

LYMPHATIC SYSTEM

INTRODUCTION

Apart from artery and vein, there exist another channel in our body, i.e. lymphatic system. Lymphatic system is accessory to venous system. It also drains tissue fluid from the tissue spaces like veins, but the difference is that it carries protein and fat macromolecules from tissue spaces. The veins carry micromolecular substance from tissue space (Fig. 1.20). Lymphatic tissue is essential for immunological defense of the body from bacteria and viruses. Lymphatic tissue starts developing in the 5th week of intrauterine life.

Lymph is the name given to the tissue fluid, once it has entered a lymphatic vessel. Composition of lymph varies from one part of body to another. Before lymph is drained into the bloodstream, it passes at

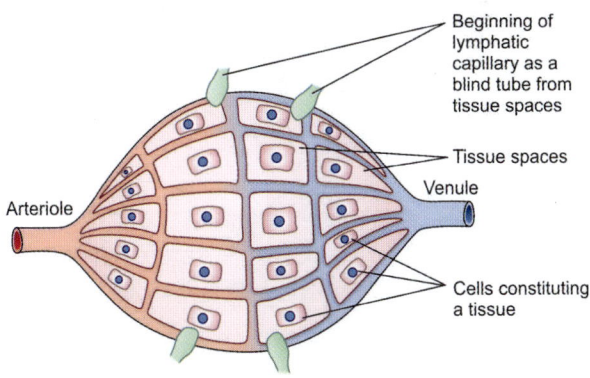

Fig. 1.20: Formation of lymph capillary

least one lymph node (small masses of lymphatic tissue), sometimes several. The lymph vessels have numerous valves. The lymph vessels which carry lymph toward the lymph node is known as afferent vessel, and that of which carries lymph away from lymph node is known as efferent vessel. The lymph reaches the bloodstream at the root of the neck by two large lymph vessels called right lymphatic duct and thoracic duct (Fig. 1.21).

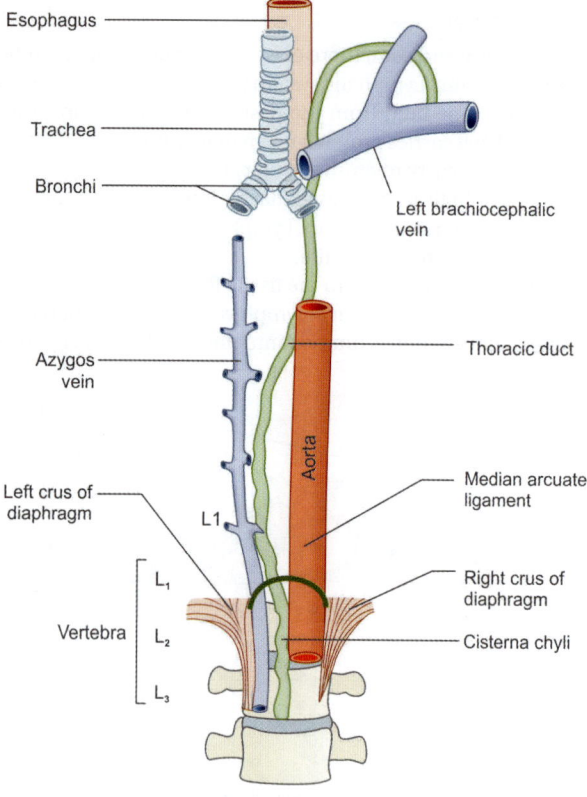

Fig. 1.21: Thoracic duct

General Anatomy

The thoracic duct (45 cm long) begins in the abdomen from a sac; cysterna chyli, and enters the thorax through an opening (aortic opening) of diaphragm. It ascends through thorax, lies in front of 7th thoracic vertebrae. At the level of T4 and T5 it bends toward left, lies between aorta on the left-hand side and azygos vein on the right-hand side in the posterior mediastinum behind the esophagus. It then ascends into neck and drains into the angle, formed by left internal jugular and left subclavian vein. *From thoracic duct lymph is pumped into venous system during inspiration.* The rate of flow of lymph is indirectly proportional to the depth of inspiration. Most of the lymph flow of the body is due to contraction of skeletal muscle like veins.

The right lymphatic duct drains lymph from the body's right upper quadrant (right side of head and neck, right upper limb and right half of thorax). The thoracic duct drains lymph from remainder of the body (Fig. 1.22). Lymph formation is directly proportional to arterial flow

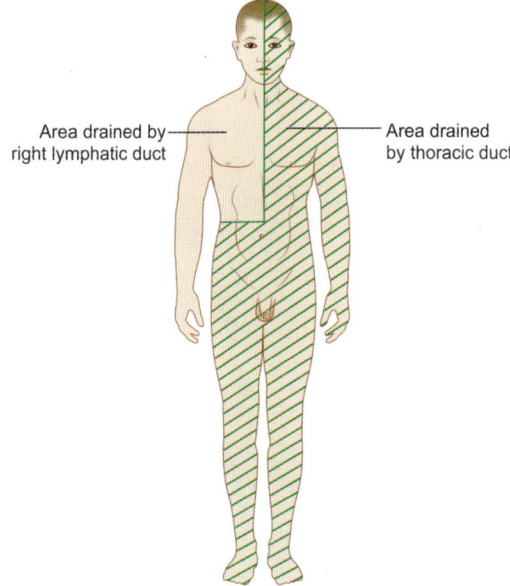

Fig. 1.22: Lymphatic drainage of whole body

and 40% of lymph is formed within skeletal muscle. In the abdomen and pelvis highest number of lymph node is present.

The central nervous system, the eyeball; the internal ear, the epidermis of skin, cartilage and bone are devoid of lymphatic vessels.

CLINICAL ANATOMY

- *Lymphangitis:* It is the inflammation of lymph vessel. When lymph vessels are severely inflamed, the vasa vasorum (vessel supplying a vessel) become congested with blood. As a result the pathway of the associated lymphatics becomes visible through skin as red line and painful to touch.
- *Lymphadenitis*: It is the inflammation of lymph node. These two phenomena may occur when the lymphatic system is involved in the spread of cancer cell.
- *Lymphedema*: The accumulation of lymph in tissue space. It occurs when lymph is not drained from an area of the body (Fig. 1.23). It is seen in coastal region of Odisha. There is repeated

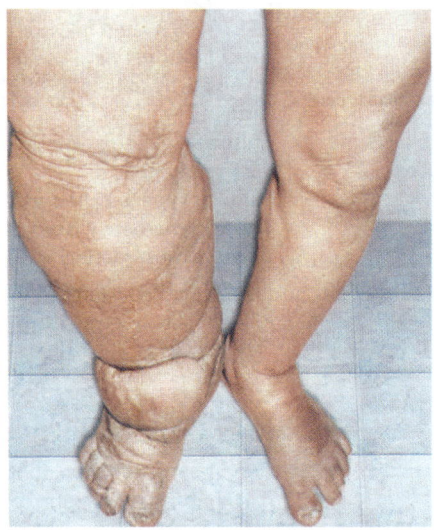

Fig. 1.23: Lymphedema (elephantiasis)

attack by filarial bacteria. The lower limb is most commonly affected and the condition is known as elephantiasis; edema of upper limb occurs due to removal of axillary lymph node for cancer of breast.
- *Lymphomas*: These are the tumor of lymph glands and are classified as Hodgkin's and non-Hodgkin's lymphomas.

> **Points to Remember**
> - Lymph nodes are sites of antigenic recognition and antigenic activation
> - Spleen is a lymphoid organ which has got abundant blood supply.

2

Superior Extremity

CHAPTER OUTLINE

Bones
- Coracoid Process
- Surgical Neck of Humerus

Muscles
- Deltoid Muscle
- Biceps Brachii Muscle
- Supinators of Forearm
- Pectoralis Major Muscles
- Rotator Cuff Muscle

Nerves
- Brachial Plexus
- Median Nerve
- Ulnar Nerve
- Radial Nerve
- Axillary Nerve
- Musculocutaneous Nerve
- Posterior Interosseous Nerve
- Anatomical Snuffbox
- Palmaris Brevis
- Dorsal Digital Expansion

Arteries
- Axillary Artery
- Radial Artery
- Anastomosis Around the Elbow Joint

Spaces
- Clavipectoral Fascia
- Cubital Fossa
- Triangular and Quadrangular Space
- Space of Parona and its Clinical Importance
- Clinical Importance of Midpalmar and Thenar Space

Others
- Pulled Elbow
- Flexor Retinaculum of Hand
- Character of Interosseous Membrane of Upper Limb
- Ulnar Paradox

SHORT NOTES

BONES

Coracoid Process (Figs 2.1 and 2.2)

- The word 'corac' means crow's beak.
- It is an example of atavistic type of epiphysis.
- It is located below the junction of lateral one-fourth and medial three-fourths of the clavicle.
- In anatomical position, it is directed forward and slightly laterally.
- Short head of biceps and coracobrachialis arise from its tip by a common tendon.
- Pectoralis minor is attached to its medial border.
- The main strong ligament the coracoclavicular ligament (which has got conoid and trapezoid part) attached to root of coracoid process and a ridge on the superior part of coracoid process.

Clinical Anatomy

- The weight is transmitted to clavicle through coracoclavicular ligament.

Surgical Neck of Humerus

- It is the narrowest part at the junction of upper end and shaft.
- It is related to axillary nerve and posterior circumflex humeral vessels.
- It forms boundary of lateral wall of axilla.
- Against it the structures present in lateral wall of axilla are palpated.

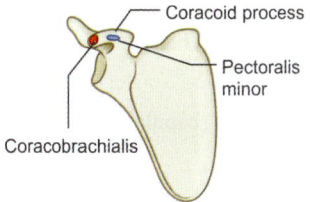

Fig. 2.1: Caracoid process of scapula

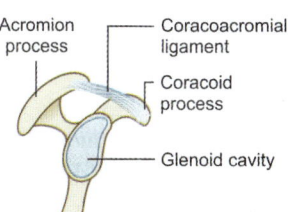

Fig. 2.2: Attachment of ligament at coracoid process

- It is vulnerable to fracture, in which case the axillary nerve and posterior circumflex humeral vessel are liable to be injured.

MUSCLES

Deltoid Muscle

- It is delta (Δ)-shaped muscle, so the name.

Origin: Anterior border lateral one-third of clavicle; acromion, lower lip of spine of scapula.

Insertion: The deltoid muscle is inserted in the deltoid tuberosity in middle of lateral surface of shaft of humerus.

Description: It is a thick, multipennate muscle, forming the rounded contour of shoulder.

Clinical Importance

It is the suitable site of intramuscular injection because it is well developed in adults and injection is given the upper part of lower half of the muscle.

Nerve supply
It is supplied by the axillary nerve.

Action
- Abducts arm
- Anterior fibers flex and medially rotate the arm
- Posterior fibers extend and laterally rotate the arm
- Action is antagonist of pectoralis major and latissimus dorsi.

Biceps Brachii Muscle

The biceps brachii muscles fall under the group of the anterior brachial muscles (Fig. 2.3).

It has two heads: (1) long head, and (2) short head.

Origin
- Long head—from supraglenoid tubercle of scapula.
- Short head—coracoid process of scapula.

Insertion
- The tendon is inserted into the posterior part of the radial tuberosity whose anterior part is separated by a bursa

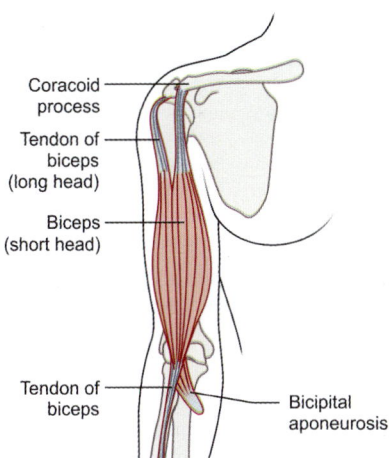

Fig. 2.3: Biceps brachii muscle

- As bicipital aponeurosis going from the tendon downward and medially to the antebrachial fascia and is attached to subcutaneous posterior border of ulna.

Description
Fusiform muscle. Two heads unite near about middle of arm.

Nerve supply
Branch of musculocutaneous nerve (C5, C6).

Action
- Flexor elbow joint and supinate the forearm.
- Long head stabilizes shoulder joint.

Clinical Importance
Tendon of biceps brachii in the cubital fossa acts as a guide to locate the brachial pulse which helps to measure the blood pressure.

Supinators of Forearm

Supination is turning of palm anteriorly from midprone position as if somebody is taking something. The supinators of forearm are: (1) biceps brachii, and (2) supinator (Table 2.1).

Table 2.1: Supinators of forearm

Muscles	Origin	Insertion	Nerve supply
Biceps brachii	By two heads: • Long head—by supraglenoid tubercle • Short head—from coracoid process	The two heads unite and form fusiform belly and inserted into tuberosity of radius and bicipital aponeurosis	Musculocutaneous nerve of forearm
Supinator	Lateral epicondyle of humerus, annular ligament	Neck and shaft of radius	Posterior interosseous nerve

Clinical Anatomy

Rupture of long head of biceps tendon occurs in intertubercular sulcus during flexion against excessive resistance like weight lifting, the tear weakens the muscle and also weakens supination.

Pectoralis Major Muscles (Table 2.2)

Table 2.2: Muscles of pectoral region

Muscle	Origin	Insertion	Description	Nerve supply	Action
Pectoralis major (pectus—chest; major—large)	Clavicle, sternum and upper six costal cartilages	Lateral lip of bicipital groove of humerus	Large, fan-shaped muscle, covering upper portion of chest, forms anterior axillary fold	Medial and lateral pectoral nerves from brachial plexus	Adducts arm and rotate it medially clavicular fibers also flex arm

Rotator Cuff Muscle

It is a musculotendinous cuff of shoulder joint. It is formed by four flattened tendons namely (Fig. 2.4 and Table 2.3):
1. Supraspinatus
2. Infraspinatus

Table 2.3: Rotator cuff muscles

Muscles	Origin	Insertion	Description	Nerve supply	Action
Supraspinatus (supra—above: a muscle lies above the spine) [rotator cuff muscle]	Supraspinous fossa of scapula	Greater tuberosity of humerus (superior facet), and shoulder joint	Lies deep to trapezius and it is a most vulnerable to injury who perform repeated throwing movements	Suprascapular nerve	Abducts and stabilizes shoulder joint. Prevent downward dislocation of shoulder while carrying a heavy suitcase
Infraspinatus (infra—below, so a muscle lies below the spine of scapula) [rotator cuff muscle]	Infraspinous fossa of scapula	Greater tuberosity of humerus, and shoulder joint	Partially covered by deltoid and trapezius	Suprascapular nerve	Laterally rotates the arm and stabilizes shoulder joint
Subscapularis (sub—under) [rotator cuff muscle]	Subscapular fossa	Lesser tuberosity of humerus	Forms part of posterior wall of axilla. Tendon passes infront of shoulder joint and separated from neck of the scapula by the sub-scapular bursa	Upper and lower sub-scapular nerve of posterior cord of brachial plexus	Chief medial rotator of arm and stabilizes shoulder joint
Teres minor (rotator cuff muscle)	Upper 2/3rd of lateral border of scapula	Greater tuberosity of humerus (lower impression)	Small muscle lies inferior to infraspinatus and may be inseparable from the infraspinatus muscle	Axillary nerve	Laterally rotate the arm and stabilizes shoulder joint

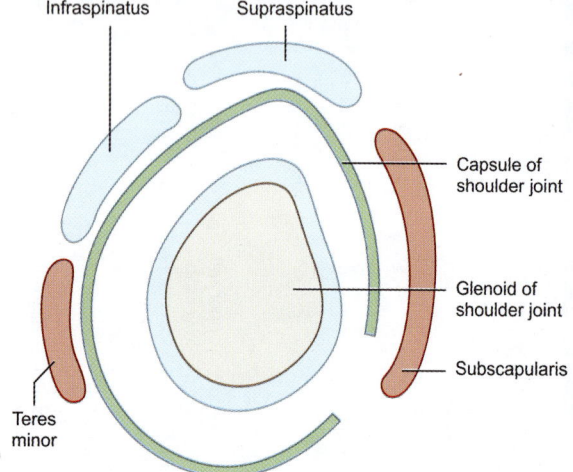

Fig. 2.4: Rotator cuff of shoulder

3. Teres minor
4. Subscapularis

Function: This cuff steadies the joint from dislocation.

NERVES

Brachial Plexus

Brachial Plexus and its Branches

The large important brachial plexus is situated partly in the neck and partly in the axilla. The plexus is formed by the ventral rami of the C5, C6, C7, C8 and the major part of T1 (Fig. 2.5).

When C_4 ventral rami contributes to the formation of brachial plexus it is known as prefixed plexus. Similarly when T_2 nerve gives branches in the formation of plexus it is known as past fixed plexus. The C_5 and C_6 root unite to born upper trunk. The C_7 is continued as middle trunk, C_8 and T_1 unite to form the lower trunk of brachial plexus. Rots and trunk are situated in the neck.

Superior Extremity

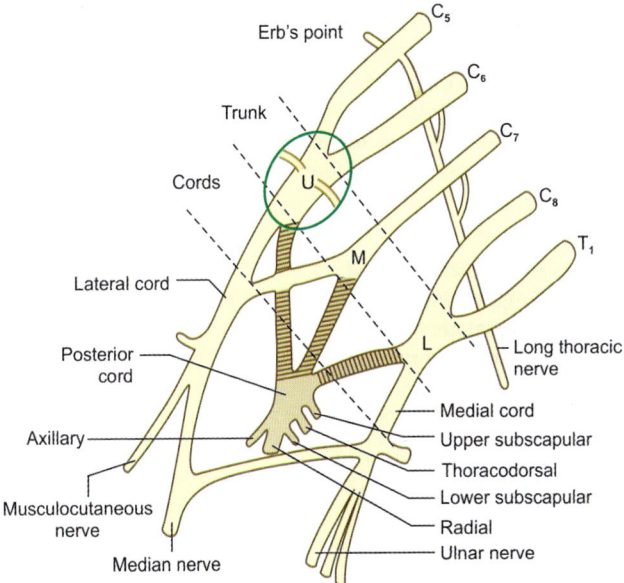

Fig. 2.5: Brachial plexus

The trunks divides into anterior (ventral) and posterior (dorsal) division. The anterior division of upper two unite and form lateral cord. The anterior division of lower trunk continued as medial cord of brachial plexus. The posterior divisions of all the three trunk unite and form the posterior cord. The name of the cord is given according to its position along the 3rd part of axillary artery. The cord and the branches of brachial plexus is located in infraclavicular region that is in axilla.

Branches from root
- Dorsal scapular
- Long thoracic
- Branches from trunk

- Nerve to subclavius
- Suprascapular nerve.

Branches from medial cord
- Medial pectoral
- Medial cutaneous nerve of arm
- Medial cutaneous nerve of forearm
- Ulnar nerve
- Medial root of median nerve.

Branches from posterior cord
- Upper subscapular nerve
- Thoracodorsal nerve
- Lower subscapular nerve
- Radial nerve
- Axillary nerve.

Branches from the lateral cord
- Musculocutaneous nerve
- Lateral pectoral nerve
- Lateral root of median nerve.

Clinical Injuries of the Brachial Plexus

- When the suprascapular nerve is injured, the supraspinatus and the infraspinatus muscles at the suprascapular notch are weakened. It results to a trauma in this region and gradually leads to muscle wasting.
    - *Nerve*: Long thoracic nerve.
    - *Site of injury*: Below in the posterior triangle of the neck or during surgical procedure.
    - *Effect*: Paralysis of the serratus anterior muscle. So there is difficulty in raising arm above head. There is winging of scapula.
- Erb-Duchenne paralysis (Figs 2.6A and B)
    - *Nerve*: Mainly C5 and partly C6 are injured.
    - *Site of injury*: In motorbike accident when there is abnormal separation of head and shoulder or during delivery (the same cause) the region of Erb's point (meeting of six nerves) is involved.

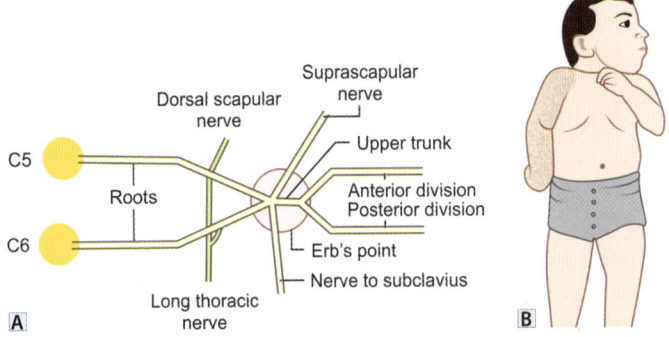

Figs 2.6A and B: Erb's point and Erb's palsy. Note the typical 'policeman receiving tip' sign

- *Effect*: Supraspinatus, infraspinatus, subclavius, biceps brachii and greater part of brachialis, coracobrachialis and deltoid are paralyzed. So the arm hangs by the side of the trunk and is rotated medially; elbow is extended and forearm is pronated.

  Movements of the wrist and fingers are not lost. It is also known as policeman's/waiter's tip position.

- Lower plexus paralysis (Klumpke's Paralysis)
  - *Nerves*: C8 and T1
  - *Site of injury*: It occurs in the lower part of the neck and axilla by cancerous infiltration from apex of lung or breast, cervical rib, etc.
  - *Effect*: Progressive weakening of small muscles hypothenar eminences. This produces claw hand (due to hyperextensions of metacarpophalangeal joint and flexions of interphalangeal joints).
- *Nerve*: Axillary nerve.
  - *Site of injury*: Fracture at the surgical neck of humerus.
  - *Effect*: Paralysis of deltoid with dropping of shoulder as first initiation of abduction is lost.

Median Nerve

Median nerve (Figs 2.7 to 2.9) of brachial plexus has been shown in Table 2.4.

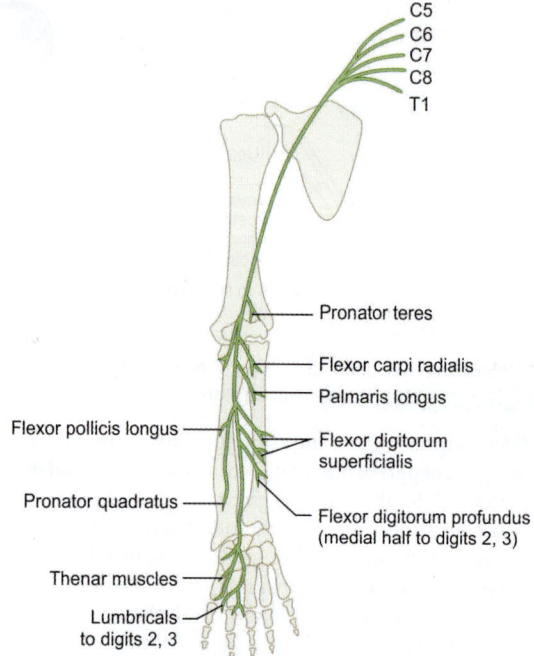

Fig. 2.7: Median nerve and its course

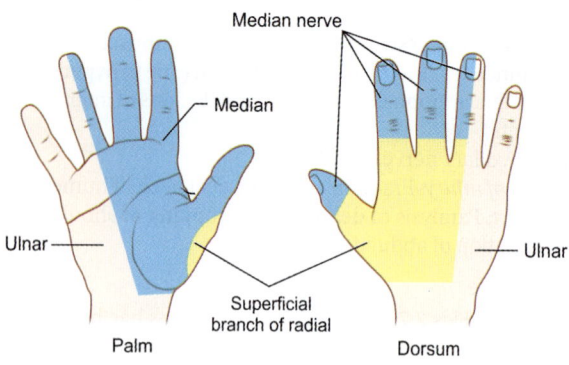

Fig. 2.8: Sensory supply of hand

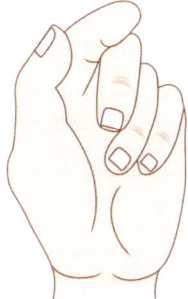

Fig. 2.9: Median nerve palsy

Table 2.4: Median nerve of brachial plexus

Origin	Course	Branches	Clinical anatomy
From lateral and medial cord of brachial plexus in axilla. Usually, it gives no branch in arm	It embraces the third part of axillary artery in the axilla. In the arm, it is lateral to brachial artery, near the insertion of coracobrachialis. It crosses in front of the artery and goes in cubital fossa and lies medial to the artery. It enters the forearm by passing between two heads of pronator teres, separated from ulnar artery by deep head of pronator teres. In the forearm, it lies deep to flexor digitorum superficialis. The nerve enters the hand by passing deep to flexor retinaculum (in the carpal tunnel) and it divides into two, to supply the lateral 3½ digits	• *Muscular* to the superficial flexor muscles of forearm except the flexor carpi ulnaris. • *Anterior interosseous* branch, supplies flexor pollicis longus and part of FDP and PQ. • *Palmar cutaneous branch*—arises above the flexor retinaculum, supplies the skin of thenar eminence. • *Articular* branches to elbow joint, the proximal radioulnar joint • *Vascular branches* to radial and ulnar artery • Branch to thenar muscles is 1st and 2nd lumbricals	Injury, above elbow (as in the supracondylar fracture)—produces paralysis of all the flexor muscles of forearm except, flexor carpi ulnaris. In the hand, thenar muscle and first and second lumbricals are paralyzed. So forearm lies in the supine position, hand is adducted; flexion at interphalangeal joints of index and middle finger is lost. When the patient tries to make a fist, the index and middle fingers tend to remain straight. The muscles of thenar eminence are paralyzed and the eminence if flattened. The thumb is adducted and laterally rotated (ape-like hand). There is sensory loss of lateral 3½ fingers

Note: There may be glass cut injury—which may involve the median nerve alone or with ulnar nerve. Involvement of median nerve occur in carpal tunnel syndrome.

Ulnar Nerve

Ulnar nerve (Figs 2.10 and 2.11) of brachial plexus has been shown in Table 2.5.

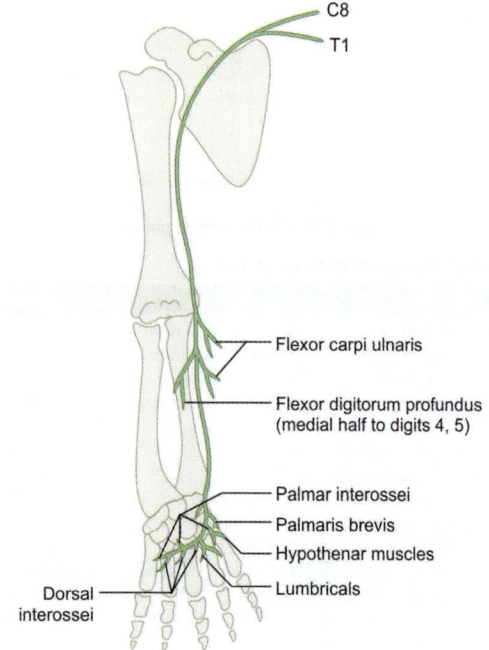

Fig. 2.10: Ulnar nerve and its course

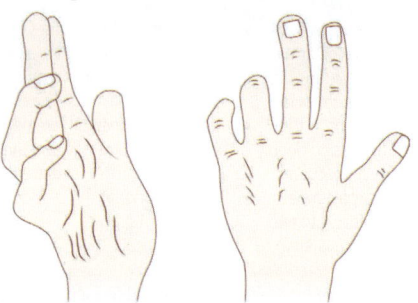

Fig. 2.11: Ulnar nerve palsy

Table 2.5: Ulnar nerve of brachial plexus

Origin	Course	Branches	Clinical anatomy
It is the continuation of medial cord of brachial plexus. It gives off no branch in axilla and arm	In the axilla, it runs downward between axillary artery and vein; then medial to brachial artery in the arm. At the middle of the arm, the nerve pierces the medial intermuscular septum, descends in the back of arm up to medial epicondyle. Here nerve can be felt against the bone. The nerve enters the forearm between two heads of flexor carpi ulnaris, runs between flexor digitorum profundus (on medial aspect) and flexor digitorum superficialis. The nerve enters the palm by passing superficial to flexor retinaculum lateral to pisiform bone	<ul><li>Articular to elbow, wrist</li><li>Muscular to flexor carpi ulnaris and part of flexor digitorum profundus</li><li>Superficial—sensory supply to medial 1½ digit and muscular to palmaris brevis</li><li>Deep terminal branch—muscular to adductor pollicis, all palmar and dorsal interossei and third and fourth lumbricals</li></ul>	Ulnar nerve paralysis commonly occurs behind the medial epicondyle of humerus. Other causes are cervical rib, thoracic outlet syndrome, osteophytes due to cervical spandylosis<ul><li>There is impairment of power of adduction at the wrist due to paralysis of flexor carpi ulnaris and medial ½ of flexor digitorum profundus flattening of medial side of forearm</li><li>Paralysis of interosseous muscle produces claw hand (hyperextension of metacarpophalangeal joint and flexion of interphalangeal joint)</li><li>Inability to adduct the thumb</li><li>Wasting of hypothenar muscle</li><li>Sensation is impaired in the ulnar 1½ fingers on both palmar and dorsal surfaces</li></ul>

Note: All muscles of hand are supplied by ulnar nerve except muscle of thenar eminence and first and second lumbricals (supplied by median nerve).

Radial Nerve

Radial nerve (Figs 2.12 and 2.13) of brachial plexus has been shown in Table 2.6.

Table 2.6: Radial nerve of brachial plexus

Origin	Course	Branches	Applied

It arises from posterior cord; largest branch of brachial plexus	In axilla, it descends behind the third part of axillary artery. In between long and lateral head of triceps, it enters the spiral groove with arteria profunda brachii. It pierces the lateral intermuscular septum to enter the anterior compartment. In front of lateral epicondyle, it divides into superficial and deep branches. The superficial branch lies in front of supinator muscle deep to brachioradialis and descends lateral to radial artery. In the middle third of arm, the artery is medially situated; it quits the artery about 7 cm above the styloid process of radius. Deep terminal branch is known as posterior interosseous nerve	• Muscular:
		  – Triceps
		  – Anconeus
		  – Brachioradialis
		  – Brachialis (lateral part)
		  – Extensor carpi radialis longus
		• Posterior interosseous nerve supplies
		  – Supinator
		  – Extensor carpi radialis brevis
		  – Extensor digitorum
		  – Extensor carpi ulnaris
		  – Extensor pollicis longus
		  – Abductor pollicis longus
		• Articular to radiocarpal joint
			Radial nerve palsy commonly occurs due to compression of nerve in axilla (malfitted crutches at armpit); arm thrown carelessly by drunkers over a chair (Saturday night palsy)
			• Elbow and wrist extension is impaired. So there is wrist drop, finger drop due to weakness of extensor tendon
			• Sensory impairment in lower part of arm, back of forearm, lateral part of dorsum of hand
			• Posterior interosseous palsy. This is due to compression of nerve within the extensor muscles
			• No sensory impairment since the superficial branch arises above this level
			• There is weakness in finger and thumb (extension and abduction)

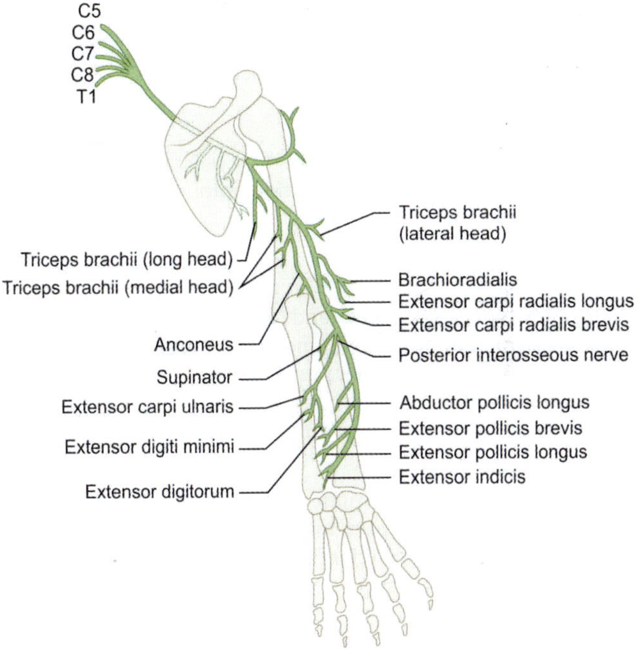

Superior Extremity

C5
C6
C7
C8
T1

Triceps brachii (lateral head)
Triceps brachii (long head)
Triceps brachii (medial head)
Brachioradialis
Extensor carpi radialis longus
Extensor carpi radialis brevis
Anconeus
Supinator
Posterior interosseous nerve
Extensor carpi ulnaris
Abductor pollicis longus
Extensor pollicis brevis
Extensor digiti minimi
Extensor pollicis longus
Extensor indicis
Extensor digitorum

Fig. 2.12: Radial nerve and its course

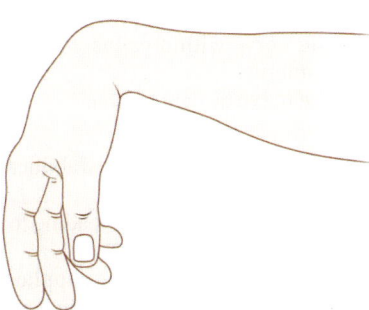

Fig. 2.13: Wrist drop due to radial nerve palsy

Axillary Nerve

- *Root value:* Ventral rami of C5-C6 course.
- It is a branch of posterior cord of brachial plexus.
- Lies behind axillary artery.
- Gives branch to shoulder joint.
- Passes through quadrangular space.

Within the quadrangular space, it divides into:
- Anterior division
- Posterior division.

Anterior Division

- It goes behind surgical neck and remains close to it.
- Accompanied by posterior humeral circumflex artery.
- Lies under cover of anterior part of deltoid.
- Pierces deltoid.
- Ends by supplying skin overlying deltoid.

Posterior Division

- It lies relatively posterior quite apart from humerus.
- Small branch forming pseudoganglion supplies teres minor.
- Lies under cover of posterior fibers of deltoid and gives branch to posterior fibers of deltoid.
- Pierces deltoid.
- Terminates as upper lateral cutaneous nerve of arm.

Applied

Causes of injury

- Fracture surgical neck of humerus.
- Entrapment of the nerve within callus, following fracture of surgical neck of humerus.
- Compression of the nerve by tight plaster.

Effect

- Paralysis of deltoid leading to almost loss of abduction of shoulder joint.
- Loss of rounded shape of the shoulder leading to asymmetry of both sides.
- Loss of cutaneous sensation of the area supplied by it but, the extent of loss will be lesser due to cutaneous overlapping from surrounding area.

Musculocutaneous Nerve

Musculocutaneous nerve of brachial plexus has been shown in Table 2.7.

Posterior Interosseous Nerve (Fig. 2.14)

It is the deep terminal branch of radial nerve and arrives in front of the lateral epicondyle. The nerve enters the back of the forearm in between superficial and deep part of the supinator muscle. It winds around the lateral side of radius. Before it passes through supinator, it provides branches to the extensor carpi radialis brevis and supinator. During its descent through the superficial and deep group of extensor muscles, the nerve divides into:

- Three short branches
- Two long branches.

Short Branches

Supply the extensor digitorum, extensor digiti minimi and extensor carpi ulnaris.

Table 2.7: Musculocutaneous nerve of brachial plexus

Origin	Course	Branches	Applied anatomy
Arises from lateral cord of brachial plexus at the level of lower border of pectoralis minor	It runs down between the axillary artery and coracobrachialis, leaves the axilla by piercing the coracobrachialis. It descends laterally between biceps and brachialis to the lateral side of the arm; just below elbow, it pierces the deep fascia, lateral to tendon of biceps, continued as lateral cutaneous nerve of forearm	• Muscular to biceps brachii • Lateral half of brachialis • Cutaneous branch to forearm • To coracobrachialis	Rarely injured, as it is protected by biceps brachii. If it is injured, high up in the arm. Biceps and coracobrachialis will be paralyzed resulting in marked weakness in elbow flexion. Sensory impairment on the extensor aspect of forearm in the lateral part

Note: The radial nerve courses with arteria profunda brachii, the median nerve courses with brachial artery and ulnar nerve courses with superior ulnar collateral artery.

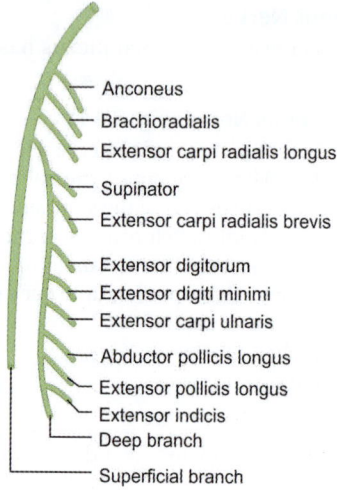

Fig. 2.14: Posterior interosseous nerve and its branches

Longer Branches

Longer branches subdivide into medial and lateral branches.
- *Medial set* supplies extensor pollicis longus and extensor indicis.
- *Lateral set* supplies the abductor pollicis longus and extensor pollicis brevis.

The nerve passes ultimately deep to extensor pollicis longus and lies on the interosseous membrane and dorsal surface of carpal bones. Here, it forms a terminal enlargement called pseudoganglion which supplies the carpal ligaments and joints.

Other branches
- Articular—to wrist; inferior radioulnar joint, intercarpal joint.
- Sensory—to interosseous membrane; radius and ulna.

Clinical Anatomy

If this nerve is injured, in lacerated wound of supinator, the extensor group of forearm muscles will be paralyzed and produce wrist drop.

Anatomical Snuffbox

It is a triangular depression proximal to dorsal aspect of thumb. It is seen well when the thumb is extended (Fig. 2.15).

Boundary
- It is bounded posteromedially by extensor pollicis longus
- Laterally by tendon of abductor pollicis longus and extensor pollicis brevis.
- Base by scaphoid and trapezium and base of 1st metatarsal bone.

Contents
- Radial artery
- Superficial branch of radial nerve
- Cephalic vein

The anatomical snuffbox is important clinically because:
- The tenderness in the box indicates fracture of scaphoid
- The pulsation of radial artery can be felt here
- The cephalic vein is commonly selected in this region for venepunture as the vein lies in the roof.

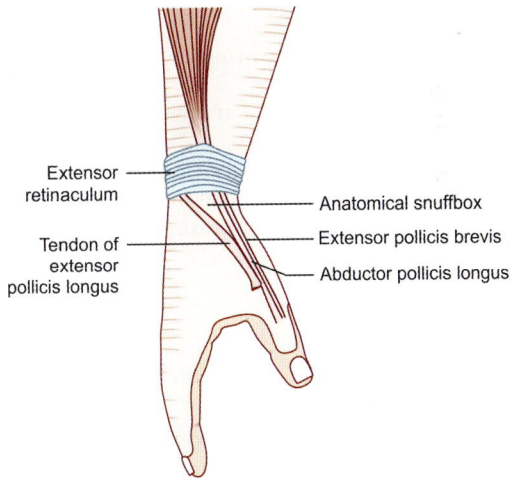

Fig. 2.15: Anatomical snuffbox

Palmaris Brevis

This is a muscle present in the superficial fascia of palm, a part of panniculus carnosus group of muscles.

Proximal Attachment
Attached to flexor retinaculum.

Distal Attachment
Attached to the skin and subcutaneous tissue on the medial side of palm.

Important Relationship
It covers the ulnar nerve and vessels running deep to it.

Nerve Supply
Superficial division of ulnar nerve.

Actions
- It fixes the skin on the medial side of the palm so that through the medial border a person can have a proper tight grip.
- It protects the ulnar nerve and vessels from compression.

Dorsal Digital Expansion

This is the mode of distal attachment of individual tendon of extensor digitorum.
- *Major tendon or body*: Tendon of extensor digitorum going to individual finger.
  - Lumbricals join from the lateral side
  - Interossei, dorsal or palmar joins from lateral or medial side.
- *Distal attachment*: At the level of proximal interphalangeal joint, it splits into three tendons.

ARTERIES

Axillary Artery (Fig. 2.16)

Beginning with level: It is the continuation of the subclavian artery from the outer border of the first rib.

Course: It enters the axilla through its apex and passes laterally deep to the clavipectoral fascia, pectoralis minor and major, along the lateral wall of the axilla up to the lower border of the teres major.

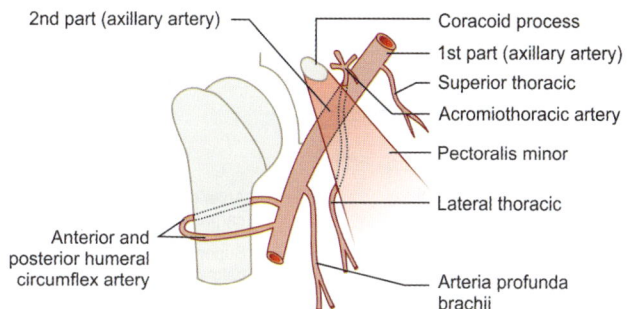

Fig. 2.16: Axillary artery and its branches

It is convex upward when arm is by the side of the body, straight when arm is at right angle to the body, concave upward when arm is raised by the side of the head.

Termination: It is continued as the brachial artery from the lower border of the teres major.

Parts and Branches

Pectoralis minor divides the artery into three parts as follows:
1. *First part:* It is the portion beyond the 1st rib up to the upper border of the pectoralis minor. One branch—superior thoracic.
2. *Second part:* Behind the pectoralis minor gives two branches—(1) lateral thoracic; and (2) acromiothoracic arteries.
3. *Third part:* Lower border of pectoralis minor up to the lower border of the teres major gives three branches:
    i. Subscapular
    ii. Anterior humeral circumflex
    iii. Posterior humeral circumflex.

Clinical Anatomy

If this artery is obstructed, collateral circulation takes place.

Radial Artery (Fig. 2.17)

- *Beginning:* It is one of the terminal branches of brachial artery forms at the level of the neck of the radius.

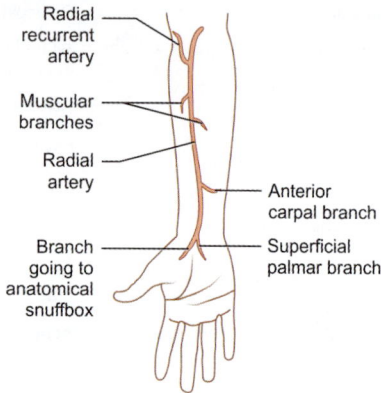

Fig. 2.17: Radial artery and its branches

- *Termination*: At the first metacarpal base, it terminates by passing through first dorsal interosseous muscle and forms the deep palmar arch.
- *Course*: In the proximal part, the radial artery is related to fleshy belly of brachioradialis and in the distal part, it is superficial, lying deep to skin and fascia.
- At the wrist, the radial artery takes a curve from the styloid process of radius, backward, across the anatomical snuffbox. At first it passes deep to the two tendons of abductor pollicis longus and extensor pollicis brevis. Then, the artery lies on the scaphoid and trapezium in the floor of the snuffbox where the cephalic vein is superficial to radial artery. Lastly the artery passes deep to the extensor pollicis longus tendon and end in the first intermetacarpal space where it enters the palm between the two heads of first dorsal interosseous muscle.
- *Branches*:
    - Radial recurrent artery in the cubital fossa
    - Muscular, anterior carpal and superficial palmar arch in the forearm
    - Posterior radial carpal and first doral metacarpal artery at the wrist.

Superior Extremity

Clinical Anatomy
- The radial pulse is felt on the anterior surface of distal end of radius lateral to the tendon of flexor carpi radialis.
- For arterial puncture, this artery is selected, since it is superficial in the distal forearm.
- The radial artery graft is used in coronary artery bypass surgery.

Anastomosis Around the Elbow Joint

If brachial artery is tied below the origin of the arteria profunda brachii, collateral circulation is carried out by anastomosis around the elbow joint (Fig. 2.18).

- In front of lateral epicondyle:
  - Radial collateral (anterior descending) branch of the arteria profunda brachii.
  - Radial recurrent artery which is a branch of the radial artery is:
    - Proximal
    - Distal to the tie

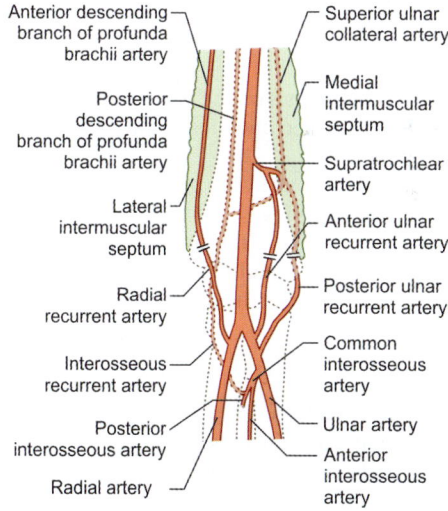

Fig. 2.18: Anastomosis around the elbow joint

- Behind the lateral epcondyle:
  - Middle collateral (posterior descending branch of the arteria profunda brachii.
  - Interosseous recurrent branch of the posterior interosseous or common interosseous artery which is a branch of the ulnar artery:
    - Proximal
    - Distal to the tie.
- In front of the medial epicondyle:
  - Anterior division of the inferior ulnar collateral artery branch of the branchial artery
  - An occasionally branch from superior ulnar collateral artery branch of the brachial artery
  - Anterior ulnar recurrent artery branch of the ulnar artery.
- Behind the medial epicondyle:
  - Superior ulnar collateral branch of the brachial artery
  - Posterior ulnar recurrent branch of the ulnar artery
    - May be proximal or distal according to the site of the tie
    - Is distal to the tie.
- Deep to the medial head of the triceps above the olecranon fossa of the humerus.

A transverse anastomosis on the posterior surface of the shaft of the humerus above the olecranon fossa and deep to medial head of the triceps.

This anastomosis is done by the posterior division of the inferior ulnar collateral artery forming.

- Middle collateral branch of the arteria profunda brachii with:
  - Superior ulnar collateral artery

In this, anastomosis ends the collateral branches of the arteria profunda brachii.

SPACES

Clavipectoral Fascia (Fig. 2.19)
- This is situated deep in the muscle plane.
- Position of body—supine, with upper limb is at right angle to the body.

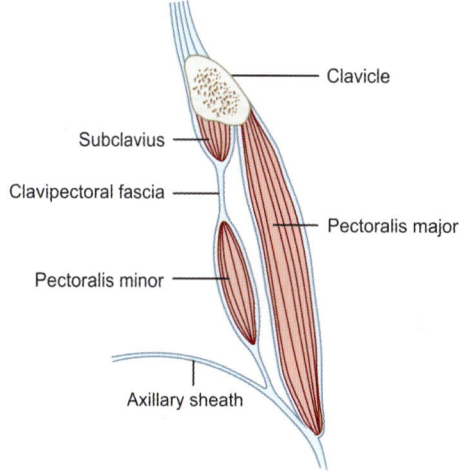

Fig. 2.19: Vertical disposition of clavipectoral fascia

Introduction

It is a strong fascia, situated deep to clavicular head of pectoralis major, and extends from lower border of subclavius to upper border of pectoralis minor. Above it splits to enclose the subclavius, below it splits again and covers the pectoralis minor and blends with axillary fascia. Medially extends up to 1st rib. Laterally extends up to coracoid process and coracoclavicular ligament.

Clavipectoral fascia and structure piercing it:
- Branches of thoracoacromial artery—a branch of 2nd part of axillary artery.
- Cephalic vein draining the lateral side of hand.
- Lateral pectoral nerve—branch of lateral cord of brachial plexus.
- Some lymphatics (Table 2.2).

How will you expose clavipectoral fascia (Fig. 2.20)?
- A transverse incision from sternal notch along the clavicle up to its acromial end.

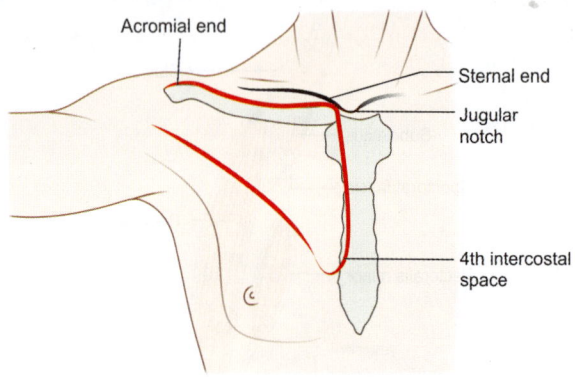

Fig. 2.20: Incision of clavipectoral fascia

- A vertical incision from sternoclavicular joint up to 4th costal cartilage.
- Another oblique incision is given extending from 4th costal cartilage upward, and along the anterior axillary fold up to upper part of humerus.
- Triangular flap of skin reflected laterally.
- Superficial fascia (containing fat) is exposed with cutaneous branches of supraclavicular nerves (lateral, intermediate and medial division). It is reflected by similar incision.
- Upper part of pectoralis major is exposed.
- Clavicular head of pectoralis major is cut and reflected laterally.
- Clavipectoral fascia is exposed.

Clinical Anatomy (Fig. 2.20)

- Cephalic vein catheterization.
- Placement of pacemaker in infraclavicular fossa.
- Developmental anomalies of breast.
- Drainage of breast abscess.

Structures piercing
- Coming out of fascia:
    - Thoracoacromial artery and its 4 branches
    - Lateral pectoral nerve.

- Going in:
  - Cephalic vein
  - Lymphatic vessels from mammary gland.

Modification
- Suspensory ligament of axilla laterally.
- Costocoracoid ligament medially.

Cubital Fossa (Fig. 2.21)

Introduction
It is a fossa in the front of the junction of arm and forearm. It is bounded:
- *Laterally:* Medial border of brachioradialis.
- *Medially:* Lateral border of pronator teres.
- *Apex:* By meeting of brachioradialis and pronator teres.
- *Base:* Imaginary like joining the two epicondyles of humerus.
- *Floor:* By supinator and brachialis.

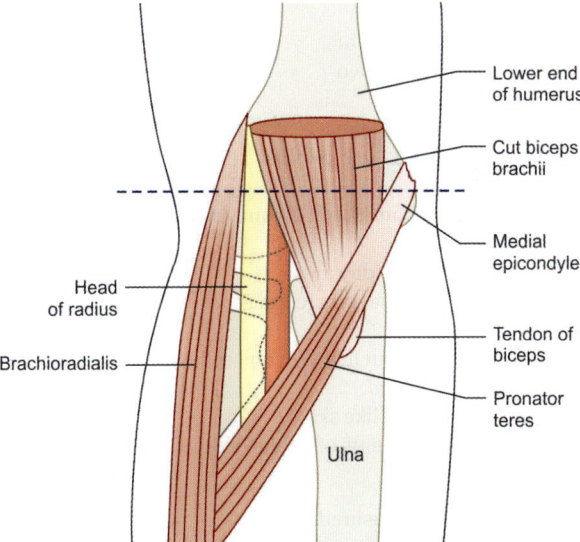

Fig. 2.21: Boundaries and floor of right cubital fossa

Identification
- Cephalic veins
- Median cubital vein
- Bicipital aponeurosis
- Brachioradialis
- Pronator teres
- Supinator
- Brachialis
- Tendon of biceps brachii
- Brachial artery and vein
- Radial blood vessels
- Ulnar artery and vein
- Superficial and deep division of radial nerve
- Nerve to pronator teres.

Exposure of the Fossa
(Fig. 2.22)

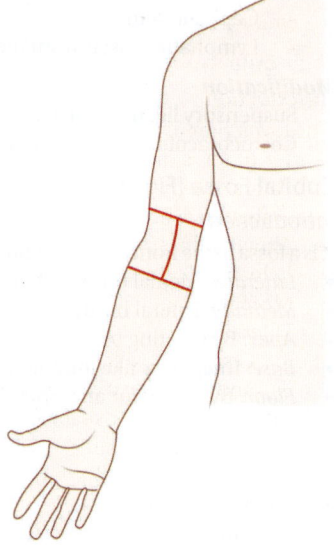

Fig. 2.22: Incision of cubital fossa

- Transverse incision at one finger above the two epicondyles.
- Transverse incision at the junction of upper 1/3rd to lower 2/3rd of the front of forearm (Fig. 2.23).
- Vertical incision from the midpoint of proximal to midpoint of distal incision.
- Reflect the skin flap sideways.
- Preserve the superficial vein (cephalic, basilic and median cubital vein).
- Superficial fascia is cut like skin and reflected.
- Deep fascia is exposed.
- It is cut and reflected like skins.
- Boundaries and contents of cubital fossa is exposed.

Clinical Anatomy
- Blood pressure is measured.
- Intravenous injection is given in medial cubital vein.

- Cubital tunnel syndrome.
- Pronator syndrome.

Triangular and Quadrangular Space (Fig. 2.23)

Introduction

The lower border of teres minor is separated by a gap from the upper border of teres major. This gap is divided by long head of triceps into lateral quadrangular and medial triangular space. Boundary of quadrangular space P.G.E.

- Above: Teres minor.
- Below: Teres major.
- Medially: Long head of triceps.
- Laterally: Surgical neck of humerus.
  - Contents: Axillary nerve, posterior humeral circumflex artery and vein above and medially.

Boundary of triangular space:
- Upper by teres minor
- Below and laterally by teres major
- Laterally: By long head of triceps.
  - Contents: Circumflex scapular vessels.

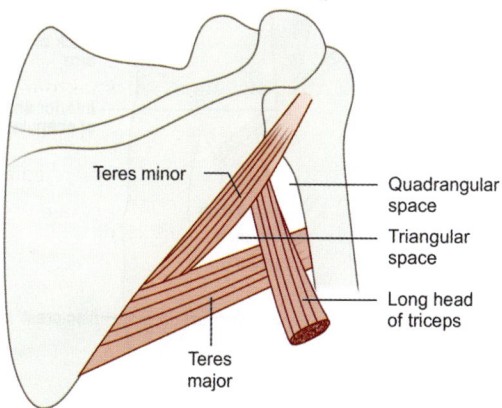

Fig. 2.23: Triangular and quadrangular space

Identification
- Muscles: Teres minor, long-head of triceps teres major, deltoid.
- Vessels: Posterior humeral circumflex vessels, circumflex scapular vessels.
- Nerves: Axillary nerve and its branches, pseudoganglion over the nerve to teres minor.

Insicion to Expose the Space (Fig. 2.24)
- Feel the spine of scapula.
- From the midpoint of spine a vertical incision extends up to inferior angle of scapula.
- Oblique incision extends from above incision along the back of the spine up to acromion and then upper part of arm.
  From it extends downwards towards the table.

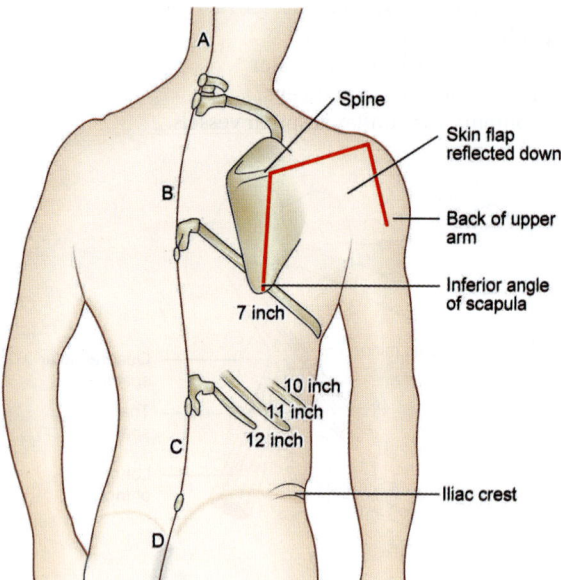

Fig. 2.24: Incisions (triangular; quadrangular space)

- Triangular flap of skin is reflected downwards and laterally.
- Superficial fascia is exposed. It lies in upper lateral cutaneous nerve of arm along the posterior fold of deltoid.
- Superficial fascia is reflected like skin. Deep fascia is exposed.
- Deep fascia is also reflected.
- Posterior part of deltoid is exposed and retracted upwards.
- Trangular and quadrangular spaces are exposed.

Clinical Anatomy

Nailing of humeral surgical neck done through this space; care should be taken during nailing, as it may damage the axillary nerve.

Space of Parona and Its Clinical Importance

Space of Parona is a space between long flexor tendons and pronator quadratus. Proximally, upward extent is limited by origin of flexor digitorum superficialis. Distally, this space extends up to flexor retinaculum. Proximal part of flexor tendon synovial sheath extends into it (Fig. 2.25).

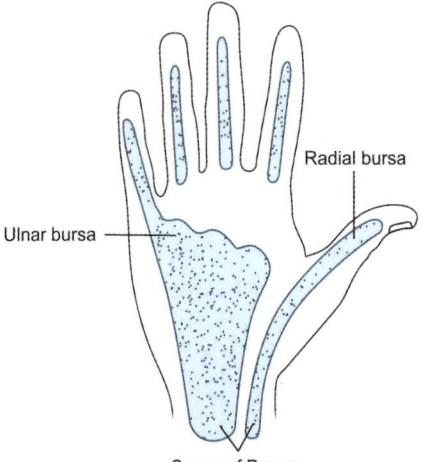

Fig. 2.25: Space of Parona

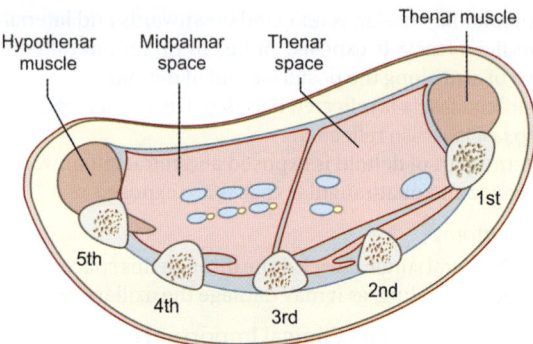

Fig. 2.26: Palmar spaces

Clinical Importance

The synovial sheath of flexor tendons or radial and ulnar bursae may be infected and pus extends into the space of Parona producing hourglass swelling.

Clinical Importance of Midpalmar and Thenar Space

Midpalmar space and thenar space are potential spaces deep to palmar aponeurosis and flexor tendons (Fig. 2.26).
- *Midpalmar space*: This space is located under inner half of hollow of palm.
- *Thenar space*: This space is located under outer half of hollow of palm.

Clinical Importance

These spaces became infected particularly in females and labors in any wound of palm, the synovial sheath infected. The spaces frequently communicate with each other. So infection can pass from one space to another.

OTHERS

Pulled Elbow

Annular ligament participates in the superior radioulnar joint in such a manner so that the head of the radius rotates within the socket formed by radial notch of ulna and annular ligament. The ligament is attached to the circumference of the head as well as upper part of the neck so it forms a tight collar preventing displacement of the head from the socket as the neck is more constricted.

In child, the head of radius is narrow like neck, so that the annular ligament is unable to prevent the displacement of it, so if forearm is pulled with a great force in a child with extended elbow, the head of radius might be dislocated out from the socket known as subluxation of superior radioulnar joint or pulled elbow. Child is unable to move the elbow joint.

Treatment the subluxation is reduced by forced supination of forearm.

Flexor Retinaculum of Hand (Fig. 2.27)
- It is the strong square-shaped fibrous band, 2 cm in length as well as in breadth.
- It is in front of the carpal bone and situated at the proximal part of hand. It is attached medially to the hook of the hamate and pisiform bone and laterally to the tubercle of scaphoid and ridge of trapezium lying between carpal and flexor retinaculum.
- There is fibro-osseous canal known as carpal tunnel.

Structure passing superficial to it (from medial to lateral):
- Ulnar nerve
- Ulnar vessels
- Palmaris longus.

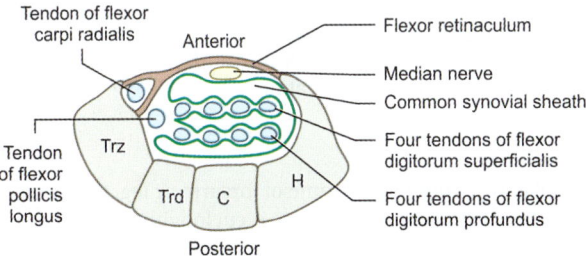

Fig. 2.27: Transverse section of carpal tunnel (left side)
Abbreviations: Trz, trapezium; Trd, trapezoid; C, capital; H, hamalte

Structure passing deep to the flexor retinaculum:
- Median nerve
- Four tendons of flexor digitorum superficialis
- Four tendon of flexor digitorum profundus
- Tendon of flexor pollicis longus (lateral most structure)
- Ulnar bursa.

Function: Its main function is to hold the flexor tendon close to wrist during flexion and prevent bowstringing.

Clinical Importance

When there is carpal tunnel syndrome, flexor retinaculum is cut to relieve the compression of median nerve and prevent weakness or wasting of thenar muscle.

Character of Interosseous Membrane of Upper Limb

- It connects the interosseous border of radius and ulna.
- The direction of the fibers is downward and medially.
- The membrane is proximally deficient. It starts 2–3 cm distal to radial tuberosity. Through the gap above the membrane passes posterior interosseous vessels.
- It has an oval aperture at distal part for passage of anterior interosseous vessels to back of forearm (Fig. 2.28).
- Interosseous membrane is taut in midprone position and relax in complete supination or pronation of forearm.

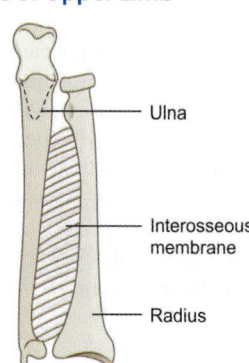

Fig. 2.28: Interosseous membrane of forearm

Clinical Anatomy

In case of compartment syndrome of forearm or leg, the fasciotomy is done (the interosseous membrane is cut longitudinally) for relieve of pain.

Ulnar Paradox

Ulnar nerve is a branch of medial cord of brachial plexus (root value C8, T1). The common site of injury or compression of ulnar nerve is behind the medial epicondyle, at wrist between the pisiform and flexor retinaculum below the hook of hamate.

Clinical Anatomy

It is seen that more distal is the lesion more clawing is there in the medial two fingers because there is more sparing of nerves. This is known as ulnar paradox.

EXPLANATORY NOTES

Q1. Biceps brachii is an important supinator muscle. Explain.

Ans. Biceps brachii arises by two heads from tip of coracoid process and supraglenoid tubercle and inserted at the radial tuberosity by a slender tendon and through bicipital aponeurosis, it is also attached with ulna.

During attachment of tendon with radius, it is twisted. So the contraction of biceps brachii leads to supination of forearm.

Q2. Basilic vein is the vein of choice for cardiac catheterization. Explain.

Ans. The basilic vein is the vein of choice for cardiac catheterization because:
- It is straighter in course without any sharp turning.
- It pierces the deep fascia in an oblique fashion.
- Size of the lumen of the vein gradually increases even after forming axillary vein.

On the contrast, cephalic vein has three sharp bendings in its course:
- At the deltopectoral groove
- While piercing deep fascia
- Before draining into the axillary vein.

Q3. Explain space of Parona and its clinical importance.

Ans. Space of Parona is a space between long flexor tendons and pronator quadratus. Proximally, upward extension is limited by origin of flexor digitorum superficialis. Distally, this space extends up to flexor retinaculum. The proximal part of flexor tendon's synovial sheath extends into it.

Clinical importance: The synovial sheath of flexor tendons or radial and ulnar bursae may be infected and pus extends into this space producing *hourglass contracture*.

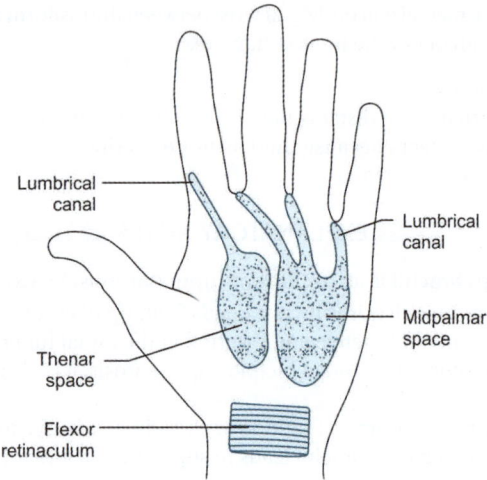

Fig. 2.29: Midpalmar and thenar spaces with lumbrical canals

Q4. Clinical importance of midpalmar and thenar space. Explain.

Ans. Midpalmar space and thenar space are potential spaces deep to palmar aponeurosis and flexor tendons (Fig. 2.29).

Midpalmar space: This space is located under inner half of hollow of palm.

Thenar space: This space is located under outer half of hollow of palm.

Clinical importance: The space becomes infected particularly in female and laborers in any wounds of palm and synovial sheath infections, they frequently communicate with each other. So infection can pass from one space to another.

Q5. Shoulder joint has gained mobility at the expense of stability. Explain.

Ans. Mobility of a joint is inversely proportional to the stability. Mobility factors of shoulder joint are:
- Shallow glenoid not matching the convexity of humeral head

- Fibrous capsule is loose and lax
- There is no strong ligament connecting scapula with humerus.

Stability factors are:
- Rotator cuff muscles fuse with the fibrous capsule of the joint from above, in front and behind to form rotator cuff
- Glenoidal labrum increases concavity of glenoid fossa.
- Long head of biceps brachii originates within the capsule from supraglenoid tubercle, runs above the head of the humerus and prevents the joint from displacing upward during abduction.

The mobility factors are more powerful than stability factor, so the shoulder joint enjoys more mobility than any other joint in the body.

Q6. Upper end of humerus is growing end.

Ans. Growing end is that end where the secondary center appears first and unites last with the diaphysis. The growing end is situated opposite the direction of nutrient foramen of that bone. The direction of nutrient foramina of long bone can be kept in mind by a dictum "to the elbow I go and from the knee I flee". Therefore, in upper limb, upper end of the humerus is the growing end.

Q7. In breast cancer peau d'orange is a condition.

Ans. This is because there is obstruction of superficial lymph vessels by cancer cells. This produces edema of skin and gives rise to an appearance like that of a skin of an orange. This is known as peau d'orange.

Q8. Why pain is felt in the medial side of the arm in cancer breast?

Ans. The mammary gland is supplied by 2nd to 6th intercostal nerves. The lateral branch of 2nd nerve known as intercostobrachial nerve supplies the medial side of arm. So pain is felt in medial side of arm in cancer breast.

Q9. Median nerve injury—manifested pointed index finger.

Ans. Injury of median nerve above elbow (as in supracondylar fracture produces paralysis of all flexor except flexor carpi ulnaris. In the hand, thenar muscles and 1st two lumbricals are paralyzed. So forearm lies in supine position, hand is adducted, flexor of interphalangeal joints of index and middle finger is lost. So when patient tries to make a fist, the index and middle fingers tend to remain straight and there is pointed index finger.

Q10. Ulnar head of pronator teres does not take part in any movement of elbow joint. Explain.

Ans. Ulnar head of pronator teres arises from coronoid process of ulna and is inserted on radius. It never crosses elbow joint, hence cannot take part in any movement of elbow joint.

Q11. Whitlow is extremely painful. Explain.

Ans. An infection of pulp space of digit is known as whitlow or felon. The pulp space is situated on distal part of thumb and all the digits. The fingers (digits) contain dense subcutaneous tissue. The dense fibrous process passes from skin to periosteum of terminal phalanx. So, there are small compartments containing fat. The vessels pass through these septa. When there is infection, these septa do not allow the swelling to expand. So there is increased tension of this space and there is severe pain.

Q12. Bone pain in case of breast carcinoma. Explain.

Ans. In breast, cancer may spread through veins. Since the azygos venous system receives intercostals veins and communicate with the vertebral venous plexus, spread of cancer can occur through this route to vertebrae (bone) and from there to cranium and brain.

Q13. Compression of brachial artery is done medial to the humerus near the middle of arm for hemostasis.

Ans. Stoppage of bleeding or blood flow is known as hemostasis. The best place to control the hemorrhage of upper limb temporarily by the tourniquet is near the middle of arm as the artery is near the humerus and no muscle lies between there two. But this compression must not be more than 4–5 hours as muscles and nerves can tolerate only 6 hours of ischemia. After that muscle tissue will be replaced by fibrous scar tissues.

Q14. Why clavicle is called a modified long bone?

Ans. Clavicle is called a modified long bone because it is horizontally place, no medullary cavity, ossifies mostly in membrane. It is sometimes pierced by cutaneous (supraclavicular) nerve.

Q15. Injury of the posterior interosseous nerve causes wrist drop/ laceration of the supinator muscle causes wrist drop. Explain.

Ans. The posterior interosseous branch of radial nerve supplies the extensor group of muscles of forearm after piercing the supinator muscle. So injury of the posterior interosseous nerve causes paralysis of extensor muscle, e.g. extensor digitorum, extensor digiti minimi, extensor carpi ulnaris, extensor pollicis longus, abductor pollicis longus, extensor pollicis brevis, extensor indicis. Thus, the flexor group of muscles lie in front of the forearm will take the upper hand and produce wrist drop.

Q16. Fracture of scaphoid produces avascular necrosis of proximal segment of bone.

Ans. The fracture of scaphoid occurs when a person falls on the outstretched hand (in motorcycle accident or falls from a height). This injury is the one of the most common injury among the upper limb bones (60–70%). Avascular necrosis of proximal segment occurs because blood supply of the proximal segment often enters entirely through the distal bone. Thus, the fracture of scaphoid disrupts its blood supply and undergoes necrosis due to loss of blood supply.

Q17. Pectoralis minor and serratus anterior play a common role in movement of shoulder girdle.

Ans. Serratus anterior arises from upper 8 ribs and attaches in medial border of scapula. It helps in binding the scapular with the thoracic wall. It protracts the scapula and acts as prime mover for all punching pushing movements.

Pectoralis minor attached in 3rd to 5th ribs anteriorly and with medial border and upper surface of coracoid process. It helps in drawing the scapula anteriorly by pulling it from front.

So, to move the scapula anteriorly, both the serratus anterior and pectoralis minor help. Serratus anterior pulls the medial border in forward and pectoralis minor pulls the coracoid process forward. So, they have common role in moving the shoulder girdle.

Q18. What is Dupuytren's contracture?

Ans. It is a partial contraction or localized thickening of palmar aponeurosis. It starts in the ring and little finger with flexion of these two fingers. There is restriction of hand function.

Q19. Claw hand. Explain.

Ans. It is the hyperextension of the metacarpophalangeal joint with flexion of interphalangeal joint of hand. It is due to injury of both median and ulnar nerve if all the fingers are affected. But if the clawing is only medial two fingers then only ulnar nerve is affected (particularly in the palm) and produce ulnar claw hand.

Q20. What is cubital tunnel syndrome?

Ans. It is one of the types of compression neuropathy. When the ulnar nerve is compressed between bands of medial collateral ligament during the coming of ulnar nerve in front from behind the medial epicondyle. There will be paresthesia (abnormal sensation) by tapping over the nerve.

Q21. What is pronator syndrome?

Ans. It is also a type of compression syndrome when median nerve is compressed between the two heads of pronator teres. Gradually anesthesia develops in the line of sensory distribution and weakness of muscle on the lateral side of forearm and palm develops. Grip strength is gradually decreased. Patient may come to normal if compression is removed.

Q22. What is cubitus valgus?

Ans. The angle formed in between long axis of arm and the forearm is known as carrying angle (10–15°). This angle is more in females than in males because of wider pelvis and forearm can move freely of hip when carrying a bucket and increase in normal carrying angle is known as cubitus valgus.

Q23. What is carpal tunnel syndrome?

Ans. It occurs usually in women between the ages 40 and 70 years. They complaint of pain in the hand in the distribution of the median nerve. There will be wasting of thenar eminence. The cause is interference of blood supply of the nerve due to compression within the flexor retinaculum due to enlarged radial bursa or ulnar bursa. It may be cured by division of retinaculum.

Q24. What is Volkmann's ischemic contracture?

Ans. Injury of the brachial artery at the level of arm or elbow results in ischemic contracture of muscles of forearm. If it lasts for more than 6 hours, the flexor digitorum profundus and flexor pollicis longus are heavily affected and their muscle fibers are replaced by fibrous tissue. The result is flexor deformity of interphalangeal joint. This contracture may occur due to tight plaster or bandages.

Q25. Dislocation of the shoulder joint almost occurs always inferiorly. Explain.

Ans. The dislocation of the shoulder joint is common due to laxity of the capsular ligament inferiorly and medially and disproportionate articular surfaces. Initially the dislocation is inferior or subglenoid and this is followed by subcoracoid. The axillary nerve may be affected in inferior dislocation.

In this position, the head of the humerus presses against the lower unsupported part of capsular ligament.

Q26. Injury to long thoracic nerve causes winging of scapula. Explain.

Ans. Long thoracic nerve supplies the serratus anterior muscle, which protracts the scapula against the chest wall. Injury to this nerve causes paralysis of serratus anterior muscle that is why protraction of scapula is lost. But due to action of rhomboideus major (which retracts the scapula) produces winging as it remains unaffected.

Q27. Injury to radial nerve in cubital fossa will not cause wrist drop. Why?

Ans. Wrist drop is pathological condition characterized by flexion at wrist joint, metacarpophalangeal joint and extension of interphalangeal joint. In cubital fossa, radial nerve is divided into superficial and deep division after piercing the lateral intermuscular septum of arm. Injury to the radial nerve in cubital fossa, deep branch may be injured. Resulting in paralysis of almost of all extensor of wrist joint except extensor carpi radialis longus which is supplied by radial nerve in the arm. So this muscle is spared which is so strong that it may alone prevent wrist drop.

Q28. Explain distal 4/5th of distal phalanx suffers from necrosis in pulp space infection.

or

Q. Explain infection of pulp space of fingers may cause necrosis of distal 4/5th of terminal phalanx.

Ans. The artery that supplies the distal 4/5th of the fingers traverses the fibrous septa present in pulp space. Infection in this area increases the tension of the distal 4/5th of the pulp space which produces occlusion of the blood supply, leading to necrosis. The proximal 1/5th escapes necrosis because the blood supply in this region does not traverse the fibrous septa.

Q29. Upper end of humerus is an example of compound epiphysis. Explain.

Ans. The upper end of humerus consists of head (epiphysis), lesser and greater tubercles (epiphysis). All the epiphyses fuse together first at 6 years then fuse with the shaft at the age of about 18–20th years. This variety is an example of compound epiphysis.

Q30. Carcinoma of the inferomedial quadrant of right mammary gland may produce secondary carcinoma of the ovary. Explain

Ans. From lower medial quadrant, the lymphatics drain into:
- Parasternal lymph node of the same side
- Parasternal lymph node of the opposite side
- Drains into lymph node in the rectus sheath liver transcelomic implantation to ovary (Krukenberg's tumor).

Carcinoma spreads to ovary as lymph vessels of breast communicate with subdiaphragmatic and subperitoneal lymph plexus after crossing the costal margin and piercing the anterior abdominal wall. The cancer cells thus reach the peritoneum through transperitoneal route and drop on the ovary resulting in secondary metastasis in ovary (Krukenberg's tumors).

Q31. Explain why the clavicle is commonly fractured at the junction of lateral one-third and medial two-thirds?

Ans. The clavicle bears weight of upper limb and transmits it to axial skeleton through coracoclavicular ligament.

The junction of lateral one-third and medial two-thirds is represented by a bend where there is sudden change of direction of force. So bend is the common fracture site. Following fracture the lateral fragment is displaced forward and medially by strong abductors. The medial fragment is tilted upward by the sternocleidomastoid (Fig. 2.30).

Q32. Why medial cubital vein is commonly used for transfusion or withdrawal of blood?

Ans. Medial cubital vein connects the cephalic vein with the basilic vein; is in the superficial fascia of elbow. It is commonly used for transfusion/withdrawal of blood because:
- It is superficial
- Very suitable position
- Fixed with deep vein by perforator.

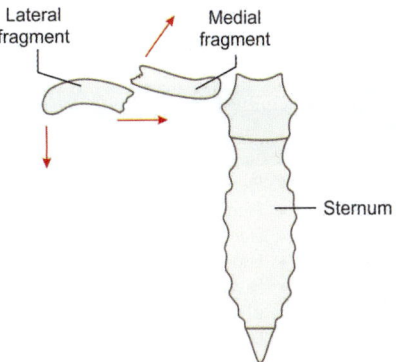

Fig. 2.30: Fracture of clavicle

Q33. Lumbrical is a linked muscle. Explain.

Ans. Lumbrical muscle is worm-like muscle which starts from the tendon of flexor digitorum profundus which is the major flexor of wrist and metacarpophalangeal joint. The other end of the muscle which is tendinous reaches the dorsum and is inserted in the dorsal digital expansion. The expansion is made by distal attachment of extensor digitorum tendon which is the major extensor of wrist, Metacarpophalangeal joint and also the interphalangeal joints.

So, the lumbricals connect the major flexor with the major extensor of hand. So, it is known as link muscle. Being a link muscle, it crosses the metacarpophalangeal joint from the flexor aspect so flexes the metacarpophalangeal joint. But, the tendon being attached to dorsal digital expansion, it extends the interphalangeal joint. So, this link muscle can flex metacarpophalangeal joint but extends interphalangeal joint.

Q34. Why 1st metacarpal is called modified phalanx?

Ans. Epiphysis of metacarpals are situated in heads and epiphysis of phalanx are situated in base. In 1st metacarpals the epiphysis is situated in base like phalanx so, it is called modified phalanx.

NERVE ENTRAPMENT OF THE UPPER LIMB AND CLINICAL ANATOMY

Nerve	Site	Cause	Muscle principally affected	Sensory loss
Median	Carpal tunnel	<ul><li>Premenstrual</li><li>Pregnancy</li><li>Fracture</li><li>Endocrine</li><li>Dislocation of lunate bone</li></ul>	Three thenar muscles:<ul><li>Abductor pollicis brevis</li><li>Flexor pollicis brevis</li><li>Opponens pollicis</li></ul>	Lateral two and a half fingers
Anterior interosseous	Elbow	<ul><li>Edema (swelling due to fluid)</li></ul>	<ul><li>Flexor pollicis longus</li><li>Flexor profundus of index + middle finger</li></ul>	None
Ulnar	Median epicondyle between heads of flexor carpi ulnaris	<ul><li>Fracture</li><li>Edema</li></ul>	<ul><li>Flexor carpi ulnaris</li><li>Flexor profundus of ring + little finger</li><li>Hypothenar muscles, interossei</li></ul>	Medial one and a half fingers
Radial	Axilla	<ul><li>"Crutch palsy" or "Saturday night palsy"</li><li>Fracture of humerus</li></ul>	Elbow and wrist	Back of hand, over first dorsal interosseous brachioradialis reflex
Posterior interosseous	Upper forearm within supinator	<ul><li>Elbow trauma</li><li>Fibrous band</li></ul>	<ul><li>Wrist + finger extensors</li><li>Wrist drop is present</li></ul>	None

SURFACE ANATOMY

INTRODUCTION

Study of anatomy in relation to body surface is known as surface anatomy. Physical examination of patient is the clinical application of surface anatomy. For this carefully selected landmark is used. These landmarks are:
1. Visible landmark
2. Palpable landmark.

Visible Landmarks

Visible landmarks are those which one can see visible with naked eye. Majority of them are produced by bones and cartilage, only nipple and umbilicus are soft tissue landmarks identified by inspection.

Palpable Landmarks (Fig. 2.31)

These landmarks are felt through skin, muscles and tendons. Artery pulsation is felt against bone (e.g. radial pulse, femoral pulse, etc.). Nerves can be rolled against bone (e.g. ulnar nerve, termination of common peroneal nerve). Superficial tendon can be felt by making the muscle prominent. Parotid duct and vas deferens can be felt through skin. During examination, it is better to use white chalk powder for points as well as for lines (because it is more prominent) as white color can be used in any type of drawings. In drawing an artery and a vein, please put a lumen inside two lines. In case of nerve, one should draw a single line.

CLINICAL IMPORTANCE (SURFACE ANATOMY)

- Physical examination of patient is the clinical application of surface anatomy.
- Determination of diminished peripheral pulse as the complication of vaso-occlusive disease (Buerger's disease).
- Prominence of some veins help in diagnosis and also therapeutic management of some condition.
- Determination of certain diseases by palpating nerves (e.g. thickening of ulnar nerve in leprosy) as well as nerve injuries due to fracture of bones.

Surgical Anatomy

Anatomical Event According to Vertebral Level (Fig. 2.31)

The anatomical event according to vertebral level has been shown in Table 2.8.

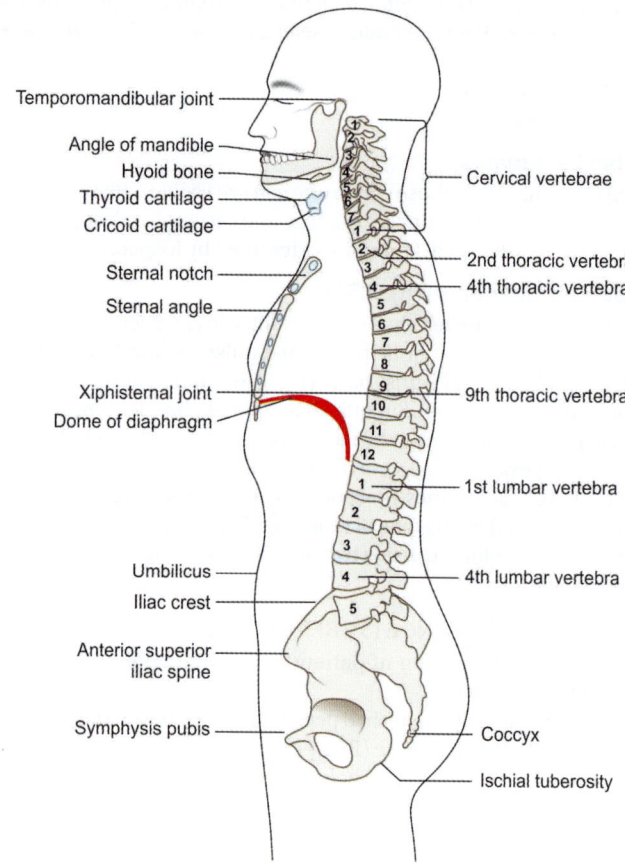

Fig. 2.31: Important visible points and palpable bony prominences used in surface marking

Table 2.8: Anatomical event according to vertebral level

Vertebral level	Anatomical event
• 1st cervical vertebra	• Commencement of spinal cord
	• Hard palate
• 2nd cervical vertebra	• Angle of mandible
• 3rd cervical vertebra	• Hyoid bone
• 4th and 5th cervical vertebra	• Thyroid cartilage
• 6th cervical vertebra	• Cricoid cartilage
	• Pharynx ends
	• Esophagus begins
	• Larynx ends
	• Trachea begins
	• Omohyoid crosses anterior to carotid sheath from medial to lateral side
	• Inferior thyroid artery crosses posterior to carotid sheath from lateral to medial side
	• Middle cervical sympathetic ganglion lies posterior to inferior thyroid artery
	• Vertebral artery enters the foramen transversarium of 6th cervical vertebra
• 7th cervical vertebra	• Isthmus of thyroid gland lies on 2nd, 3rd and 4th tracheal rings
	• Maximum height of thoracic duct
• 2nd thoracic vertebra P.G.E.	• Corresponds with superior angle of scapula
• Disk between 2nd and 3rd thoracic vertebrae	• Suprasternal notch/jugular notch
• 3rd thoracic vertebra P.G.E.	• Root of spine of scapula

Contd...

Surgical Anatomy

Contd...

Vertebral level	Anatomical event
• Sternal angle of Louis (disk between 4th and 5th thoracic vertebrae) P.G.E.	• The imaginary line division into superior and inferior mediastinum, passes through this level
	• Articulation of 2nd costal cartilage. It helps in counting of ribs
	• Ascending aorta ends
	• Descending thoracic aorta begins
	• Arch of aorta begins and ends
	• Bifurcation of trachea
	• Bifurcation of pulmonary trunk
	• Azygos vein ends in superior vena cava
	• Thoracic duct passes from right to left across the front of vertebral column
	• Position of deep cardiac plexus
	• Junction of intra- and extrapericardial parts of superior vena cava
	• Pleurae meet in the midline
• 7th thoracic vertebra P.G.E.	• Inferior angle of scapula
• 8th thoracic vertebra P.G.E.	• Inferior vena cava pierces the diaphragm
• 9th thoracic vertebra	• Xiphisternal joint
	• Inferior border of heart
• 10th thoracic vertebra P.G.E.	• Esophagus pierces the diaphragm
• 12th thoracic vertebra P.G.E.	• Aortic opening of diaphragm
	• Origin of celiac trunk

Contd...

Contd...

Vertebral level	Anatomical event
• 1st lumbar vertebra (lower border)—transpyloric plane P.G.E.	• Tip of 9th costal cartilage • Hilum of both kidney
	• Pylorus of stomach
	• Termination of spinal cord
	• Neck of pancreas
	• Formation of portal vein
	• Fundus of gallbladder
	• Origin of superior mesenteric artery
• 2nd lumbar vertebra	• Duodenojejunal flexure
	• Opening of bile duct in the second part of duodenum
• 3rd lumbar vertebra (upper border) P.G.E.	• Level of subcostal plane
	• Origin of inferior mesenteric artery
• 4th lumbar vertebra	• Highest point of the iliac crest
• 5th lumbar vertebra	• Level of transtubercular plane
	• Commencement of inferior vena cava
• 1st sacral vertebra	• Ileocecal orifice
	• Appendicular orifice
• 2nd sacral vertebra P.G.E.	• Posterior superior iliac spine
	• Spinal dura mater, arachnoid mater, spinal subarachnoid space ends
• 3rd sacral vertebra	• Sigmoid colon ends
	• Rectum begins
• Coccygeal 1	• Filum terminale ends

Surface Anatomy of Upper Limb

Surface anatomy of upper limb which is helpful in clinical practice. Dark area palpable features of superior extremity have been shown in Figure 2.32.

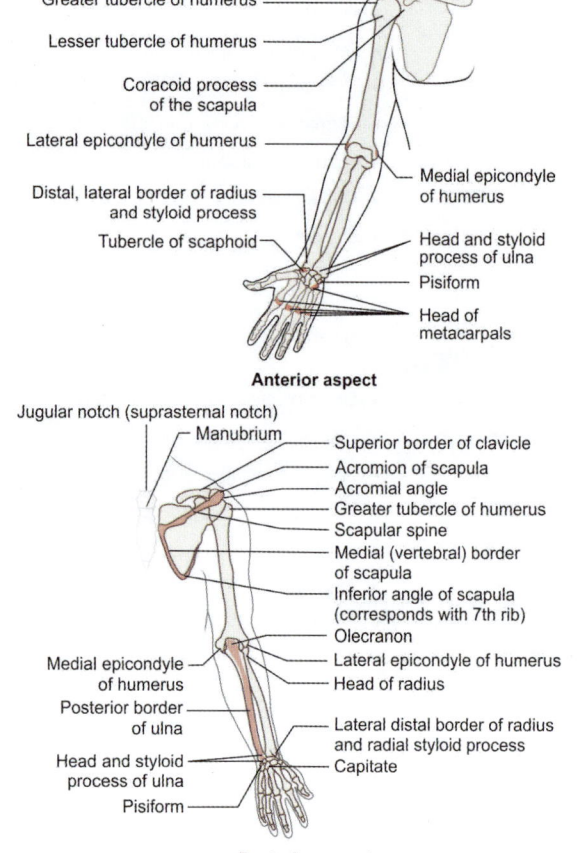

Fig. 2.32: Dark area palpable features of superior extremity

Lines

Left axillary artery *(Fig. 2.33):* Arm is abducted at right angles to the body. The points are:
- At the lower border of midpoint of the clavicle (Please identify the sternal end and then trace acromial end of clavicle and then assess the midpoint of clavicle).
- At the junction of anterior two-thirds and posterior one-third of the line joining the distal ends of anterior and posterior axillary folds (Anterior axillary fold is formed by pectoralis major and later by teres major and latissimus dorsi).

Two parallel lines joining the above points represent the axillary artery.

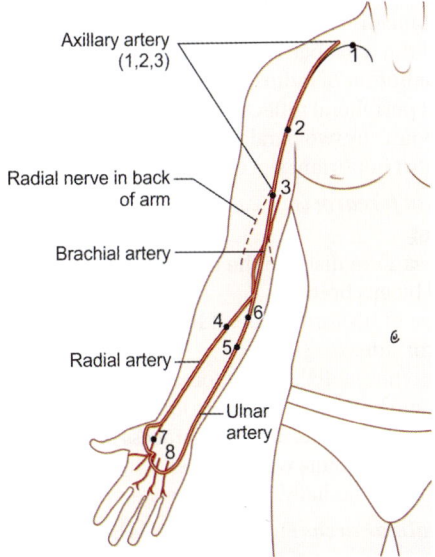

Fig. 2.33: Axillary artery, brachial artery (in arm), radial artery, ulnar artery (in forearm) and superficial palmar arch (in palm)

Surgical Anatomy

Brachial artery *(Fig. 2.33)*:

The points are:
- At the junction of anterior two-thirds and posterior one-third of the line joining the distal ends of anterior and posterior axillary folds.
- The point is 1 cm distal to the elbow joint at the level of neck of radius. The point lies on the medial aspect of tendon of biceps brachii.

Two parallel lines joining the above points represent brachial artery.
- Brachial artery is compressed on the medial aspect of tendon of biceps during blood pressure recording.

Radial artery in the forearm *(Fig. 2.33)*:

The points are:
- A point 1 cm below the elbow joint on the medial side of tendon of biceps brachii.
- In front of the wrist between flexor carpi radialis and lower part of anterior border of radius, where pulsation is felt. It is the most important peripheral reflection of cardiac action.

Join the two points by two parallel lines.
- It is the most important site of recording pulse.

Ulnar artery in forearm *(Fig. 2.33)*:

The points are:
- The point is 1 cm distal to the elbow joint on the medial side of tendon of biceps brachii.
- At the base of pisiform bone. It has a very superficial course in the forearm side.
- A point on the medial part of forearm at the junction of upper one-third and lower two-thirds of a line drawn from base of medial epicondyle of humerus to styloid process of ulna.

  Join these three points with a lumen within. The line between 1 and 3 is convex medially. The line between 2 and 3 is straight.

Superficial palmar arch *(Figs 2.33 and 2.34)*:

The points are:
- Lateral side of pisiform bone.
- Center of thenar eminence in a line with the web between middle and index finger.

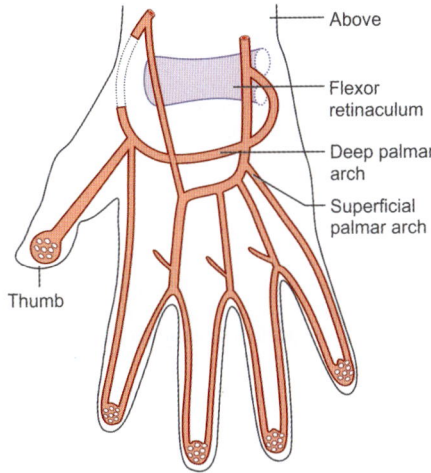

Fig. 2.34: Superficial and deep palmar arch

The points are joined by two curved lines the summit passing along the distal border of outstretched thumb.
- Due to superficial and deep palmar arches the palm is more warmer than dorsum.

Radial nerve in the back of the arm *(Fig. 2.33)*:

The points are:
- At the termination of axillary artery, i.e. at the junction of anterior two-thirds and posterior one-third of the line joining the distal ends of anterior and posterior axillary folds.
- Junction of upper and middle third of the line joining insertion of deltoid to lateral epicondyle.

Join the two points by a single line.

Ulnar nerve in forearm:

The points are:
- Behind medial epicondyle of humerus.
- Lateral to pisiform bone.

Join these two points with a single line.

Points to Remember

- Variation of brachial plexus is common
- During axillary node dissection (as in removal during breast surgery), two nerves are at risk of injury, long thoracic nerve (supplies serratus anterior muscle) and thoracodorsal nerve (supplies latissimus dorsi)
- Commonly chosen intravenous route is median cubital vein. Next is dorsal venous arch of hand, cephalic vein (Figs 2.35 to 2.37)
- Hazards of venepuncture are:
  - Air embolism
  - Infection may be induced
  - Discoloration at the area of injection and formation of hematoma
- Compression of third part of axillary artery is done in the inferior part of lateral wall of axilla to stop profuse bleeding resulting from stab or bullet wound at axilla
- There are some potential spaces within the palm. These are: (1) thenar space, (2) midpalmar space and (3) hypothenar space. They are the common sites of palmar abscess
- Thenar muscles are essential for gripping
- Four muscles (supraspinatus, infraspinatus, teres minor and subscapularis) form rotator cuff which help to stabilize multiaxial shoulder joint.

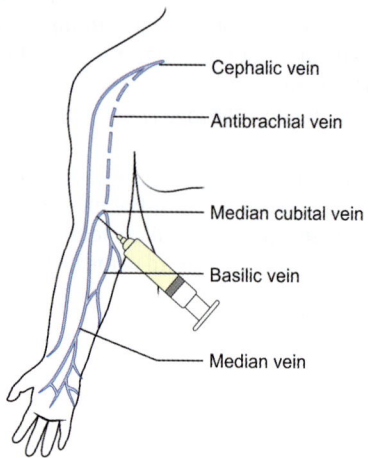

Fig. 2.35: Intravenous injection in median cubital vein

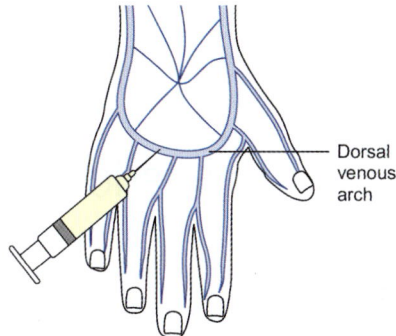

Fig. 2.36: Intravenous injection into dorsal venous arch

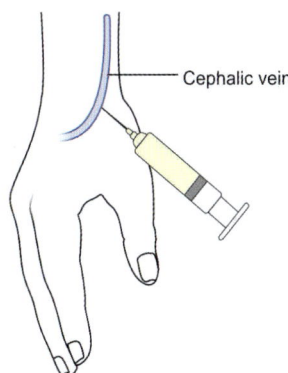

Fig. 2.37: Intravenous injection into cephalic vein

3
CHAPTER

Inferior Extremity

CHAPTER OUTLINE

- Femoral Triangle
- Saphenous Opening
- Great Saphenous Vein
- Perforating Veins
- Iliotibial Tract
- Profunda Femoris Artery
- Interosseous Membrane (Lower Limb)
- Acetabular Labrum
- Popliteus Muscle
- Locking and Unlocking of the Knee Joint
- Superficial Peroneal Nerve
- Deep Peroneal Nerve
- Obturator Nerve
- Trendelenburg Test
- Factors that Increase the Stability of Hip Joint
- Extra-articular Ligament of Knee Joint
- Deltoid Ligament
- Spring Ligament
- Greater Sciatic Foramen
- Medial Longitudinal Arch of Foot
- Inguinal Lymph Nodes

SHORT NOTES

FEMORAL TRIANGLE (FIG. 3.1)

The triangle is situated in front of the thigh. One can observe a depression over the upper and front of thigh in the region of femoral triangles.

Boundary
- *Base*—inguinal ligament
- *Apex*—meeting of the medial border of adductor longus with the medial border of sartorius
- *Laterally*—medial border of sartorius
- *Medially*—medial border of adductor longus.

Floor (Lateral to Medial)
- Iliacus
- Psoas major
- Pectineus
- Adductor longus.

Roof
It is formed by skin, superficial fascia [containing superficial inguinal lymph nodes (LN) and deep fascia].

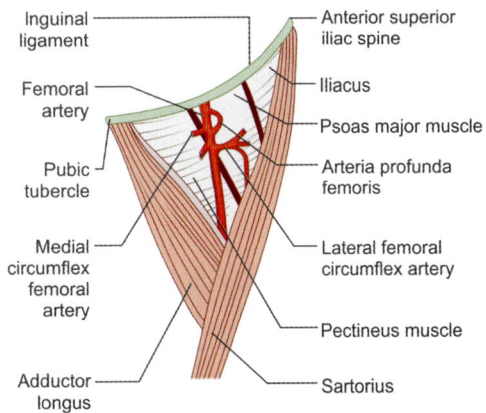

Fig. 3.1: Femoral triangle

Content (Lateral to Medial)
- *Lateral femoral cutaneous nerve*: It lies close to anterior superior iliac spine
- Femoral nerve (lies in the iliopsoas groove) with branches
- Femoral sheath (which cover upper 4 cm of femoral vessels) with its contents (femoral artery in lateral compartment, femoral vein in intermediate compartment, femoral canal in medial compartment)
- Profunda femoris vessels
- *Femoral nerve*: It lies in the groove between iliacus and psoas major. It sends a branch called nerve to pectineus, which passes behind the femoral sheath. Femoral artery gives three superficial and three deep branches in the femoral triangle. They are:
  1. Superficial external pudendal
  2. Superficial epigastric
  3. Superficial circumflex iliac artery.

Clinical Anatomy
- *Femoral hernia*: The femoral canal is a potential weak area through which abdominal viscus or part of a viscus may come out forming hernia
- The femoral artery can be compressed at mid-inguinal point against head of femur or superior ramus of pubis to control bleeding of lower limb
- Femoral artery is quite superficial in femoral triangle. So, catheters are passed upwards up to the heart for certain minor operation
- Stab wound at the apex of femoral triangle may cut all the large vessels of lower limb because they are in one line from before backwards at this point.

SAPHENOUS OPENING
Introduction
It is an oval opening in the fascia lata on the upper part of the medial side of the thigh (Fig. 3.2).

Measurement
Length: 3 cm; and breadth: 1.5 cm.

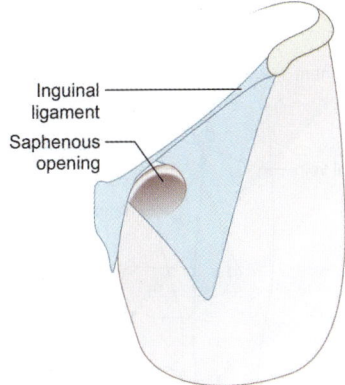

Fig. 3.2: Deep fascia (left thigh)

Description

It has sharp falciform margin, which bounds on the superior, lateral and inferior aspect. The medial margin is smooth and merges with fascia covering the anterior surface of pectineus. The falciform margin lies anterior to the femoral sheath whereas, the medial margin passes posterior to the sheath. The opening is blocked by cribriform fascia. It is known as cribriform fascia because of its sieve-like appearance. The structures pierces saphenous opening—long saphenous vein, lymph vessels and superficial external pudendal, superficial epigastric and superficial circumflex iliac arteries.

Clinical Anatomy

The saphenous opening is very important surgically.

GREAT SAPHENOUS VEIN (FIG. 3.3)

Formation

It is the continuation of the medial marginal vein of the foot.

End

In the femoral vein, about 3 cm below the inguinal ligament.

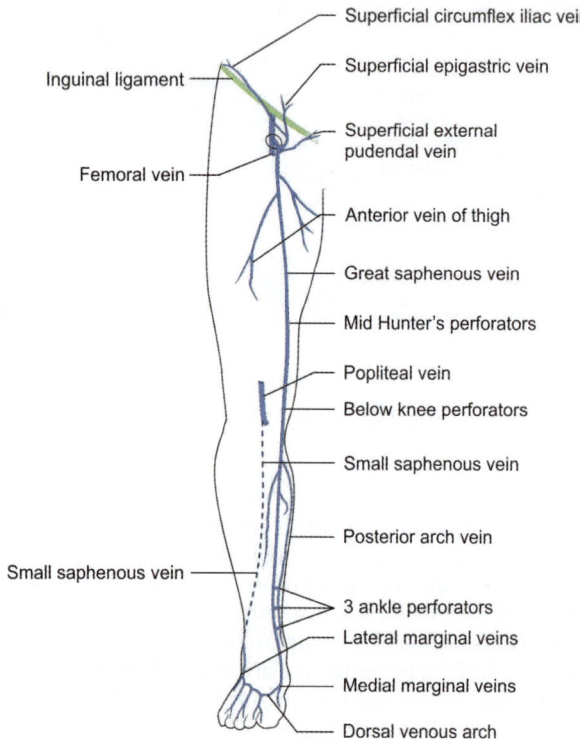

Fig. 3.3: Great saphenous vein

Course

- It is the longest vein in the body
- It ascends in front of the medial malleolus and ascends upwards and backwards on the medial surface of tibia to reach its medial border along which it ascends to the knee
- It runs upwards then ascends behind medial condyle of tibia and femur. And then along with medial part of the front of thigh. It finally passes through the saphenous opening piercing the cribriform fascia and end in the femoral vein about 3.25 cm below and lateral to the pubic tubercle.

Relations
- *In the thigh*: It is accompanied by the some branches of the medial femoral cutaneous nerve
- *On the medial side of the knee*: It is accompanied by the saphenous branch of the descending genicular artery
- On the medial side of the leg and in front of the medial malleolus and in foot, it is accompanied by the saphenous nerve, which lies in front of the vein.

Valves
10–20 in number they are more in the leg than in the thigh.

Two valves are constant:
1. Just before piercing the cribriform fascia
2. At its end in the femoral vein.

Tributaries
- From sole of the foot through the medial marginal vein
- Communicating veins with:
  - Small saphenous vein
  - Anterior tibial vein
  - Posterior tibial vein
- Cutaneous veins
- Veins of the thigh
- Accessory saphenous vein
- Superficial epigastric vein
- Superficial circumflex iliac vein
- Superficial external pudendal vein
- Deep external pudendal vein.

Clinical Anatomy

Venesection

When patient is in collapse state as in shock, it is not easy to get superficial veins. So, saphenous vein is cut in front of ankle for treatment purpose (Fig. 3.4).

Varicosity

Dilation and tortuosity of vein are known as varicosity. It is seen in long-saphenous vein in person with long-standing habit.

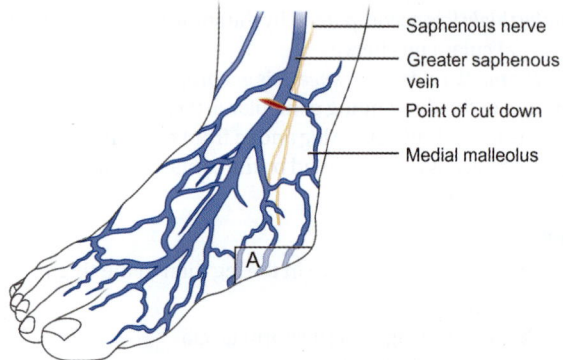

Fig. 3.4: Dorsal venous network and level of venesection

PERFORATING VEINS

The superficial and deep veins of the lower limb are connected by perforating veins. Perforating veins are of two types:
1. *Indirect*: The superficial vein pierces the deep fascia and end in veins within the muscles, which in turn connect the veins
2. *Direct*: The superficial veins after piercing the deep fascia directly connect the deep veins. These are great saphenous vein, small saphenous vein and smaller perforating veins. The communications are as follows:
   – In thigh
   – In femoral region—great saphenous vein ending in femoral vein
   – In adductor canal—a communicating vein in between the great saphenous with the femoral vein
   – A little above the knee—small saphenous vein ending in popliteal vein
   – In the leg (just distal to knee)—a communicating vein between the great saphenous and posterior tibial.

Ankle Perforating Vein

There are upper, middle and lower perforating veins. These perforating veins have valves, which are so arranged that venous blood will not go from deep to superficial. When this valve become defective, venous blood will enter the superficial veins causing dilatation and tortuosity. This is called varicose vein.

Normally through superficial vein, little blood is carried because they have to drain the blood against gravity. Though the deep veins drain the blood against gravity but the blood is pushed towards the heart by means of muscular action.

ILIOTIBIAL TRACT

Introduction
It is the condensed lateral part of fascia lata (Fig. 3.5).

Attachments
- *Above*: To the anterior part of iliac crest
- *Below*: To the anterior surface of lateral condyle of tibia on a tubercle (Gerdy's tubercle).

Importance
- The iliotibial tract provides insertion to tensor fasciae latae and gluteus maximus muscle. The tract extends their insertion to tibia
- It plays an important role to stabilize the knee joint particularly in extended knee especially during running.

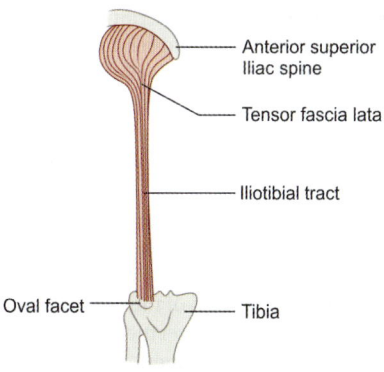

Fig. 3.5: Iliotibial tract

Clinical Anatomy

The long-distance runner or excessive cycling develops inflammation near its insertion and produces pain. It is relieved by cortisol injection or by surgical sectioning of the tract.

PROFUNDA FEMORIS ARTERY

It is the biggest branch of femoral artery. It supplies the extensor, adductor and flexor muscles of the thigh. It arises from lateral side of the femoral artery 3.5 cm below the inguinal ligament. It then goes medially behind the femoral vessels. It leaves the femoral triangle by passing through the pectineus and adductor longus. Then it passes through the adductor brevis and adductor longus, and after that it passes through adductor longus and adductor magnus. It finally pierces adductor magnus as fourth perforating artery and ultimately anastomoses with the superior muscular branch of the popliteal artery. In femoral triangle, it gives two branches:
1. Lateral circumflex femoral
2. Medial circumflex femoral.

During rest of the course, it gives muscular branches and three perforating branches.

Branches of Profunda Femoris

Lateral Circumflex Femoral

It passes through the anterior and posterior division of femoral nerve and passes beneath the sartorius and rectus femoris and ultimately dividing into: (1) ascending; (2) transverse; and (3) descending branches.

- *Ascending branch*: It ascends up to anterior-superior iliac spine and takes part in formation of spinous anastomosis with superficial and deep circumflex iliac artery, iliac branch of iliolumbar artery and superior gluteal artery.
- *Transverse branch*: It goes laterally over the vastus medialis muscle and pierces the vastus lateralis muscle and then winds the greater trochanter and forms one limb of the cruciate anastomosis.
- *Descending branch*: It descends over the anterior border of the vastus lateralis and anastomosis with superior lateral genicular artery.

Medial Circumflex Femoral Artery

It goes medially in between the psoas and pectineus and then adductor brevis and obturator externus and over the upper border of adductor magnus. It divides into transverse and ascending branches. The transverse branch forms cruciate anastomosis with transverse branch of lateral femoral circumflex artery ascending branch of the first perforating artery and descending branch of inferior gluteal artery.

Ascending branch goes over the quadratus femoris and takes part in trochanteric anastomosis (which is chief blood supply of head and neck of femur). An acetabulum branch arises from the medial circumflex femoral artery at the upper border of the adductor brevis and it enters inside the hip joint. It supplies the acetabular fat, limited area if head of femur and ligamentum teres femoris.

Perforating Arteries

There are four in number and the last one is the continuation of the profunda femoris artery. The perforating arteries pierces the adductor magnus and supplies the adductor and hamstring muscles and vastus lateralis muscles and here they are interconnected with each other through a series of anastomosis. The first perforating artery lies above the adductor brevis, second in front of the brevis and third just below the brevis. The second pierces the adductor brevis and magnus, provides a nutrient artery to femur. At the back of the thigh, each perforating artery branches into ascending and descending branches near to the insertion of the adductor magnus. They anastomoses with each other and the highest branch go in formation of the cruciate anastomosis and the lowest goes to anastomose with popliteal artery.

INTEROSSEOUS MEMBRANE (LOWER LIMB) (FIG. 3.6)

- It connects the interosseous border of tibia and fibula
- Proximal end has large oval opening for passage of anterior tibial artery
- Distally perforating branch of peroneal artery pierce it
- Direction of fibers—downward and laterally
- Distally it is continuous with fibers of distal talofibular joint.

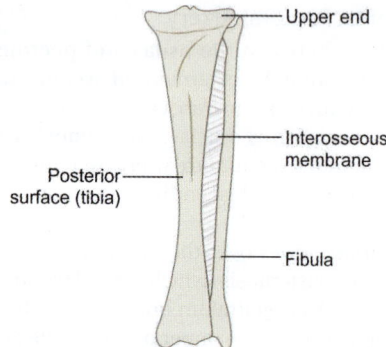

Fig. 3.6: Interosseous membrane (lower limb)

ACETABULAR LABRUM

It is a cartilaginous disc, triangular in shape, which lies along the acetabulum and thus increases the stability of hip joint, by making the articulating bone more congruent. A part of the acetabular labrum bridges the acetabular notch as transverse acetabular ligament. Part of ligament of head of femur fuses with transverse acetabular ligament.

POPLITEUS MUSCLE

It is a flat triangular muscle (Fig. 3.7).

Origin

- Anterior part of the popliteal groove on the lateral surface of the lateral condyle of the femur
- Outer margin of the lateral meniscus
- Arcuate popliteal ligament.

Course and Direction

Fibers descend downwards and medially forming the floor of the popliteal fossa.

Insertion

- Medial two-thirds of the popliteal surface of the tibia above the soleal line
- Fascia covering the popliteus.

Inferior Extremity

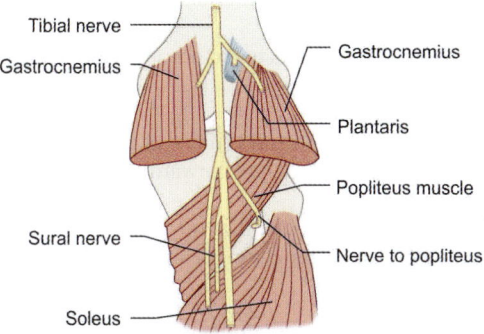

Fig. 3.7: Popliteus muscle

Nerve Supply

Nerve to popliteus [branch of tibial (medial popliteal) nerve], which supplies the muscle from its anterior deep surface by hooking the lower border of popliteus.

Action

Flexion of knee joint (by doing medial and lateral rotation of the leg, which causes unlocking of the knee joint).

Clinical Anatomy

Injury to tibial nerve may result in inability of unlocking.

LOCKING AND UNLOCKING OF THE KNEE JOINT

Locking

- Knee joint is fully flexed
  ↓
- Lateral and medial condyle rest on menisci at the posterior end of posterior horn
  ↓
- Condyles begin to move forward
  ↓
- Initiation of extension
  ↓
- Condyles run on menisci, along the evolute of profile
  ↓
- Lateral menisci is smaller

- Lateral condyle reaches the anterior horn of lateral menisci earlier than medial meniscus
- Further extension is restricted as the anterior cruciate ligament is taut
- 30° short of extension
- So, there is rotation of lateral condyle of femur forward
- Medial condyle rotates to come forward and get the anterior horn of medial meniscus
- This position is locked by further movement
- No skeletal muscle contraction, so person can stand prolonged.

Unlocking
- Tendon of popliteus starts contracting
- Beginning of flexion
- Lateral condyle moves forwards and it is unlocked and further flexion occurs.

SUPERFICIAL PERONEAL NERVE

It is the nerve of the lateral (peroneal) compartment of the leg (Fig. 3.8).

Origin with Level

It is one of the terminal division of common peroneal nerve at the lateral surface of the neck of the fibula between the two heads of the peroneus longus.

Component

It is a mixed nerve.

Course with End

Within lateral compartment of the leg:
- It lies at first deep to the peroneus longus; then between it and extensor digitorum longus separated by anterior intermuscular septum
- It then passes downwards and forwards between the peroneus brevis and extensor digitorum longus pierces the deep fascia of the leg at the junction of upper two-thirds and lower one-thirds
- It gives off muscular branches to the peroneus longus, peroneus brevis, skin of lower part of the leg.

Inferior Extremity

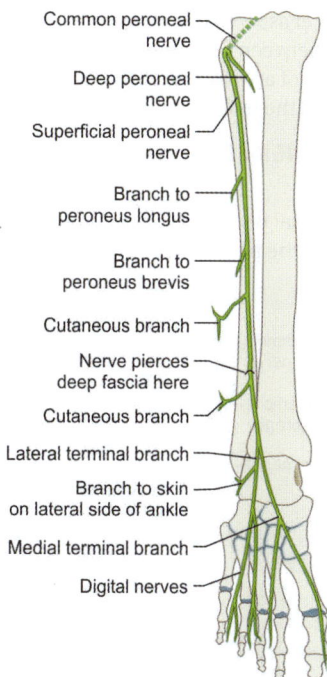

Fig. 3.8: Superficial peroneal nerve

Rest of its course: It lies in the subcutaneous tissue in front of the leg and divides into a medial and a lateral branch.

Both the divisions reach the dorsum of the foot in front of the superior and inferior extensor retinaculum and supply skin on dorsum except a small triangular area in between first and second toe and lateral border of dorsum of foot.

Clinical Importance

This nerve and also deep peroneal nerve generally involved in fracture of neck of fibula. The effects due to injury of this nerve area as follows:

- Sensation of outer aspect of leg and whole of dorsum of foot except the web space between first and second toes are lost
- Evertors of the foot are paralyzed. So, the man has to walk on the medial border of the foot.

DEEP PERONEAL NERVE (FIG. 3.9)

Origin

It is one of the terminal divisions of the common peroneal nerve on the lateral surface of the neck of the fibula between the two heads of peroneus longus.

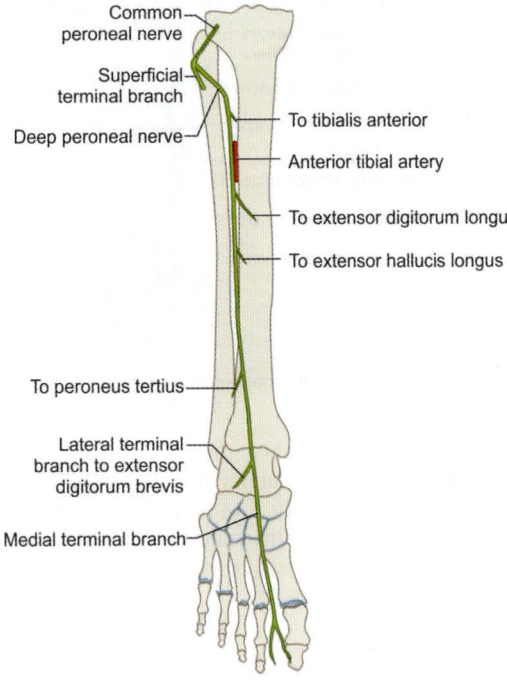

Fig. 3.9: Deep peroneal nerve

Course

It passes obliquely forwards and enters the anterior compartment of the leg by piercing the anterior intermuscular septum and deep to the origin of the extensor digitorum longus.

It then descends on the interosseous membrane along with anterior tibial artery.

Branches

- *Muscular branches* to tibialis anterior, extensor digitorum longus and extensor hallucis longus
- *Cutaneous branch* to the interdigital cleft between first and second toe.

Clinical Anatomy

Lesion of this nerve produces foot drop (foot is fully plantar flexed) due to paralysis of all the muscles of anterior compartment of leg, extension of toes is lost due to paralysis of extensor digitorum longus and hallucis longus.

OBTURATOR NERVE (FIG. 3.10)

Origin

From the ventral division of the anterior rami of L_2, L_3 and L_4 nerves; L_3 nerve is the largest.

Course with Relations

- *In posterior abdominal wall*: It descends through psoas up to the sacroiliac joint where it emerges from the medial border of the psoas major and its sheath
- *Entrance into the pelvis*: At the sacroiliac joint, it passes behind the bifurcation of common iliac vessels. It supplies the sacroiliac joint by a small twig
- *On lateral wall of the pelvis*: It descends first lying on the fascia covering the obturator internus underneath the ovarian fossa and then below the superior ramus pubis, lying between the pelvic brim and upper attachment of the obturator fascia. It finally reaches the obturator canal.

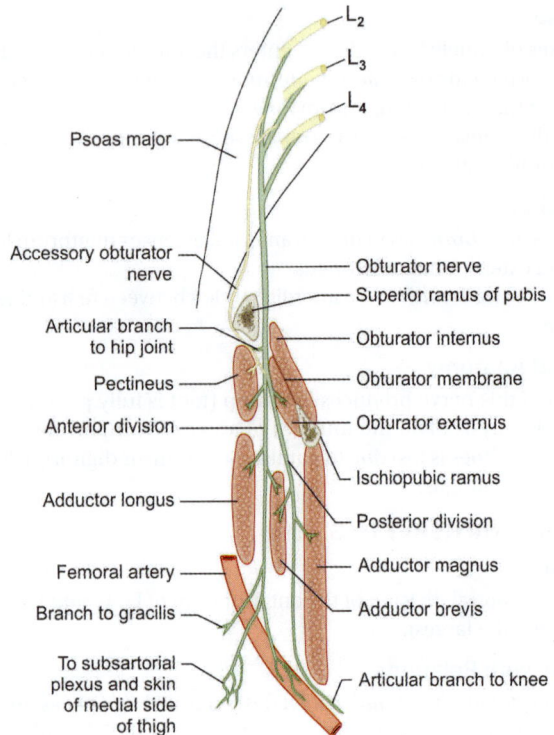

Fig. 3.10: Obturator nerve

Relations of this part:
- *Above*: Obliterated umbilical artery
- *Below*: Obturator artery and vein
- Laterally:
  - Obturator muscle and its fascia in the upper part.

Clinical Anatomy

The obturator nerve may be damaged as a result of anterior dislocation of hip joint. The adduction is lost due to paralysis of adductor muscles and sensory loss on the medial aspect of thigh.

TRENDELENBURG TEST

This test is done to note the stability of hip joint. A positive test confirms a defect in osseomuscular stability, especially abductors of hip joint and a patient has a lurching gait. If the patient is asked to stand on one leg, if abductors of thigh (gluteus medius and minimus) are paralyzed on that side, they will be unable to sustain the pelvis against body weight and pelvis tilts downward on the unsupported side.

FACTORS THAT INCREASE THE STABILITY OF HIP JOINT

The stability of the hip joint is maintained by the following factors:
- Depth of acetabulum with narrow mouth, made by acetabular labrum
- Strength of surrounding ligaments
- Strength of surrounding muscles
- Length and obliquity of neck of femur.

The wide range of mobility depends upon the neck of the femur, which is narrower than equatorial diameter of head.

EXTRA-ARTICULAR LIGAMENT OF KNEE JOINT

The extra-articular ligaments of knee joint are as discused follows:
- *Capsular ligament:* It covers the knee joint but there are gaps in two sides.
    - Anteriorly the fibrous capsule is deficient over patellar area. Though this gap suprapatellar bursa may communicate with the joint cavity. The capsule is blend with the ligamentum patellae in other places.
    - Posteriorly and above it is attached to the articular margin of femoral condyles and posterior intercondylar fossa.
      Below it is attached to tibial condyles and intercondylar. But there is a gap in the lateral aspect for the passage of tendon of popliteus.
- *Tibial collateral ligament:* It is Y-shaped ligament. Stem or upper part is attached to the medial epicondyle of femur.
    - Anterior or superficial part is attached to the medial margins encroaching the medial surface of shaft of tibia. It is 10 cm long. It is the degenerated part of serial fiber of adductor magnus.

- Posterior (Deep part) is attached to bellow to the medial condyle of tibia above groove for semi-membranosus. It also blends with capsular ligament and medial semilunar cartilage.
- *Fibular collateral ligament:* It is a strong cord-like ligament attached above—to the lateral epicondyle of femur above the groove of popliteus.

  Below—it is attached to the styloid process of head of fibula. This ligament pierces the insertion of bifemoris and it is separated from lateral semilunar cartilage by tendon of popliteus.
- *Oblique popliteal ligament:* This ligament is situated at the back of knee. It is an expansion of semi-membranosus. It extends upwards and laterally and attached to the lateral inter condylar line and lateral condyle of femur. The ligament is pierced by (i) Middle genicular vessels and nerve (ii) Posterior division obturator nerve.

DELTOID LIGAMENT (FIG. 3.11)

It is triangular or delta-shaped ligament (Δ).

Nature

Very strong.

Parts

Superficial (Attachment)

- *Above*: Tip of medial malleolus
- *Below*: It splits into three bands, namely:
  1. *Anterior/tibionavicular*—attached to tuberosity of navicular bone and blends with spring ligament
  2. *Middle/tibiocalcaneal*—attached to sustentaculum tali of calcaneum
  3. *Posterior or talotibial*—attached to posterior tubercle of talus.

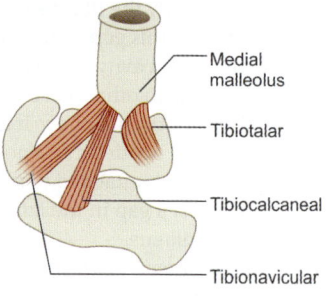

Fig. 3.11: Superficial part of deltoid ligament P.G.E.

Deep (Attachment)
- *Above*: Just inside the tip of medial malleolus
- *Below*: Rough area just below the comma-shaped facet on medial surface of body of talus.

Functions
- Major ligament of ankle joint
- Prevents excessive eversion.

Clinical Anatomy
Forceful eversion produces injury to deltoid ligament producing ankle sprain.

SPRING LIGAMENT
It is also known as plantar calcaneonavicular ligament. The name spring ligament is misnomer in the sense that it does not contain any elastic tissue. But, as it maintains the dynamic platform during walking like spring, it is known as spring ligament.

Attachments
- *Behind*—in front of sustentaculum tali
- *In front*—tuberosity of navicular bone
- *Surfaces*:
  - *Superior*—it is fibrocartilaginous, coming in contact with head of talus
  - *Inferior*—supported by tibialis posterior.

Borders
- *Medial*—blends with deltoid ligament
- *Lateral*—with fibrous capsule of talocalcaneonavicular joint.

Importance
- Major ligament of talocalcaneonavicular joint
- Supports head of talus from below
- Maintains medial longitudinal arch
- When this ligament is weak due to long-standing or congenitally it produces flat foot.

GREATER SCIATIC FORAMEN (FIG. 3.12)

- Greater sciatic notch is converted into greater sciatic foramen by the attachment of the sacrotuberous and sacrospinous ligament
- Structures coming out through the greater sciatic foramen:
  - Piriformis muscle
- *Above piriformis:*
  - Passes superior gluteal vessels and nerves
- *Below piriformis:*
  - Passes inferior gluteal vessels and nerves
- Sciatic nerve
- Posterior cutaneous nerve of thigh
- *Structures over the ischial spine:* They comes out through greater sciatic foramen and lie over the ischial spine
  - Internal pudendal vessels, pudendal nerve
  - Nerve to obturator internus
  - Nerve to quadratus femoris.

Clinical Anatomy

Piriformis Syndrome

Sometimes sciatic nerve divides earlier. Then one branch of it comes through piriformis muscle. Entrapment of the division of sciatic nerve occurs and causes pain during the external rotation of the hip joint. This is known as piriformis syndrome.

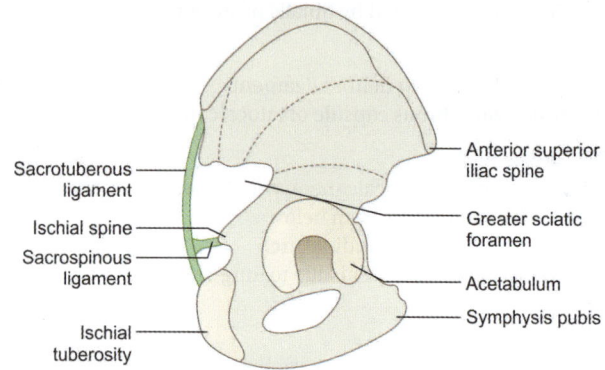

Fig. 3.12: Greater sciatic foramen

MEDIAL LONGITUDINAL ARCH OF FOOT

Arch of foot acts as an elastic platform, which helps to carry the weight of body to the ground efficiently and economically. It also protects plantar vessels and nerve from compression (Fig. 3.13).

INGUINAL LYMPH NODES (FIG. 3.14)

They lie below the inguinal ligaments and divided into two groups—(1) superficial and (2) deep.

1. *Superficial group*: It lies in superficial fascia like letter T. It is divided into a horizontal (lies below and parallel to inguinal ligament) and vertical group (lies along the upper part of great saphenous vein).

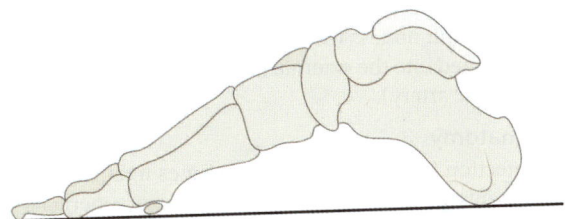

Fig. 3.13: Medial longitudinal arch

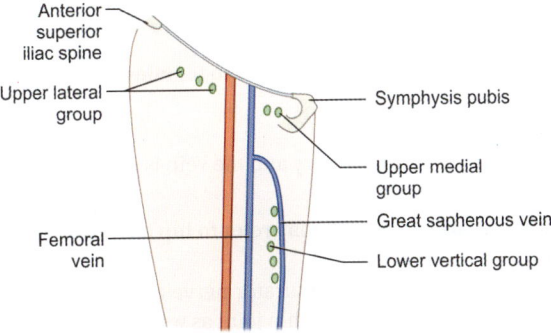

Fig. 3.14: Distribution of inguinal lymph nodes

The superficial inguinal lymph node (LN) drain the following area:
- Superficial lymphatics from skin and subcutaneous tissue of lower limb (Fig. 3.14)
- Gluteal region
- Anterior abdominal wall below the level of umbilicus
- Perineum and external genitalia except glans penis
- Vagina below hymen and lower part of anal canal below pectinate line.

2. *Deep inguinal lymph nodes*: They are few lymph nodes lying along the upper part of femoral vein. One of them lies within femoral canal known as gland of Cloquet. All the vessels from superficial nodes drain into deep group; in addition, they receive deep lymphatics from the deeper structure of lower limb via popliteal lymph nodes. The lymphatics of glans penis also drained into deep inguinal lymph nodes. The efferents from deep inguinal lymph nodes drained into the external iliac lymph nodes (lies along the external iliac artery).

Clinical Anatomy

- Any infection in the foot, even sometimes tight shoes produce (blister) enlargement of inguinal lymph nodes (superficial group)
- In cancer of glans penis, deep inguinal lymph nodes are enlarged
- In carcinoma of body of uterus superficial inguinal lymph nodes (medial group) will be enlarged.

EXPLANATORY NOTES

Q1. Femoral hernia is more common in females because.

Ans.
1. Broader pelvic cavity
2. Caliber of the femoral artery and the vein is much less in case of females than the males.

Q2. Pain in ovarian diseases may refer to hip as well as knee joint. Explain.

Ans. Ovarian fossa contains obturator nerve and obturator vessels, obturator nerve also supply the hip joint as well as the knee joint. So pain in ovarian disease may refer to hip as well as knee.

Q3. Intracapsular fracture of the neck of the femur may cause avascular necrosis of its head. Explain.

Ans. Intracapsular fracture of the neck of the femur may cause avascular necrosis of its head because there is the presence of retinacular fibers, which ascend in front of the neck of the femur. Now when there is a fracture, it causes tear of the retinacular artery. Hence, head of femur does not get adequate blood supply resulting in avascular necrosis.

Q4. What are the anatomical factors that stabilizing the hip joint?

Ans.
1. Deep acetabulum
2. Acetabular labrum keeps the head within the cavity
3. Attachment of fibrous capsule and ligamentum teres femoris between the head of the femur and acetabulum
4. Fibrous capsule is strong.

Q5. Congenital dislocation of hip is common in girls. Explain.

Ans. This is a condition of spontaneous dislocation of the hip joint often bilateral, occurring before, during or shortly after birth.

Present evidence suggests that there are two distinct types of congenital dislocation of hip (CDH)—those already dislocated at birth, the classic CDH and the other type, dislocatable after birth. In either case, CDH is 5–9 times more common in girls.

The etiology origin is yet not well-understood but the following factors appear to be important:

- *Hereditary predisposition* to joint laxity, which makes the joint prone to dislocation in some positions of the fetus in uterus specially during the third trimester or faulty child handling
- *Hormone-induced joint laxity*: A ligament relaxing hormone called relaxin is secreted the gravid uterus of the mother crosses the placental barrier and enters the fetus. If the hormonal status of the fetus is a female, relaxin acts on the fetal joints and produces joint laxity and thus the dislocation.

This explains why girls are common sufferers of CDH.

Q6. Medial meniscus is more prone to injury than the lateral one. Explain.

Ans. It is connected with the tibial collateral ligament while lateral meniscus is not attached to fibular collateral ligament.

The medial meniscus is tightly adherent to the superior surface of condyle of the tibia but the lateral meniscus is free. So in rotational injury medial meniscus is more prone to injury than lateral.

Q7. Ligamentum patellae are a part of a tendon. Explain.

Ans. We know muscles are usually inserted into the bone by means of a tendon.

The quadriceps femoris comprises of:
- Vastus medialis
- Vastus lateralis
- Vastus intermedius
- Rectus femoris.

They form an expansion, which is attached around the margin of the patella and contains plenty of fibrous tissue (tendon).

From this expansion, ligamentum patellae are formed and therefore it is a part of the tendon of quadriceps femoris.

Q8. Epiphysis around the knee joint is important, medicolegally.

Ans.
- Usually, the epiphysis appear after birth of baby
- But lower end of femur, which is an epiphysis around knee joint, violates the law. It appears before birth at 9 month of intrauterine life
- This has tremendous importance to forensic experts to determine the child age and detect cases of infanticide.

Q9. Sciatic nerve is damaged in dislocation of hip joint, explain.

Ans. The sciatic nerve is likely to be damaged due to posterior dislocation of hip joint, associated with fracture of posterior lip of acetabulum. In this region, the sciatic nerve is closely related. That is the reason sciatic nerve is damaged in dislocation of hip joint.

Q10. A patient having pathology of hip joint complains of pain in both hip and knee joint.

Ans.
- Both hip and knee joint are supplied by obturator nerve. So in pathology of hip joint, patient complains of pain both in hip and knee joint.

Q11. Patella is usually fractured due to indirect violence. Explain.

Ans. Indirect violence means fracture due to pull of muscle. When an elderly person slips, then he/she may try to prevent himself/herself from falling down. So, there is severe contraction of quadriceps producing fracture of patella.

Q12. Fracture of talus at neck may cause avascular necrosis. Explain.

Ans. The fracture of talus is rare but forceful dorsiflexion of foot may cause fracture along the neck of talus. The arteries enter through the neck of the talus and supply the bone. So, in fracture of neck of talus, the posterior segment, i.e. the body undergoes avascular necrosis (Fig. 3.15).

Q13. Piriformis is the key muscle of the gluteal region. Explain.

Ans. The piriformis divides the gluteal region into two parts—(1) the structure above the piriformis and (2) the structures below the piriformis.

Not only that, the piriformis acts as an external rotator of the hip.

Sometimes, there may be entrapment neuropathy of sciatic nerve and that is known as "piriformis syndrome". So piriformis is known as key muscle of the gluteal region.

Q14. Injury to the superior gluteal nerve shows positive trendelenburg's sign. Explain.

Ans. The stability of the hip joint while standing on one leg with raised opposite foot depends on few factors:

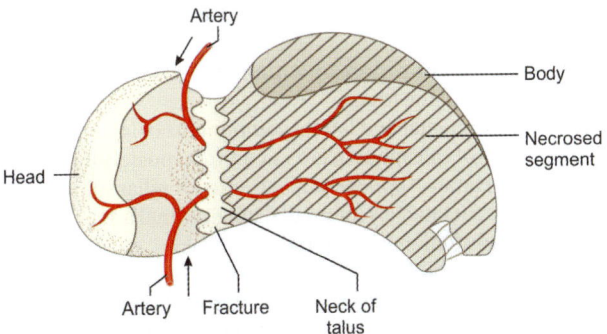

Fig. 3.15: Avascular necrosis of talus following fracture across its neck

- Functioning gluteus medius and minimus (supplied by superior gluteal nerve)
- Head of femur must be located inside acetabulum
- Intact neck of femur and normal neck-shaft angle
- Defect in any one factor may lead to Trendelenburg's sign, i.e. pelvis sinks downwards in unsupported healthy side
- Gluteus, medius and minimus is abductor of hip joint and they are supplied by superior gluteal nerve.

In injury of superior gluteal nerve, the gluteus, medius and minimus are affected. So, they cannot support to opposite-sided unsupported pelvis and it sinks down and shows positive Trendelenburg's sign.

Q15. Fracture of the neck of fibula results in foot drop.

Ans. After the fracture of the neck of the fibula, common peroneal nerve is damaged. When the nerve is completely damaged, the following manifestation is observed. Motor paralysis affects all muscles of peroneal and extensor group of leg including extensor digitorum brevis. This results in foot drop.

Q16. Injury to spring ligament causes flat foot. Explain.

Ans. In order to carry the body weight efficiently and economically, foot is made up of the arches. Acting as segmental lever contributed by the tarsal and metatarsal bones and strengthened by ligaments, muscles, tendons, etc.

The foot has a longitudinal arch system subdivided into medial and lateral arches. One-half of transverse arch in each foot that form a half dome and completed when both feet are brought in contact with each other.

Flat foot is a condition in which there is flattening of the longitudinal arch of the foot.

For both the medial and lateral components of longitudinal arch medial tubercle of calcaneus acts as a common posterior pillar while heads of five metatarsal bones complete anterior pillar support (heads of medial three metatarsals for medial longitudinal arch, fourth, fifth metatarsal heads for lateral longitudinal arch).

The most vulnerable part of the medial arch is represented by the head of talus, acting as the keystone and the most important ligament supporting the medial arch in the plantar calcaneus navicular or the spring ligament (on the upper surfaces of which there is a cartilaginous tissue) on which lies the unsupported part of the head of talus, spring ligament goes from sustentaculum tali to the under surface of the tuberosity of the navicular bone. Its medial margin blends with the deltoid ligament. The ligament itself is supported from below by a slip from the tendon of tibialis posterior. In traumatic flat foot, mostly due to fracture of calcaneum, thin ligament in either weakened or permanently stretched, which ultimately forms flat foot.

Q17. Spring ligament is a misnomer.

Ans. The plantar calcaneonavicular ligament is called the spring ligament. It extends from sustentaculum tali of calcaneum up to tuberosity of navicular bone. It has no elastic tissue, so it has no spring-like properties. But the action is such when the weight of the person falls on the ground, there is flattening of medial longitudinal arch and pressure on the spring ligament. When the person's foot is off the ground, the foot comes back to its original position by spring-like action of the ligament. So by action it is spring like but by property it is misnomer.

Q18. Explain anterior compartment of leg syndrome.

Ans.
- If a person walks rapidly in a very short time to reach the destination, the person accumulates fluid within the anterior compartment of leg due to less drainage of fluid through vein and lymphatics. This may cause severe pain that the person may unable to walk temporarily
- *Treatment*:
    - Rest
    - Massaging
    - In severe cases, incision is given to deep fascia to relieve its tension.

Q19. Soleus is also called peripheral heart. Explain.

Ans.
- Soleus is bulky muscle forming the bulk of calf along with two heads of gastrocnemius
- Multiple perforating veins pass through it. This perforating vein connects superficial vein with deep veins. Some of the perforators form venous sinuses, which store huge amount of blood

- During walking, there is contraction of soleus, which stores the huge amount of blood toward deep vein and it is compared with heart and there is pumping of blood in the circulation. So, soleus is known as peripheral heart
- So, when there is prolonged immobilization, there may be deep vein thrombosis, for that reason patient has to walk on the same day of operation.

Q20. Caries spine of lumbar vertebra may produce swelling of femoral triangle.

Ans.
- Caries spine is also known as tuberculosis of lumbar vertebrae. It produces careation (a type of sticky pus) and that descends through psoas sheath
- The psoas sheath extends up to femoral triangle and so carries spine produces swelling in femoral triangle.

Q21. Which form of dancing is insecured and risky—heel dancing or tip-toe dancing?

Ans. Tip-toe or ballet dancing is risky and insecured because ankle joint has a high risk of coming out of tallus (body) from tibiofibular mortis. So, stability is less. Sprain of the ankle is very common in this position.

Q22. Tibialis anterior maintains the medial longitudinal arch whereas peroneus longus maintains the lateral longitudinal arch.

Ans. Tibialis anterior is inserted into inferior surface of medial cuneiform and base of first metacarpal bone and arises from anterolateral surface of tibia, so it maintains the medial longitudinal arch by sling action.

Q23. Peroneus longus tendon maintains both transverse and longitudinal arches of foot.

Ans. This crosses below the lateral malleolus and goes up to the groove on the lateral border of cuboid. This part maintains the lateral longitudinal arch by sling action.

From the groove on the cuboid bone, it passes obliquely along the plantar aspect of foot and inserted into the base of first metatarsal bone. It crosses the bone obliquely and thus maintains in the transverse arch of foot by bowstring/tie beam arrangement.

Q24. Talipes equinovarus (club foot). Explain.

Ans. It is probably the most common type of foot deformity in which the patient walks on the lateral border of the front part of the foot with heel raised. Combination of the primary deformities may take place in the form of talipes equinovarus. Factors involved in the development of the congenital clubbed foot may be due to failure of muscle growth to keep pace with skeletal growth and imbalance in the growth of different muscles or tendons.

SURFACE ANATOMY OF LOWER LIMB

1. *Tip of medial malleolus*: It is formed by lower projecting part of tibia.
2. *Tip of lateral malleolus*: It is formed by lower end of fibula. It is 0.5 cm lower than the medial malleolus.
3. *Tubercle of navicular bone*: 2 cm below the tip of medial malleolus and 2-cm in front of it.
4. *Adductor tubercle (Figs 3.16 and 3.17)*: Thigh is abducted and laterally rotated; hip and knee are slightly flexed. A small

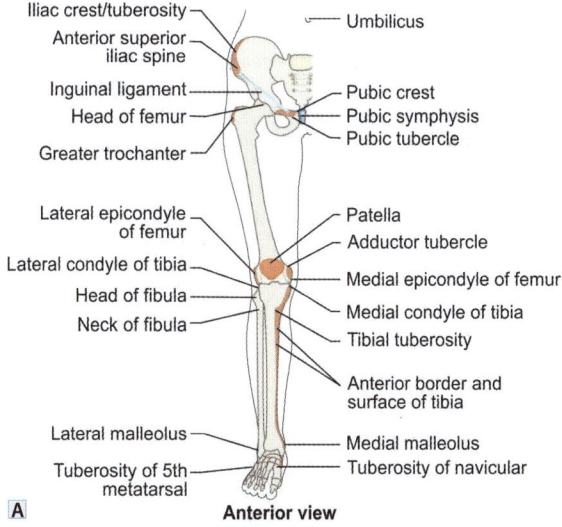

Fig. 3.16A: *Contd...*

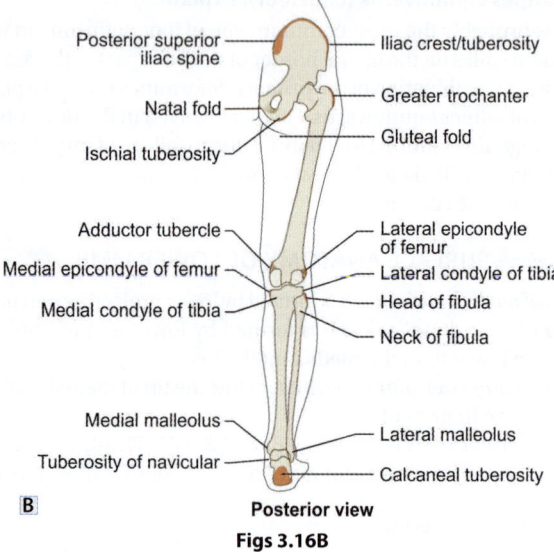

Figs 3.16A and B: Palpable features of inferior extremity

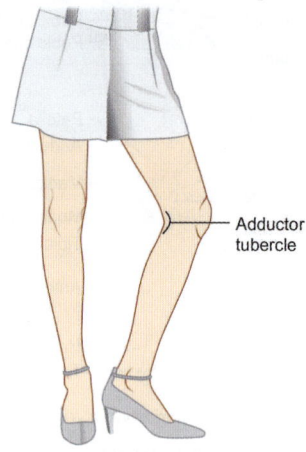

Fig. 3.17: Adductor tubercle (in semiflexed hip and knee)

projection at the upper part of medial condyle of femur is palpated by tracing the tendon of adductor magnus from above.
- *Importance*:
    - Insertion of adductor magnus
    - Junction of epiphysis and diaphysis.

> **Points to Remember**
>
> - *Peroneal muscle atrophy*: It is a common muscle disorder occurs in the age group 20–30. This disorder is slow progressive and gradually spread to calf muscles Number of valves in great saphenous vein is 15–20, whereas in short saphenous vein is only 1
> - During removal of superficial vein, vein should be ligated deep to the deep fascia
> - Doppler ultrasound can detect the deep vein thrombosis and incompetence of saphenofemoral and saphenopopliteal junction
> - *Tibial nerve entrapment or tarsal tunnel syndrome*:
>   - The tibial nerve leaves the posterior compartment of leg and passes deep to flexor retinaculum (which extends from medial malleolus to calcaneus.) Entrapment or compression of tibial nerve occurs (tarsal tunnel syndrome) when there is edema and tightness in the ankle due to involvement of synovial sheath of tendon and muscles of posterior compartment of leg. There is heel pain
> - Postural muscles are at work when person is in rest
> - *Flat foot (pes planus)*—it can be congenital or acquired (due to overweight) and prolong standing
> - *High arch (pes cavus)*—height of arch is more
> - *Talipes equinus*—heal raised; person walks on toes
> - *Talipes calcaneus*—person walks on heel
> - *Talipes varus*—person walks on lateral border of foot
> - *Talipes valgus*—person walks on medial border of foot
> - *Talipes equinovarus*—most common combination. It is also called clubfoot Above all deformities produce impairment of movements and pain.

4 CHAPTER

Abdomen

CHAPTER OUTLINE

Short Notes
- Rectus Sheath
- Inguinal Canal
- Hesselbach's Triangle
- Gastric Triangle
- Stomach Bed
- Bare Area of Liver
- Common Bile Duct
- Calot's Triangle
- Extrahepatic Biliary Apparatus
- Portal Vein
- Peyer's Patches
- Esophageal Varices
- Second Part of Duodenum
- Renal Fascia
- Hepatorenal Pouch of Morison
- Porta Hepatis
- Epiploic Foramen
- Pelvic Mesocolon
- The Mesentery
- Lesser Omentum
- Coronal Section of Kidney
- Base of Urinary Bladder
- Membranous Urethra
- Ectopic Testis
- Ovarian Fossa of Lateral Pelvic Wall
- Celiac Trunk
- Pudendal Canal
- Ischioanal/Ischiorectal Fossa
- Fallopian Tube
- True Ligaments of Uterus
- Superficial Perineal Pouch
- Deep Perineal Pouch
- Pelvic Diaphragm
- Ileocecal Orifice
- Ligaments of Spleen
- Fascia of Colles
- Blood Supply of Vermiform Appendix
- Phimosis
- Bicornuate Uterus
- Cremasteric Reflex

SHORT NOTES

RECTUS SHEATH (FIG. 4.1)

It is an aponeurotic envelope for the rectus abdominis muscle on each side of linea alba. This aponeurotic envelop is derived from three flat muscles present on anterolateral abdominal wall namely: (1) external oblique, (2) internal oblique and (3) transversus abdominis.

Anterior Wall

- *Above the costal margin:* Wall is thin and formed by external oblique aponeurosis
- *From costal margin to midway between umbilicus and symphysis pubis:* The wall is thicker. It is formed by anterior lamella of internal oblique aponeurosis with external oblique aponeurosis
- From rest part (midway between umbilicus and symphysis pubis) to symphysis pubis

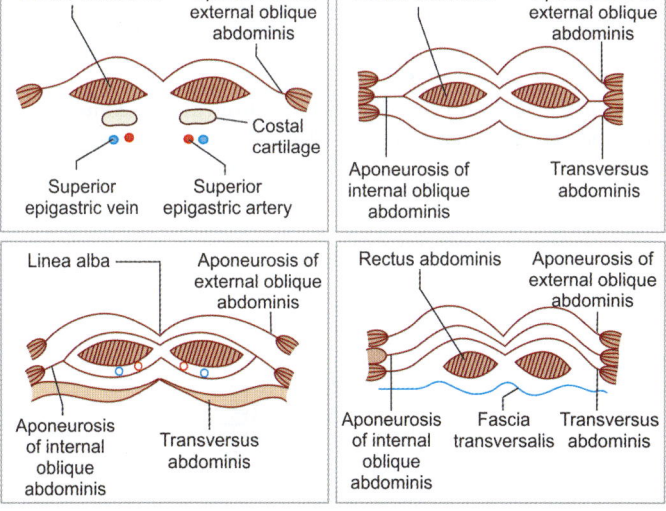

Fig. 4.1: Formation of rectus sheath at different level

Wall is thickest and formed by fusion of aponeurosis of the three muscles: (1) external, (2) internal oblique and (3) abdominis transversus.

Posterior Wall
1. *Above costal margin:* The wall is deficient and muscles rest on 5th, 6th, 7th costal cartilage
2. From the costal margin to midway between umbilicus and symphysis pubis. It is complete rectus sheath. Posterior layer is formed by posterior layer of internal oblique and transversus abdominis
   - *Medial margin:* It is formed by linea alba
   - *Lateral margin:* It is formed by linea semilunaris.
3. *Below the arcuate line:* The rectus muscle is covered posteriorly by fascia transversalis only.

Content
- Rectus abdominis
- Pyramidalis, if present
- Inferior epigastric and superior epigastric vessels
- Lower five intercostal nerves and the subcostal nerve.

INGUINAL CANAL

It is a muscular canal 4 cm long extending from deep inguinal ring to the superficial inguinal ring (Figs 4.2 and 4.3).

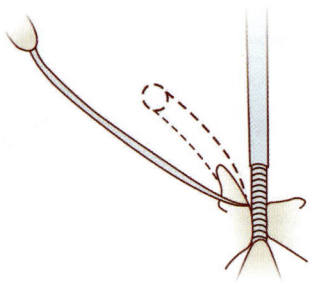

Fig. 4.2: Inguinal canal

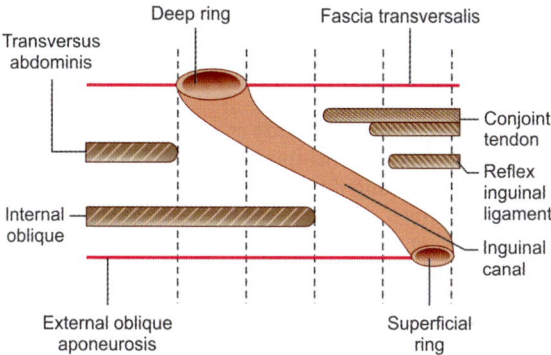

Fig. 4.3: Inguinal canal: Schematic representation of structures forming the anterior and posterior walls

Direction

Downwards, forwards and medially.

Boundary (Box 4.1)

Box 4.1: Inguinal canal boundaries

This canal is 4 cm long and extends from deep ring to superficial inguinal ring.
- *Anterior wall:*
  - Throughout its whole extent formed by external oblique aponeurosis
  - Anterolaterally reinforced by internal oblique and transversus abdominis
- *Posterior wall:* Throughout its whole extent, it is formed by fascia transversalis. Medial part of this wall is reinforced by conjoint tendon
- *Roof:* Formed by arched fibers of internal oblique and transversus abdominis
- *Floor:* Inguinal ligament

Contents

- The spermatic cord in male and round ligament of uterus in female
- *Ilioinguinal nerve:* (Partial content) enters the canal through roof and comes out through superficial inguinal ring, so the nerve is the partial content.

Development

The inguinal canal is formed in the intrauterine life during the descend of gonads. The gonads are developed in lumbar region of the posterior abdominal wall. It descends with gubernaculum (rudder) and in male, it reaches the scrotum and in females it descends up to lesser pelvis. The processus vaginalis is a peritoneal sac that follows the course of gubernaculum.

- *Shutter mechanism or protection of inguinal canal:* It is the weak part of abdominal wall. So, there are some natural mechanisms, which protect the inguinal canal from developing hernia. The mechanisms are:
  - *Obliquity of inguinal canal:* Facilitates the closure during raised of intra-abdominal pressure
  - The contraction of cremaster provides an effective plug to the superficial inguinal ring
  - The internal oblique muscle lies in front, above and posterior wall and hence its contraction obliterate the canal.

HESSELBACH'S TRIANGLE

It is a triangular area situated in lower part of anterior abdominal wall (Fig. 4.4).

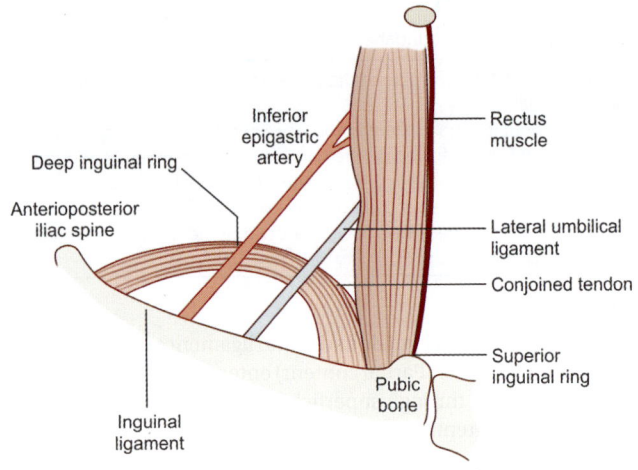

Fig. 4.4: Direct hernia arises through Hesselbach's triangle

Boundary
- Inferior epigastric artery (laterally)
- Lateral border of rectus abdominis (medially)
- Inguinal ligament (below).

Subdivisions
This triangle is also divided into medial and lateral parts by passage of obliterated umbilical artery. So, direct hernia is also divided into medial direct hernia and lateral direct hernia.

Clinical Importance
Direct inguinal hernia enters into inguinal canal through this triangle. So, the neck of direct inguinal hernia lies medial to inferior epigastric artery. By this, direct inguinal hernia is differentiated from indirect inguinal hernia.

GASTRIC TRIANGLE
This is an area overlying anterosuperior surface of stomach, which is not in relation with any viscera.

Boundary
- Above and to the right—inferior border of the liver
- Above and to the left—left costal margin
- Below—transverse colon.

Importance
This part of the anterosuperior surface the stomach is not in relation with any viscera and directly in relation with anterior abdominal wall.

Applied Anatomy
In gastrostomy operation, a Ryle's tube is introduced through this triangle into the stomach under local anesthesia to maintain nutrition in case of malignancy esophagus where the lumen is irreversibly obstructed.

STOMACH BED
Stomach bed is defined as the collection of structures on which stomach rests in supine posture separated by a cavity of lesser sac.

Structures
- Left crus of diaphragm
- Left suprarenal gland
- Anterior surface of left kidney
- Anterior surface of body of pancreas
- Tortuous splenic artery
- Transverse mesocolon
- *Spleen*—but always separated from stomach by a cavity of greater sac.

BARE AREA OF LIVER
It is the largest nonperitoneal area on the posterior surface of the right lobe of liver (Fig. 4.5).

Boundary
- Base is formed by groove for inferior vena caval
- Apex is formed by meeting of the two layers of the coronary ligament forming the right triangular ligament
- Above by superior layer of coronary ligament
- Below by inferior layer of coronary ligament.

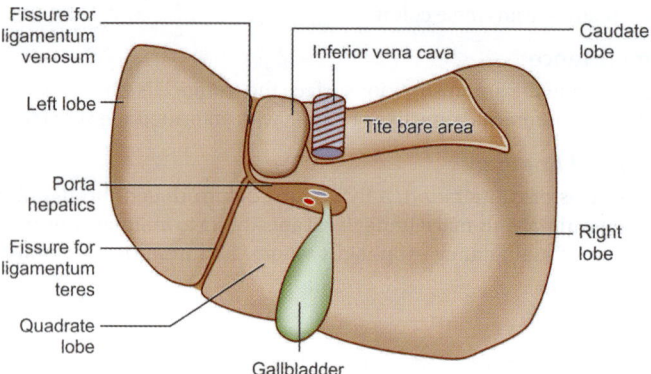

Fig. 4.5: Bare area of liver

Relations

- Part of right suprarenal gland comes to the relation with the bare area
- *Clinical importance:* Anastomosis between portal vein with the veins of diaphragm (systemic).

COMMON BILE DUCT (FIG. 4.6)

Formation

Common hepatic duct after joining with the cystic duct forms the common bile duct (CBD).

Length

It is 8 cm long and has a diameter of 6 mm.

Structures

It has four parts:
1. Supraduodenal
2. Retroduodenal
3. Infraduodenal
4. Intraduodenal.

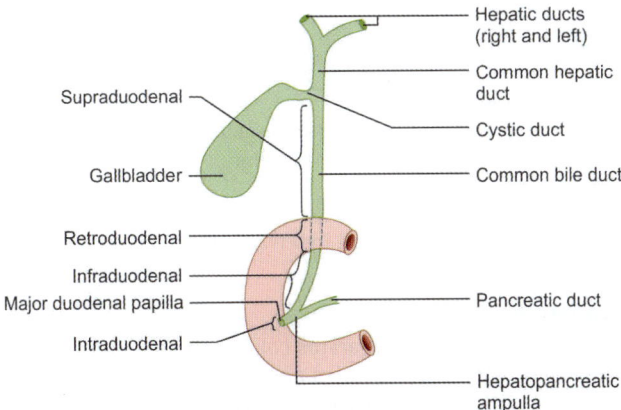

Fig. 4.6: Common bile duct

Draining At
Ampulla of Vater in the major duodenal papilla of second part of duodenum.

Blood Supply
Cystic artery

Clinical Anatomy
- *Cholangitis*—infection of CBD
- Bile duct obstruction causes obstructive jaundice
- *Choledocolithiasis*—stone in the CBD
- Stricture of CBD may occurs during cholecystectomy.
- Bile duct can be assessed by ERCP (endoscopic retrograde cholangiography).

CALOT'S TRIANGLE
The triangle presents in the abdomen in relation to billiary system.
This triangle is very important for surgeons during cholecystectomy.

Boundary
- Above—inferior border of liver
- Below—cystic duct
- Medially—common hepatic duct.

Contents
- Cystic artery
- Cystic lymph node
- Autonomic fibrous supplying in the gallbladder.

Triangle present in the right lumbar region.

EXTRAHEPATIC BILIARY APPARATUS (FIG. 4.7)
Biliary apparatus is subdivided into two parts: (1) intrahepatic and (2) extrahepatic.

Extrahepatic
The extrahepatic biliary apparatus collects the bile from the liver, by common hepatic duct, stores and concentrate the bile in the gallbladder and then transmit it to second part of duodenum by CBD. It consists of:

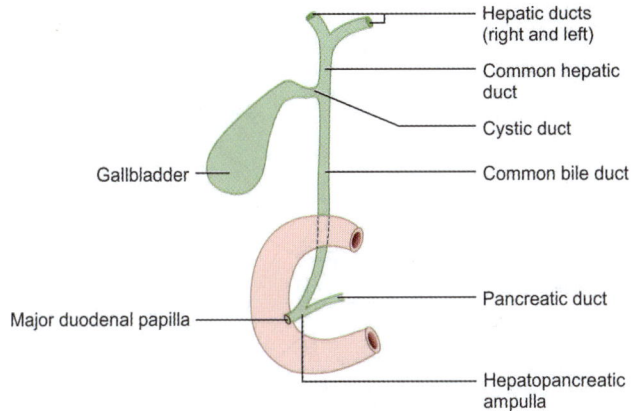

Fig. 4.7: Extrahepatic biliary apparatus

- Common hepatic duct
- Gallbladder
- Cystic duct
- CBD.

Clinical Importance
- Gallstone is very common. Stone may be impacted within cystic duct or CBD. Obstruction of CBD by gallstone produces obstructive jaundice
- Ultrasound is the widely used imaging technique for the diagnosis of a suspected gallstones and biliary tract disease.

PORTAL VEIN
The hepatic portal system collects blood from digestive tract and is valveless. The superior mesenteric vein unite with splenic vein and form a trunk—the portal vein, which enter into the liver and breaks up into capillaries (Fig. 4.8).

Important Portosystemic Anastomosis
Under normal condition, portal blood passes through the liver and drains in the inferior vena cava, by hepatic veins. But when this route is blocked some communication exists at:

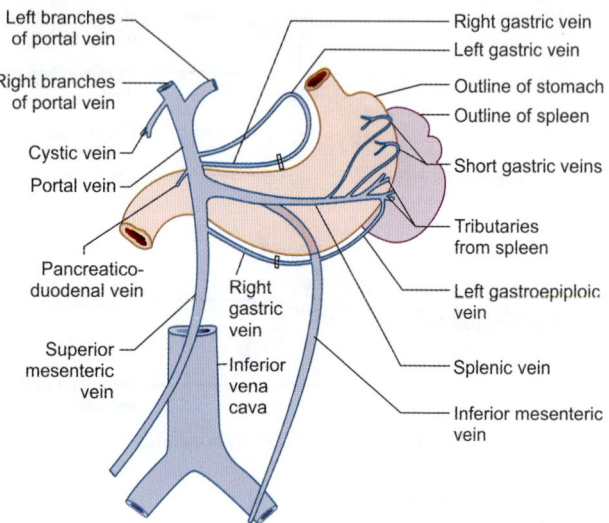

Fig. 4.8: Scheme to show the tributaries of the portal vein

- *Lower end of esophagus:* Communication between esophageal branch of left gastric (portal system) and esophageal branch of azygos system
- *In the distal part of analcanal:* The superior rectal vein (portal system) anastomoses between the middle and inferior rectal vein (systemic)
- *In umbilical region:* Paraumbilical vein connects left branch of portal vein with the superficial vein of abdomen (systemic).

Clinical Anatomy

The anastomotic channels may be distended and ruptures and produces severe hemorrhage. It may be treated with sclerotherapy.

PEYER'S PATCHES

These are the aggregations of lymphatic tissue within the ileum of small gut. Previously, in the enteric fever (typhoid) the Peyer's patches were infected. Previously, it produced perforation of gut and peritonitis. Nowadays, this perforation is prevented by the drug chloramphenicol.

ESOPHAGEAL VARICES

Normal pressure of portal vein is 5-15 mm Hg. When the pressure rises above 40 mm Hg is known as portal hypertension. It is due to cirrhosis of liver, Banti's disease and portal vein thrombosis. In this case, the venous blood can reach the heart via important portacaval anastomosis (Fig. 4.9) described below:

This communication exists at:

- *Lower end of esophagus:* Communication of esophageal branch of left gastric (portal system) with esophageal veins of azygos system (systemic). An abnormally large amount of blood passes through these channels and forms esophageal varices. Channels may rupture and produce severe hemorrhage. It may be corrected by giving sclerosing agent
- *In the distal part of analcanal:* The superior rectal vein (portal system) anastomoses with the middle and inferior rectal vein (systemic). In portal hypertension, these veins dilated and protruded through mucosa and form internal piles (hemorrhoids), which may rupture during passage of stool. It may be corrected by sclerosing agent

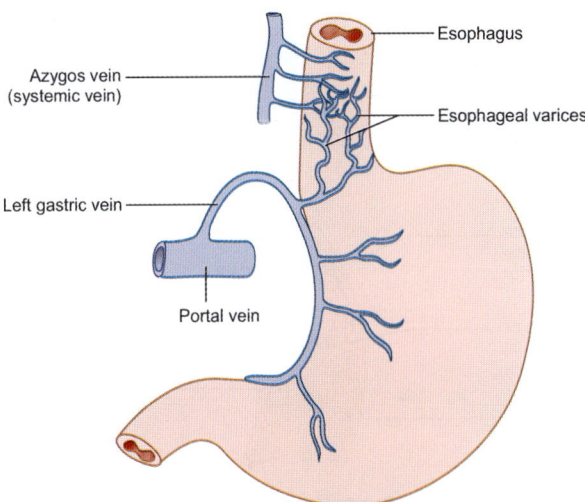

Fig. 4.9: Communication of blood via different veins

- *In umbilical region:* The paraumbilical vein connects with left branch of portal vein with the superficial vein of abdomen (systemic circulation). In portal hypertension, these veins are enlarged and radiates around the umbilicus and form caput medusa.

SECOND PART OF DUODENUM (FIGS 4.10A AND B)

Beginning
From superior duodenal flexure at the level of the neck of gallbladder.

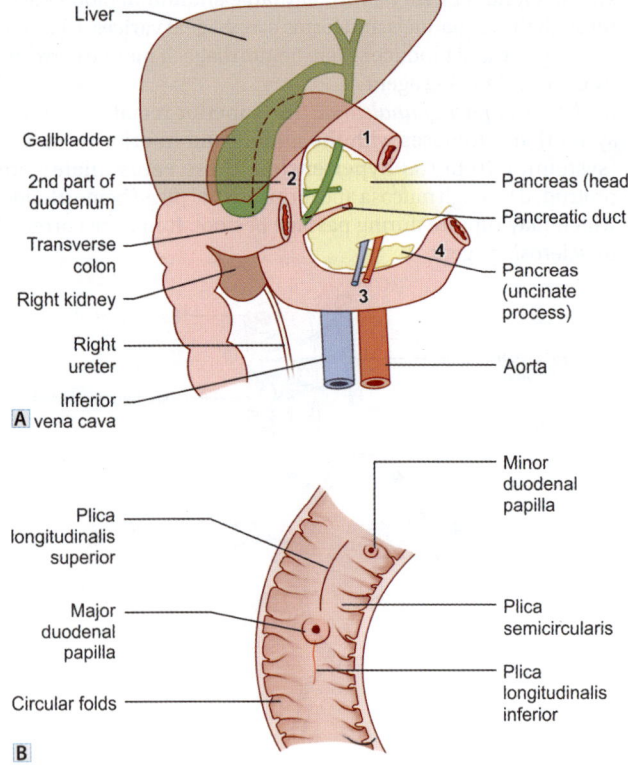

Figs 4.10A and B: (A) Relations of the second and third parts of the duodenum; (B) Interior of the second part of the duodenum

End
It is continuous with third part at inferior duodenal flexure.

Length
About 3 inches.

Peritoneal Relation
In the middle, it is crossed by transverse colon and that part is nonperitoneal. The remaining part of anterior surface is peritoneal. Posterior surface is nonperitoneal.

Features within the Second Part of Duodenum
There is circular mucous fold and in posteromedial aspect there lies major duodenal papilla over which open the ampulla of bile duct. Left border is related with head of pancreas and superior and inferior pancreatico duodenal artery. It lies 8–10 cm away from pylorus. 2 cm proximal to this major papilla lies minor duodenal papilla, over which accessory pancreatic duct open (when present).

Artery Supply and Development
Part above the major duodenal papilla is developed from foregut, so this part is supplied by superior pancreaticoduodenal branch of gastroduodenal artery, which is branch from celiac trunk. The part below the major duodenal papilla is developed from midgut. So, it is supplied by inferior pancreaticoduodenal artery—branch of superior mesenteric artery.

Clinical Importance
In endoscopic examination of second part of duodenum bile is seen to comes out as soap bubble in appearance.

RENAL FASCIA
It is the outermost covering of kidney. It consists of anterior and posterior layers. Upper part fuses above the kidney and encloses suprarenal gland in separate compartment. The two layers remain separated in lower part. Laterally they are fused and become continuous with fascia transversalis. Medially the anterior layer blends with the fascia sheath of the aorta and inferior vena cava. Posterior layer blends with the psoas fascia. Within the renal fascia lies perinephric fat. If the amount of perinephric fat is reduced (due to debilitating disease), the kidney becomes hypermobile and may produce symptoms of renal colic caused by kinking of ureter (Figs 4.11A and B).

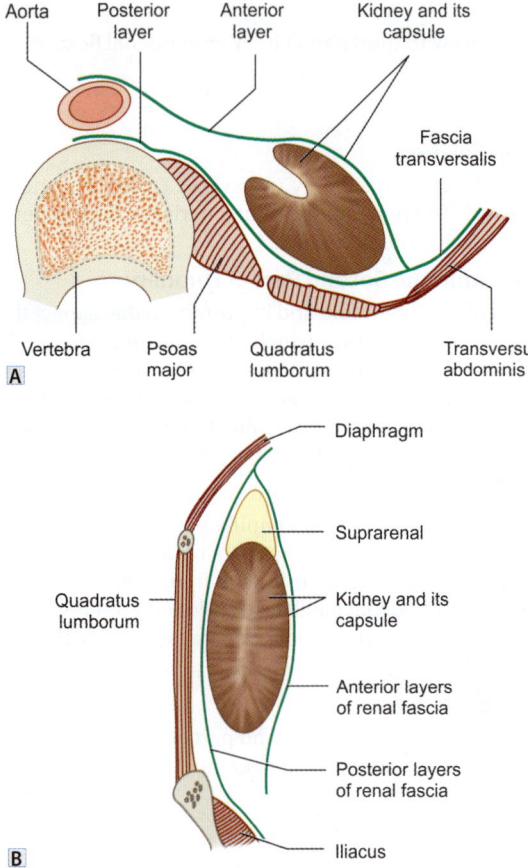

Figs 4.11A and B: Renal fascia

HEPATORENAL POUCH OF MORISON

It is the peritoneal recess situated behind the right lobe of the liver and in front of the right kidney. It is the most dependent part in lying down position. Pathological material gets collected in this pouch (Fig. 4.12). Boundaries of the pouch are as follows:

Abdomen

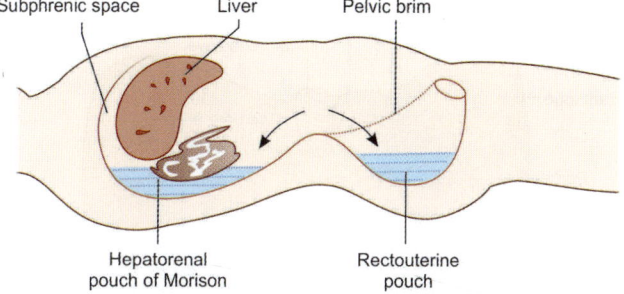

Fig. 4.12: Hepatorenal pouch of Morison

- *Superiorly*: By the inferior layer of coronary ligament of liver
- *Anteriorly*: By the visceral surface of the right lobe of liver
- *Posteriorly*: By the parietal peritoneum that covers the right suprarenal gland and the right kidney
- *Inferiorly*: The space communicates with right paracolic gutter, and hence it ultimately communicates with pelvic cavity
- *On the left side*: The space communicates with the lesser sac through the epiploic foramen.

Thus, the space is connected with the pelvic cavity, so any collection in pelvic cavity (like pouch of Douglas) gets collected in this space and vice-versa.

PORTA HEPATIS

Introduction
It is a transversely situated bare area on the inferior surface of the liver (Fig. 4.13).

Length
About 2–3 cm.

Boundary
- Anteriorly by the quadrate lobe of the liver
- Posteriorly by the lower part of caudate lobe and caudate process
- Right side by neck of gallbladder
- Left side by the meeting of fissure for ligamentum venosum and ligamentum teres.

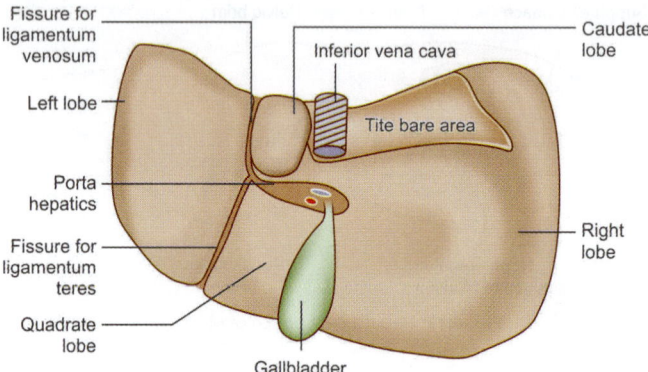

Fig. 4.13: Liver—posteroinferior surface showing the bare area and porta hepatis

Structures

Passing Through

Going in:
- Two division of hepatic artery with sympathetic plexus
- Two divisions of portal veins

Coming out:
- Two hepatic ducts
- Lymph vessels

Relation of these structures from:

From before—backwards:
- Two hepatic duct
- Hepatic artery
- Hepatic vein.

EPIPLOIC FORAMEN

It is a space (foramen), through which greater sac communicates with lesser sac. Its space is like vertical slit 2.5–3 cm in size, bounded anteriorly by free margin of lesser omentum-containing hepatic artery, bile duct and portal vein, behind—by inferior vena cava, below—by first part of duodenum and above—by caudate process of liver (Fig. 4.14).

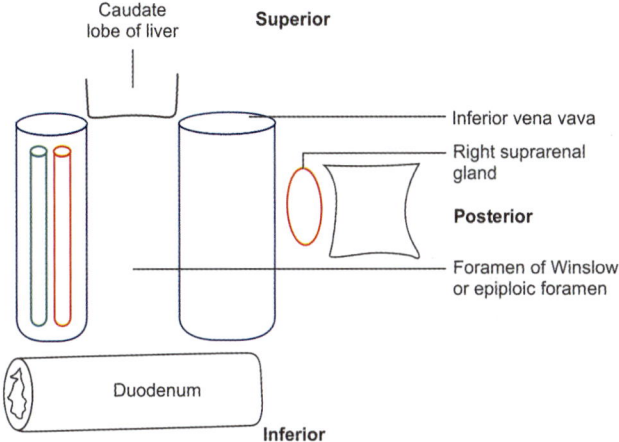

Fig. 4.14: Boundaries of foramen

Clinical Anatomy

Herniated intestinal loop may pass through epiploic foramen and produce internal hernia.

PELVIC MESOCOLON

It is a mesentery of sigmoid/pelvic colon (Fig. 4.15).

Shape

Triangular.

Attachments

- *Apex*: At the left sacroiliac joint. Behind the apex passes the left ureter
- *Left limb*: At the pelvic brim
- *Right limb*: On the pelvic surface of sacrum.

Contents

- Pelvic colon
- Blood vessels for pelvic colon
- Fat
- Lymphatics.

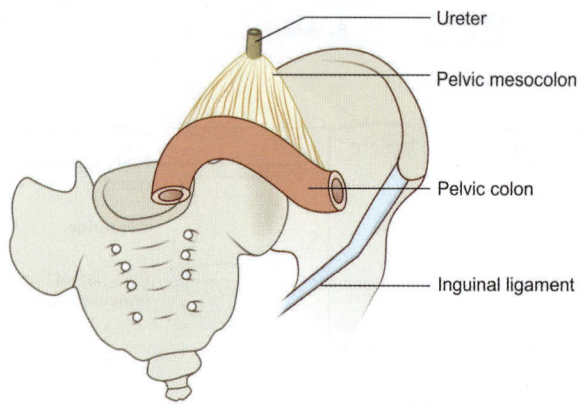

Fig. 4.15: Attachment of the pelvic mesocolon

Development

It is the original dorsal mesentery of the gut.

THE MESENTERY

The mesentery is a fold of peritoneum and has two borders:
1. Vertebral is about 15-cm long extends from duodenojejunal flexure at the level of L_2 vertebra to right sacroiliac joint at the ileocecal junction (Fig. 4.16).
   Structures crossed by the root of the mesentery (vertebral border of the mesentery):
   - Third part of duodenum
   - Abdominal aorta
   - Inferior vena cava
   - Right gonadal vessels
   - Right ureter at sacroiliac joint
   - Right psoas major
   - Right genitofemoral nerve
   - Right sacroiliac joint.
2. Intestinal border—about 5 meters in length.

Contents

- Jejunum and ileum
- Jejunal and ileal branches of superior mesenteric vessels

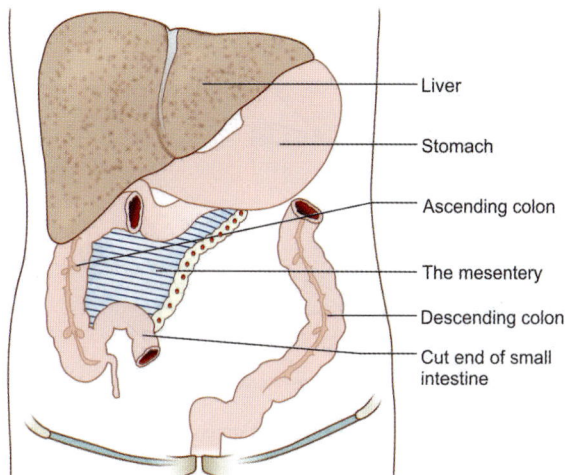

Fig. 4.16: The mesentery

- Lacteals and mesenteric lymph nodes
- Loose areolar tissue
- Fat
- Nerve fibers.

Clinical Anatomy
- Transverse tear of the mesentery is common and effects part of small intestine, whereas longitudinal tear causes more damage to small gut
- Volvulus is also common in the mesentery
- Mesenteric lymph node may enlarge in lymphoma.

LESSER OMENTUM (FIG. 4.17)
- It is a fold of peritoneum extends from lesser curvature of stomach and first 1 inch of duodenum to liver
- It has two parts: (1) hepatogastric—the portion of lesser omentum between lesser curvature of stomach and liver, (2) hepatoduodenal—the portion between first 1 inch of duodenum to the liver.

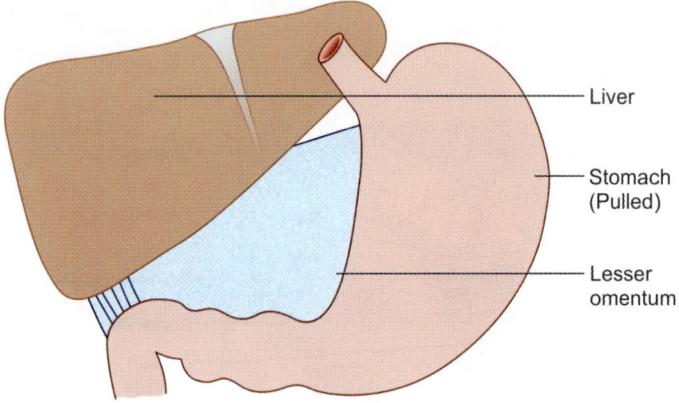

Fig. 4.17: Lesser omentum

- Behind the lesser omentum lies the part of lesser sac
- Its right-free margin contains hepatic duct, hepatic artery proper and portal vein
- Right margin forms the anterior boundary of epiploic foramen
- Along the lesser curvature of stomach and adjoining 1 inch of first part of duodenum, the following structure lies:
    - The right and left gastric vessels
    - The gastric group of lymph nodes and lymphatics
    - The branches of gastric nerves.

CORONAL SECTION OF KIDNEY

Coronal section of kidney presents in two distinct area: (1) Outer cortex and (2) inner medulla, and a space known as renal sinus (Fig. 4.18). Outer cortex composed of glomeruli, proximal and distal convoluted tubules and collecting ducts. Inner medulla is composed of straight portion of tubules, loop of Henle, vasa recta and terminal collecting duct. In medulla, few conical structures are seen, which are renal pyramids. In apices of pyramid, 16–20 duct of Bellini open. The papilla is received by a cup-like tube known as calices minor. In between two pyramids, there is cortical tissue, known as renal column;

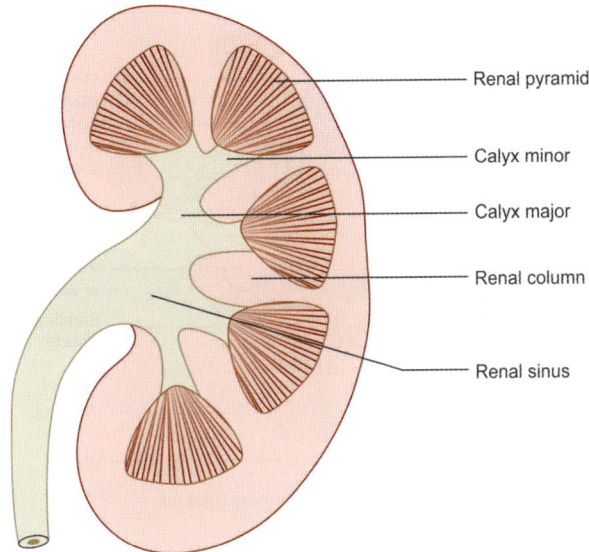

Fig. 4.18: Coronal section of kidney

over the base of pyramid the cortical tissue is known as cortical arches. Several minor calices join and form major calyx. Two to three major calices join to form pelvis of ureter.

BASE OF URINARY BLADDER (FIG. 4.19)

Situated behind the bladder, and it is nonperitoneal. In male, this surface is related to seminal vesicle and ampulla of vas. The two ureters open in this surface. In female, it is related to upper part of anterior vaginal wall, anterior surface of supravaginal part of cervix.

In the interior of bladder near the region of base, there is smooth triangular region known as internal trigone. It is bounded on either side by opening of both ureters and below by internal urethral orifice.

Clinical Importance

Infection in the region of internal trigone tends to persist.

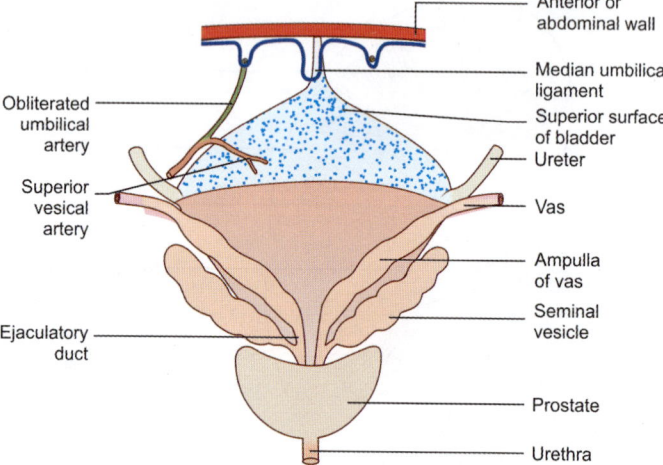

Fig. 4.19: Base of urinary bladder

MEMBRANOUS URETHRA

- This part of urethra lies within deep perineal pouch. It begins at the apex of prostate and passes through anterior part of levator ani to deep perineal pouch
- This is the narrowest part of urethra with star-shaped lumen
- The urethra is surrounded on all sides by a strong muscle known as sphincter urethral membranosus
- Its anterior wall is longer than the posterior wall
- This is the least dilatable part of male urethra
- The rigid perineal membrane fixes the urethra firmly to pelvis
- So, this part is vulnerable to injury and collection of urine with deep perineal pouch.

ECTOPIC TESTIS

It is also called maldescent of testis. In this case, testis successfully completes its intra-abdominal descent up to superficial inguinal ring but thereafter it deviates from its normal path, and fails to reach the scrotum. It is found in the following regions (Fig. 4.20):

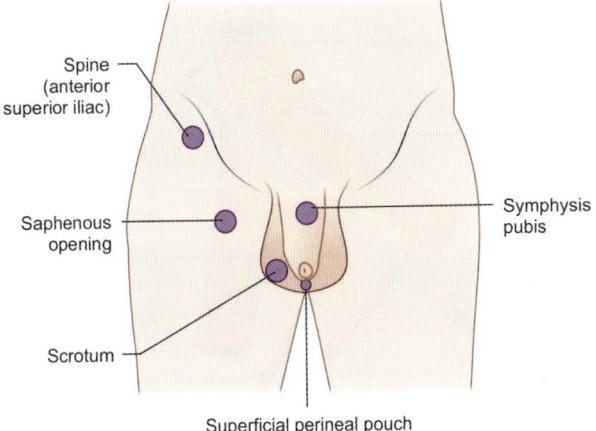

Fig. 4.20: Five sites of ectopic testis starting from letter "S"

- In the superficial fascia of abdominal wall above the superficial inguinal ring
- At the root of penis
- In the perineum
- In the upper and medial side of thigh.

Clinical Anatomy
It may be corrected and taken back to normal position by operation.

OVARIAN FOSSA OF LATERAL PELVIC WALL
It is a fossa present in the true pelvis, which contains ovary. The ovarian fossa is bounded (Fig. 4.21):
- Above by external iliac vessels
- Anteriorly by the upturned end of the obliterated umbilical artery
- Posteriorly by ureter and internal iliac vessels
- Laterally by the peritoneum covering the following structures:
    - Obliterated umbilical artery
    - Obturator nerve, obturator artery, obturator vein
    - Fascia covering the obturator internus.

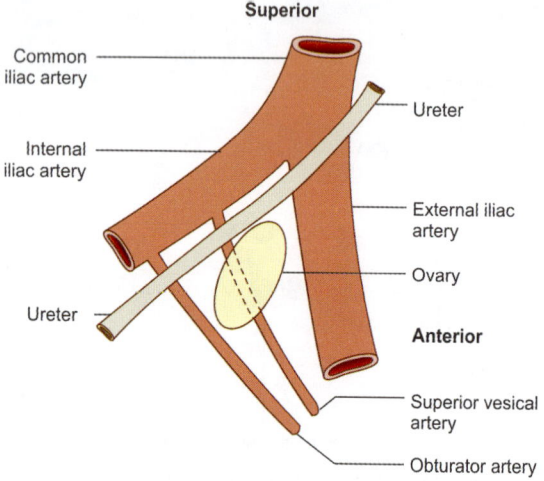

Fig. 4.21: Ovarian fossa of lateral pelvic wall

Clinical Anatomy

The inflammation of the ovary produces localized peritonitis of the fossa, and it leads pain on the medial side of thigh.

CELIAC TRUNK (FIG. 4.22)

Beginning

Wide, unpaired ventral branch of abdominal aorta lies 1.25 cm above the transpyloric plane slightly left to the midline (at the level of intervertebral disc present between T_2 and L_1).

Termination

Passes almost horizontally forward and slightly right, above pancreas and splenic vein, divides into three branches. It is surrounded by celiac plexus of nerves.

Branches

- Left gastric
- Common hepatic
- Splenic.

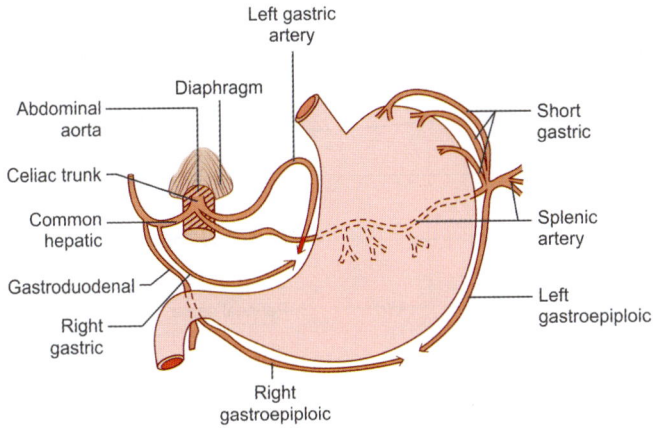

Fig. 4.22: Celiac trunk

Area Supplied
Stomach, liver and spleen and part of the duodenum (proximal part) up to major duodenal papilla.

Clinical Anatomy
Obstruction of common hepatic artery proximal to right gastric artery may save liver because of establishment of collateral circulation between gastric and gastroepiploic arteries. But if occlusion affects hepatic artery properly, then there is liver necrosis.

PUDENDAL CANAL

Introduction
It is a connective tissue canal situated in the lower and lateral part of ischioanal (or ischiorectal) fossa (Fig. 4.23).

Situation
Lies 2.5 cm above the ischial tuberosity.

Contents
- Pudendal nerve
- Internal pudendal vessels.

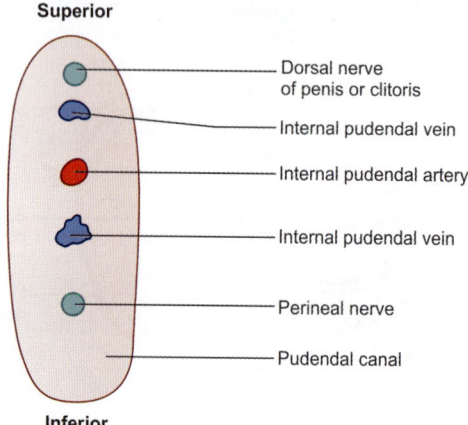

Fig. 4.23: Arrangement of structures in pudendal canal

The pudendal nerve divides within the canal into dorsal nerve of penis or clitoris and perineal nerve.

Clinical Anatomy

The pudendal nerve is blocked to anesthetize the perineum to perform any operation in perineum and for painless delivery.

It is done by two methods:
1. Transvaginal route
2. *Perineal method*: This is easier method. The ischial tuberosity is felt subcutaneously and injection is given on medial side of the tuberosity, 1 inch above the tuberosity.

ISCHIOANAL/ISCHIORECTAL FOSSA

It is located on either side of anal-canal, below the levator ani and underneath perianal skin (Fig. 4.24).

Boundary

- *Anterior wall (base)*:
  - Base of fascia of Colles
  - Transversus perinei superficialis
  - Urogenital diaphragm

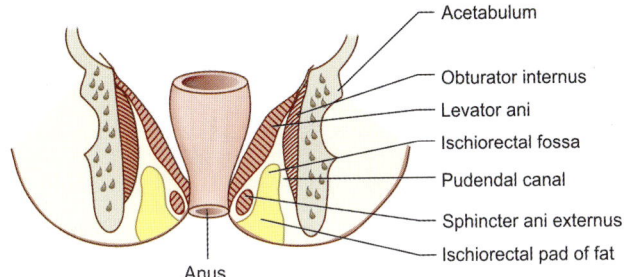

Fig. 4.24: Ischioanal fossa with its boundaries and contents

- *Posterior wall*:
  - Sacrotuberous ligament
  - Lower fibers of gluteus maximus
- *Lateral wall*:
  - Obturator internus
  - Ischial tuberosity (medial surface)
- *Medial wall*:
  - Levator ani with and fascia
  - Sphincter ani externus
- *Apex*: Meeting of anal fascia with obturator fascia
- *Base*: Base is formed by skin.

Contents
- Ischioanal pad of fat
- Ischioanal vessels and nerves
- Transverse perineal vessels
- Scrotal or labial vessels.

Clinical Importance
This fossa has got high tendency to become infected and infection of one fossa may spread readily to other fossa behind the oral canal and forms horseshoe-shaped abscess.

FALLOPIAN TUBE
It is the tube for the passage of ovum from ovary into the cavity of the uterus (Fig. 4.25).

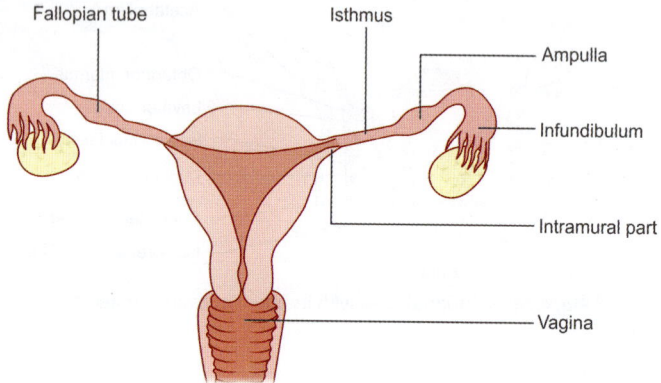

Fig. 4.25: Fallopian tube

Extent
- *Laterally*—it opens into pelvic ostium
- *Medially*—it opens into uterine ostium.

Situation
- Some part lies within the muscle of uterus
- The rest lies in the free border of broad ligament.

Length
- About 10 cm.

Parts (from Medial to Lateral)
- Pars uterina (1 cm) tubae or intramural part
- Isthmus (3 cm)
- Ampulla (5 cm)
- Infundibulum (1 cm).

Relations
- Below and in front of the tube lies round ligament of uterus
- *Below and behind*—it lies ligament of ovary and ovary
- Below the tube:
  - Anastomosis between uterine vessels and ovarian vessels.

Clinical Importance
- Fertilization occurs in the ampullary part of uterine tube
- *Tubectomy*: It is sterilization operation. When family is complete, patient is advised to go for this operation for permanent contraception. Here, the ampullary part of the tube is cut and ligated
- *Ectopic pregnancy*: In this case, fertilized ovum is implanted in ampulla of uterine tube. The embryo cannot grow beyond 2 months. There is severe pain and rupture of uterine tube producing alarming hemorrhage. It is corrected by surgery.

TRUE LIGAMENTS OF UTERUS

True ligaments are usually embryological remnant or condensation of pelvic cellular tissue (Fig. 4.26).

- *Round ligaments of uterus (embryological remnant)*: Each ligament is about 10–12 cm long. It is attached proximally to the lateral angle of uterus, below and in front of uterine tube.
    - *Function*: It pulls the fundus forwards and maintains the anteversion and anteflexion of uterus.
- *Mackenrodt's ligament*: It is fan-shaped. It extends laterally from the cervicovaginal junction to the fascia covering levator ani.
    - *Function*: Each ligament keeps the cervix in position and prevents downwards displacement.

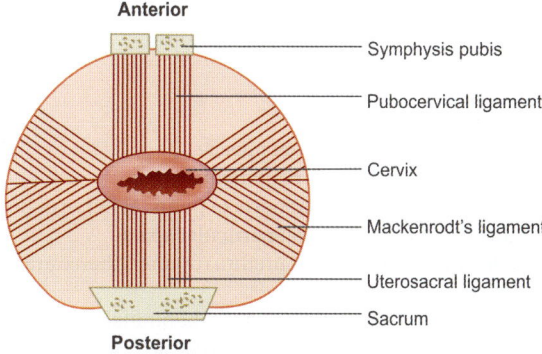

Fig. 4.26: Ligamentous supports of uterus

- *Uterosacral ligaments*: Each ligament extends from the cervix to the third sacral vertebra.
  - *Function*: It maintains anteflexion and anteversion.
- *Pubocervical ligaments*: These ligaments extend from cervix to the pubic bones.
  - *Function*: It pulls the cervix forward.

Clinical Importance
- The prolapse of uterus is most commonly seen after menopause as the pelvic fascia tends to atrophy.
- All these ligaments maintain support of uterus and damage to the ligaments, particularly Mackenrodt's ligament due to repeated childbirth, produces prolapsed uterus.

SUPERFICIAL PERINEAL POUCH (FIG. 4.27)

Boundary
- *Superiorly*: By the inferior layer of urogenital diaphragm or perineal membrane.
- *Inferiorly*: The membranous layer of superficial fascia of perineum (Colles fascia).
- *Posteriorly*: The pouch is closed by fusion of superior and inferior walls.
- *Anteriorly*: Pouches open and it communicates with the anterior abdominal wall—via scrotum and penis.

Contents
- Base of penis (bulb of penis with two crura)
- Corpus spongiosum
- Corpus cavernosus
- Ischiocavernosus
- Superficial transverses perinei muscle
- Perineal branch of posterior cutaneous nerve
- Posterior scrotal vessels + transverse perineal nerve of posterior scrotal vessel one seen in that particular space.

In saddle injury, when bulbar urethra ruptures, then extravasation of urine occurs.

The urine may ascend in the anterior abdominal wall in the space between membranous layer of superficial fascia (fascia of Scarpa) and aponeurosis of external oblique muscle.

The urine cannot enter the thigh due to fusion of superficial fascia (membranous layers) with the fascia lata of thigh.

DEEP PERINEAL POUCH

This is a space between perineal membrane and superior layer of urogenital diaphragm. Deep pouch contains a paired transverse perinei profundus muscle (lies beneath transverse perinei superficialis). In the middle lies sphincter urethrae membranosa. This muscle surrounds the membranous part of urethra. In female, vagina also lies here (Fig. 4.27).

Nerve lies in this space—(1) in male dorsal nerve of penis and in female dorsal nerve of clitoris (branch of internal pudendal nerve), and (2) muscular branches of perineal nerve.

Vessels

Artery to penis branch of internal pudendal artery.

Clinical Anatomy

If rupture of urethra occurs in the deep pouch, the extravasated urine remains within the closed pouch and there will be tremendous pain.

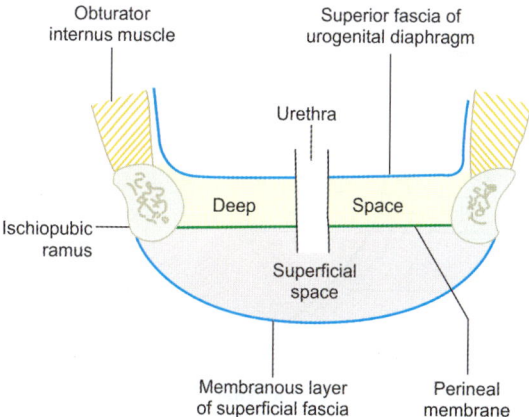

Fig. 4.27: Schematic coronal section through urogenital triangle to show formation of superficial and deep perineal spaces

PELVIC DIAPHRAGM

It is a transverse muscular partition, voluntary in nature, between the pelvic cavity and the perineum. It slopes downwards and medially. Its upper surface supports the pelvic viscera like urinary bladder and prostate and rectum in male; and urinary bladder, uterus with its appendages, rectum in female. It steadies the perineal body. It is covered by fascia on both sides (Fig. 4.28).

Structures passing through it:
- From anterior to posterior:
    - *In male*: Urethra and anal canal
    - *In female*: Urethra, vagina and anal canal.

Parts of pelvic diaphragm are (anatomical): Anteriorly levator ani muscle and posteriorly coccygeus.

Origin

- *Levator ani*: Posterior surface of body of the pubis, arcus tendinosis (white line of the pelvis)
- *Coccygeus*—From internal surface of coccyx.

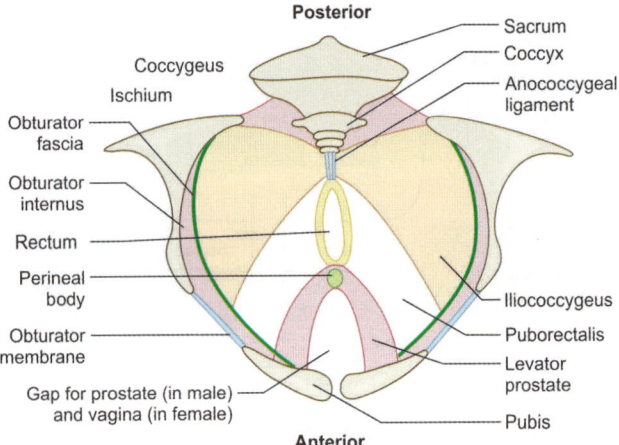

Fig. 4.28: Scheme to show the arrangement of the levator ani and coccygeus muscles (pelvic diaphragm)

Clinical Anatomy

The levator ani may be injured during childbirth. When the perineal body is torn and cannot be repaired, satisfactorily results in prolapse of the uterus is not attained.

ILEOCECAL ORIFICE

Terminal part of ileum opens into cecum through ileocecal orifice (Fig. 4.29). It is guarded by ileocecal valves, which are formed by duplication of mucous membrane and muscle of ileum. The valves have two lips and two frenula. The upper lip is horizontal. The lower lip is longer and concave.

Clinical Anatomy

Some people feel urge of defecation after taking meals. This is known as gastrocolic reflex.
- Material from the ileum passes in small amount within the large gut.
- It is commonly involved in amebiasis, intestinal tuberculosis (TB) and carcinoma.

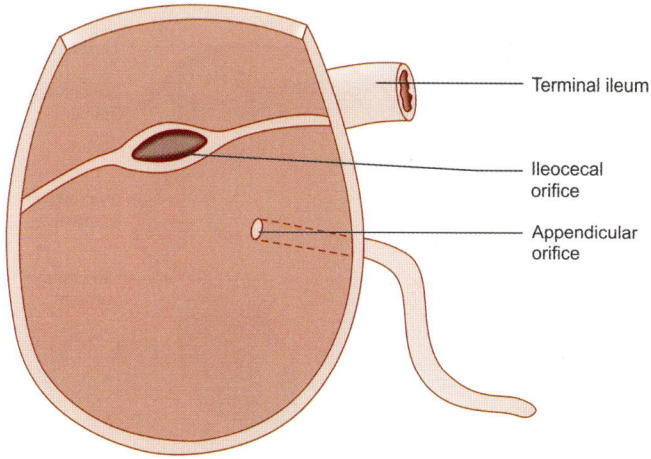

Fig. 4.29: Ileocecal orifice

LIGAMENTS OF SPLEEN

Spleen has three ligamentous supports (Fig. 4.30):
1. Gastrosplenic ligament
2. Lienorenal ligament
3. Lienophrenic ligament.

In addition to phrenicocolic ligament extending from the left colic flexure to the diaphragm supports the spleen from below, known as sustentaculum (shelf) lienis.

These ligaments are false ligaments or peritoneal folds.

Gastrosplenic Ligament

Gastrosplenic ligament having two layers connects fundus of stomach with the anterior lip of hilum of the spleen. Its anterior layer is derived from the greater sac and posterior layer from lesser sac.

Contents
- Short gastric and left gastroepiploic vessels.

Lienorenal Ligament

It extends from anterior surface of the left kidney to the posterior lip of the hilum of spleen. Anterior layer of gastrosplenic ligament after covering the spleen becomes posterior layer of gastrosplenic ligament.

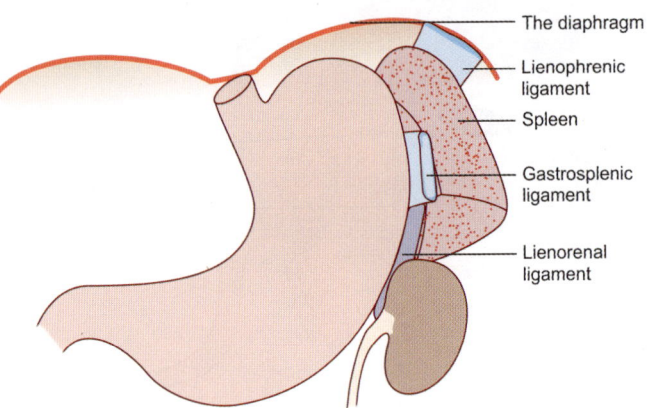

Fig. 4.30: Schematic diagram of ligaments of spleen

Again, the posterior layer of gastrosplenic ligament is continuous with the anterior layer of lienorenal ligament.

Contents
- Splenic vessels, nerves, lymphatics and, sometimes, the tail of pancreas.

Lienophrenic Ligament

It is the upward continuation of lienorenal ligament extending from hilum to the diaphragm. It suspends spleen from above, so also known as suspensory ligament of spleen.

Clinical Anatomy

In splenectomy, ligation of the pedicle of the spleen is important. The pedicle is being formed by gastrosplenic and lienorenal ligament, where tail of the pancreas should be searched for.

FASCIA OF COLLES

The superficial fascia of the anterior abdominal wall just deep to skin splits into two layers below the umbilicus—the superficial fatty layer or fascia of Camper and deeper membranous layer, fascia of Scarpa. Fascia of Scarpa is continuous below with a similar membranous layer of superficial fascia of the perineum known as fascia of Colles. The attachment of Colles fascia is as follows:

- Below Holden's line (begins a little lateral to pubic tubercle and extends horizontally laterally 8 cm)
- Pubic tubercle
- Body of the pubis, deep fascia on adductor longus and gracilis
- Margins of the pubic arch below the crus penis
- Posterior border of the perineal membrane.

The space in between Colles fascia superficially and perineal membrane in a deeper plane is known as superficial perineal space/pouch. In case of rupture of urethra, urine extravasates either superficially (or deep) in a space deep to fascia of Colles and extension of this extravasated urine is prevented into the thigh and ischioanal fossa by the above mentioned attachment.

BLOOD SUPPLY OF VERMIFORM APPENDIX

It is supplied by the inferior division of the ileocolic artery. The artery goes behind the terminal part of the ileum and supplies the whole organ. A recurrent artery arises from it near the base and anastomoses with posterior cecal artery. The appendicular artery is an end artery. The tip of the appendix is least vascular and obstruction of the artery (as seen in appendicitis) can lead to gangrene formation at the tip of appendix.

PHIMOSIS

It is a condition where the foreskin of penis is so tight that it cannot be retracted over the glans penis fully. Normally, it may be present up to 3 years and progressively it is nonadherent by the age of 6 years. Children above 6 years suffer from balanitis and ballooning of foreskin during voiding.

Clinical Anatomy
- Surgical removal of foreskin is known as circumcision and is advised above 7 years of age.

BICORNUATE UTERUS (FIG. 4.31)
- It is the developmental anomaly of uterus
- In this condition, uterus has two horns entering into common vagina
- This condition is normal in many mammals below primates

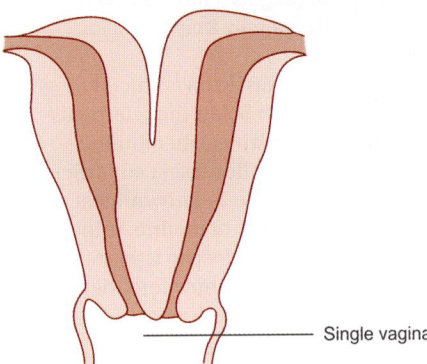

Fig. 4.31: Bicornuate uterus

- It is due to lack of fusion of paramesonephric ducts in a local area through their normal line of fusion
- It may result in infertility or may lead to recurrent abortion
- Treated surgically.

CREMASTERIC REFLEX

Skin over the medial side of the thigh and that over the femoral triangle is supplied by ilioinguinal nerve (root value of L1) and genitofemoral nerve (root value—ventral rami of L1, L2). So, if those parts of the thigh are irritated, they can produce a local spinal reflex at the level of L1 segment of spinal cord.

Genital branch of genitofemoral nerve (L1, L2) supplies cremaster. So if medial part of the thigh is irritated via the local spinal reflex, contraction of cremaster, it will lead to pulling up of testis. This is known as cremasteric reflex.

EXPLANATORY NOTES

Q1. Cremasteric reflex is a protective reflex. Explain?

Ans. The cremasteric muscle is "U"-shaped loop of muscle is derived from internal oblique. So, when internal oblique contracts, cremasteric fibers are also pulled. As a result, spermatic cord is pulled up, lower end of which has testis, so superficial ring is blocked by the testis. This is also known as ball valve mechanism. So, cremasteric reflex is a protective reflex.

Q2. False ligaments are peritoneal fold and do not play a supportive role. Explain.

Ans. They are:
- Median umbilical fold due to medial umbilical ligament
- Medial umbilical folds—due to obliterated umbilical arteries
- Lateral false ligament—it is formed due to reflection of peritoneum from urinary bladder to lateral pelvic wall
- Posterior false ligaments are sacrogenital folds.

Q3. Explain nerve supply of urinary bladder.

Ans.
- Both sympathetic and parasympathetic nerves supply the urinary bladder through the vesical plexus.

- The parasympathetic supply is via pelvic splanchnic nerve (S1, S2 and S3) and they are constrictor of detrusor muscle and relaxing of internal sphincter. So, parasympathetic is nerve of voiding.
- The sympathetic fiber arises from T11, T12, L1 and L2 segment of spinal cord. It has action on internal sphincter and muscle surrounding bladder neck. Spinal micturition center is controlled by higher cortical center (paracentral lobule).

Q4. Explain basivertebral Foramen and its Importance.

Ans.

- It indicates the junction between two somites, so that the upper part of the body of vertebra ossifies from the lower part of the upper somite and lower part of the body ossifies from upper part of lower somite.
- Through basivertebral foramen passes basivertebral vein, which drains into basivertebral venous plexus, this vein is valveless. So when malignant cell reaches vertebral venous plexus can produce secondary deposit in the vertebral body. For example, cancer prostate and cancer breast.

Q5. Urine leaks through umbilicus of a newborn baby. Explain.

Ans. Allantois goes from apex of the developing urinary bladder to the umbilicus. It obliterates to form the median umbilical ligament after birth. When it is not obliterated and persists as a hollow tube, called urachus and urine comes out through umbilicus in a newborn.

Q6. Varicocele occurs on left side.

Ans. Varicocele occurs when valves within the veins along the cord do not work properly. This results in backflow of blood into pampiniform plexus and causes increased pressure, ultimately leading to permanent damage of testicular tissue.

About 98% idiopathic varicocele occurs on left side, apparently because the left testicular vein connects to the renal vein at 90° angle while the right testicular vein drains at acute angle directly into the inferior vena cava.

More causes:

- Left testicular vein is longer
- Valves are less competent
- It passes behind the sigmoid colon-containing solid fecal matter, which may press the vein

- As it opens at 90° to the left renal vein, so stagnation of blood in the left testicular is more leading to its dilatation.

Q7. Carcinoma of prostate can rapidly metastasize to the brain. Explain.

Ans. Prostatic venous plexus communicates with vertebral venous plexus through some valveless veins (veins of Batson). During malignancy of prostate the malignant cells, while straining during coughing, sneezing, micturition, defecation, may pass via the backward route due to absence of valves. By moving into vertebral venous plexus, the malignant cells may go to internal jugular vein and communicate with intracranial venous sinuses. So, malignant cells can reach the cranial cavity and affect the meninges and the brain.

Q8. Complete perineal tear is associated with fecal and urinary incontinence.

Ans. If perineal tear occurs, urethra is ruptured. So, urine can accumulate in the superficial perineal pouch and continued upwards in the anterior abdominal wall and can go up to axilla, as this pouch is opened in front.

Q9. Pain in ureteric colic is Felt from loin to groin.

Ans. When a stone passes down the ureter, this results in ureteric colic. The renal pelvis and ureter send their afferent nerves into the spinal cord at segments:

- T_{11}
- T_{12}
- L_1
- L_2.

So in ureteric colic referred to loin and groin due to involvement of the nerves:

- Subcostal
- Iliohypogastric
- Ilioinguinal
- Genitofemoral.

The upper ureteric colic referred to loin and groin is carried by iliohypogastric and ilioinguinal nerve.

When ureteric colic is referred to testicles/thigh, the genitofemoral nerve is involved.

Q10. Incision of the lacunar ligament is to be done carefully while reducing a strangulated femoral hernia.

Ans. If there is presence of abnormal obturator artery, it may be damaged during incision of lacunar ligament. So, the incision must be done carefully.

Q11. Elderly female (38 years) gave birth to a baby who is examined to have a rounded face, epicanthic folds and a characteristic single palmar crease. Explain the genetic cause of the event.

Ans. The condition is known as Down's syndrome or Mongolism. It occurs due to numerical abnormality of the autosomes. There is an extrachromosome in number 21 and it is known as trisomy 21. It occurs due to nondisjunction of the chromosomes during meiosis.

Q12. A middle-aged woman with recurrent attack of salpingo-oophoritis presents with pain in the hip and knee joints.

Ans. In case of salpingo-oophoritis, the inflammation also affects the obturator nerve—as there is peritonitis. As the obturator nerve supplies both the hip and knee joint. So, there will be pain in the said two joints.

Q13. After cholecystectomy drain is inserted into the hepatorenal pouch of Morison.

Ans. Hepatorenal pouch of Morison is the most dependent part during lying down position. So, if there is collection of fluid, it will accumulate in this pouch. For this reason, drain must be inserted in the hepatorenal pouch after cholecystectomy.

Q14. Surgical removal of uterus may involve ureter. Explain.

Ans. During hysterectomy operations, when clamp is placed at the cervicovaginal junction, the ureter is placed very near. So, there may be cutting of the ureter in this time.

Q15. Male baby was diagnosed to be a case of "ectopic testis" when he was detected to have one side of the scrotum empty.

Ans. Ectopic testis: It is maldescended testis. The testis descends up to superficial inguinal ring but thereafter in spite of descent in the scrotum, it descends in the following sites:

- At the superficial fascia over the superficial inguinal ring

- At the root of the penis
- At the upper and medial side of thigh
- In the perineum.

Q16. Portal hypertension causes hemorrhoids.

Ans. When the pressure of the portal vein increases there is dilatation of veins in the region of pectinate line of anal canal. These dilated veins protrude through the mucous membrane.

Hemorrhoids produce soft swelling and are not visible unless they prolapsed through the anus. They are supplied by the autonomic nerve. Hence, do not cause any discomfort unless they are thrombosed prolapsed or infected.

They are usually seen at 3, 7 and 11 o'clock position when patient is examined in lithotomy position.

Q17. Patient is detected to have horseshoe-shaped kidney.

Ans. During development, kidney ascends from pelvis. If the kidneys are very close together, lower poles fuses and form a single horseshoe-shaped kidney. It is in lower position than normal kidney. This condition is usually asymptomatic and no treatment is required.

Q18. Cannula for rectal washing is usually passed in left lateral position.

Ans. The interior of rectum possess four valves, which are horizontally placed, semilunar in shape and situated along the lateral concavities of rectum. Out of these valves, third is the most important because it lies in middle lateral curve and may prevent the passage of the instrument, if passed in patient with supine of right lateral position and may be injured in doing so.

So, to avoid injury to third valve, the instrument must pass carefully with patient in left lateral positions.

Q19. A middle-aged man suffering from caries spine (TB of vertebral bodies) may present a swelling in the groin.

Ans. Tuberculosis of vertebral body produces pus within the psoas sheath and that pus follows the sheath and ends in the groin that is the base of femoral triangle. So, swelling may present in groin in caries spine.

Q20. Highly stressed individuals are susceptible to suffer from duodenal ulcer.

Ans. Highly stressed person secretes more HCl in the stomach, which is controlled by the higher centers in the brain. This acid chyme passes to the first 1 inch of the first part of the duodenum. So, the duodenal mucous membrane is always irritated with acid chyme. Duodenal ulcer is common in higher socioeconomic group duodenal glands of bruner secret less mucous in highly stressed individual. So, the acid chyme easily, comes in contact with the first part of the duodenum as there is less mucous barrier.

Q21. Direct inguinal hernia occurs in old age.

Ans. When the herniation occurs through the Hesselbach's triangle, it is known as direct inguinal hernia. It usually occurs in old age because:
- Abdominal muscles become weak
- There may be chronic constipation, chronic cough and chronic strain in passing urine. It gives pressure over the viscus (particularly the small intestine)
- Indirect inguinal hernia passes through the inguinal canal, which is oblique and this indirect hernia occurs in case of child as there is persistence of processus vaginalis. So, in case of old age stressed occur in the region of the anterior abdominal wall directly, the superficial inguinal ring is laxed.

Q22. Duodenal ulcer commonly occurs in the first part of the duodenum.

Ans. Ulcer commonly occurs in the first part of the duodenum because:
- It is supplied by end artery (supraduodenal artery of Wilkie)
- Acidic chymes come from the stomach irritate this first part
- Decrease bicarbonate production in the mucosal layer
- Hypermotility.

Q23. Dribbling of urine and frequent urge of micturition in elderly male.

Ans. Hyperplasia of prostate affects the median lobe, the median lobe enlarged and blocks the internal urethral orifice, so, less urine is coming out through the urinary bladder, this causes frequent urge of micturition and dribbling of urine.

Q24. Suprarenal gland does not follow the kidney when the latter drops down.

Ans. Kidney is retained in position by renal fascia, paranephric fat, renal vessels. During extreme starvation or emaciation, kidney drops down as the paranephric fat is absorbed.

Renal fascia forms a separate compartment for the suprarenal gland. So, when kidney drops down, it prevents the dropping down of suprarenal gland along with the kidney.

Q25. Pain in acute appendicitis is felt first in the umbilical region and then in the McBurney's point.

Ans. Pathway of pain of appendicitis to umbilicus is a referred pain.

Pathway: Afferent fibers from appendix accompanies the sympathetic nerves, enters the t10 through superior mesenteric plexus, so, pain is referred to umbilicus.

Then inflammatory process extended beyond the appendix and involved in the parietal peritoneum. So, there is severe localized pain and tenderness.

Q26. Pain from the gallbladder is referred to the right shoulder region.

Ans. Gallbladder is mainly supplied by sympathetic celiac plexus that passes along the hepatic artery to reach the gallbladder. When the parietal peritoneum is involved, it also irritates the diaphragm, which is supplied by phrenic nerve (c3, c4 and c5) so, pain is referred to shoulder region due to supply of c3, c4 and c5 in the shoulder region.

Q27. Which position of appendix is most dangerous?

Ans. The preileal position of appendix is the most dangerous because this position is nearest to parietal peritoneum. So, peritoneum gets easily involved and there is quick peritonitis.

Q28. Spleen moves with respiration, but kidney does not. Explain.

Ans. Kidney also moves with respiration but the range of movement is proportionately, less than that of the spleen. Spleen is more near the anterior abdominal wall, whereas kidney is situated in the posterior abdominal wall and hence during respiration, spleen moves more as it is in the anterior abdominal wall.

Q29. Renal angle and its importance.

Ans. It is the angulation formed by the lower border of 12th rib and the lateral border of erector spinae muscle.

- Tenderness (pain on palpation) at this point is seen in the diseased condition of lower part of the kidney.
- Ultrasound-guided renal biopsy also taken from here.

Q30. Where do you palpate the vas? What precaution will you take during vasectomy?

Ans. The vas is felt between upper part of scrotum and superficial inguinal ring, with index finger and thumb. Its feeling is cord like because the muscular coat is very thick and lumen is very narrow. Vasectomy should be done bilaterally and care must be taken not to damage the superficial external pudendal artery, which crosses in front of the vas.

Q31. Development of diabetes mellitus after splenectomy operation.

Ans. The tail of the pancreas lies within the lienorenal ligament. The tail contains plenty of islets of Langerhans. During splenectomy operation, if the surgeon is not careful to preserve the tail of pancreas then the patient suffers from diabetes mellitus.

Q32. Cancer stomach may cause esophageal stricture.

Ans.

- Cancer of stomach usually affects the greater curvature. From here, there is lymphatic spread to esophagus
- There is abrupt change of epithelium from stratified squamous to columnar. So, there may be metaplasia of epithelium from stomach to esophagus, which produces esophageal stricture.

Q33. Why lesser curvature of stomach is prone to ulceration?

Ans. The lesser curvature of stomach is prone to ulceration because:

- Here lies the gastric canal through which the irritant fluid (like very hot milk) passes
- The epithelial layer is very thin
- Blood supply is less because of straight arteries arises from left and right gastric artery without any submucous plexus
- Has less mucous secretion.

Abdomen

Q34. A newborn is suffering from swelling of scrotum while crying or straining during passing of stool.

Ans.
- Gubernaculum is attached to the lower pole of testis acts as an guiding force to descent the testis in scrotum
- During the descent of testis, a peritoneal pouch known as processus vaginalis is dragged by testis and gubernaculum
- Later, the upper part of the processus vaginalis disappears, but lower part presents as tunica vaginalis, which covers the anterior and sides of testis
- If the processus vaginalis persists, it may give rise to congenital hernia or hydrocele, so during crying or straining, some of the contents may descend through processus vaginalis and produces swelling in scrotum.

Q35. First part of duodenum resembles more like stomach than duodenum.

Ans.
- Like the lesser and greater curvature of stomach, the 1st inch of duodenum is attached to lesser and greater omentum. Rest of the duodenum is devoid of peritoneal folds
- First part of duodenum is mobile-like stomach, rest part of duodenum is immobile
- Stomach as well as the first part of duodenum suffers from peptic ulcer
- First part of duodenum is supplied by end artery whereas rest of the duodenum is supplied by superior and inferior pancreaticoduodenal artery.

Q36. Why is the gallbladder pain felt in the inferior angle of right scapula?

Ans. The sympathetic supply of the gallbladder is from C7 to T9 segment. This explains, why the gallbladder pain is referred to the inferior angle of right scapula.

Q37. An elderly female is having progressive deepening of jaundice. Explain anatomically.

Ans. This is due to blockage of the CBD; either due to stone or carcinoma of the head of pancreas. The bile, which contains bilirubin, accumulates in the biliary tree leading to stasis in the biliary canaliculi. So, there is deepening of jaundice.

Q38. Cecum is an important organ for a surgeon to detect intestinal obstruction.

Ans.
- In a case of intestinal obstruction, the abdomen is usually opened through a paramedian or midline (right) incision. Its normal downward extent is not enough to look for carcinoma, neither it is easy to mobilize cecum in front as it is a fixed structure on iliac (right) fossa
- If distended loops of small or large gut hinders the site to be looked for to identify the reason of intestinal obstruction, incision line may be extended downwards for better exposure and handling. In that situation, if you see a collapsed cecum, it indicates small intestinal obstruction and it is dilated usually a large intestinal obstruction is suspected.

Q39. Pain in ovarian diseases may refer to hip and knee joint.

Ans. It is because:
- Ovary is situated in ovarian fossa of lateral pelvic wall
- Laterally, this fossa is related to the following structures covered by peritoneum:
    - Obliterated umbilical artery
    - Obturator nerve and vessels
    - Fascia covering obturator internus.
- The inflammation of the ovary produces localized peritonitis of the fossa, which may irritate the obturator nerve and the obturator nerve supplies the hip and knee joint. So, the pain is referred to hip and knee joint.

Q40. Females are more prone to peritonitis.

Ans. The peritoneal cavity of female is open to exterior because of pelvic ostium open to perineal cavity. If the female is not maintaining the proper hygiene ascending infection from vagina enters the peritoneum through pelvic ostium-producing peritonitis.

Q41. A male child with abdominal testis.

Ans. During birth, testis descends up to scrotal sac. This is required for normal spermatogenesis, as abdominal temperature is 4° higher than scrotal temperature. As the male child has abdominal testis bilaterally, the child will be sterile. There may be also development of cancer in the testis.

Q42. Why femoral hernia is more common in females?

Ans. When a part of the viscera comes out through the femoral ring into the femoral canal, it is known as femoral hernia.

Causes:
- Wider pelvis
- Narrow femoral vessels
- Pressure due to repeated childbirth.

Sex difference: It is more common in females. It lies below and lateral to pubic tubercle and does not descend below the Holden's line.

Q43. Unilateral hydronephrosis following hysterectomy?

Ans. During hysterectomy operation, uterine arteries are ligated closed to the isthmus of uterine tube. In this region, ureter the uterine artery crosses the ureter. So, during ligation of uterine artery ureter may be ligated and is sided and this causes hydronephrosis following hysterectomy operation.

Q44. Position of inferior epigastric vessels to distinguish between oblique and direct inguinal hernia?

Ans.
- Oblique inguinal hernia is defined as hernia, which passes through deep ring and comes out through superficial inguinal ring
- Congenital due to persistence of processus vaginalis
- It lies lateral to inferior epigastric artery
- Direst hernia occurs in old age due to weakness of muscle
- *Origin*: Due to persistent cough, constipation, repeated pregnancy, etc.

When the hernia develops, it lies medial to inferior epigastric artery, so the position of inferior epigastric vessels distinguishes between oblique and direct inguinal hernia.

Q45. Highly selective vagotomy produces avascular necrosis of lesser curvature of stomach?

Ans. Highly selective vagotomy is very delicate operation.

During its operation, the surgeon goes through the lesser omentum dissecting the finer branch of anterior gastric nerve.

During the dissection, there may be cutting of multiple straight branches from left and right gastric arteries that supplies the lesser curvature of stomach. So, highly selective vagotomy avascular necrosis of lesser curvature of stomach.

Q46. Incisions along the linea semilunaris is contraindicated because.

Ans. The lower six intercostal nerve, which supplies and rectus abdominis muscle and enters the rectus sheath from lateral aspect near linear semilunaris. So, there will be damage if there is incision along the linea semilunaris.

Q47. Ilioinguinal nerve is a collateral branch of hypogastric nerve?

Ans.
- Because both are having same root value (L1) and both are branch of thick nerve
- Courses of them are parallel
- Both supply the skin at the end
- Iioinguinal nerve is not having any lateral cutaneous branch, but iliohypogastric is having one.

Q48. An elderly person following a heavy meal is complaining of chest discomfort.

Ans.
- Fundus of stomach after cardiac notch ascends upwards, backwards and to the left and its summit reaches up to the apex of the heart, which is situated in the left 5th intercostal space 9 cm away from midline
- So, this part of stomach is separated from heart only by diaphragm. Fundus contains gas, which swallows during ingestion of food
- So, when a person swallows food very quickly, he/she swallows large amount of gas
- Also, gas accumulates in fundus after partial digestion of heavy meal
- This huge amount of gas pushes the heart and produces chest discomfort.

Q49. Carcinoma of stomach presents enlarged Virchow's lymph gland in the neck.

Ans.
- Carcinoma of stomach spread through lymphatics
- From local lymph vessels, it goes to thoracic duct.

The thoracic duct opens at the angle of left subclavian vein and internal jugular vein and in this region, one of the supraclavicular glands is enlarged and stony hard. This is known as Virchow's gland. So, in carcinoma stomach, there is enlarged Virchow's gland.

Q50. The pectinate line of anal canal is called watershed line?

Ans. The pectinate line forms the mucocutaneous junction of the anal canal. The upper and lower region of which are different developmentally and anatomically (Table 4.1).

Table 4.1: Developmental and anatomical difference between above and below pectinate line

Name	Above the pectinate line	Below the pectinate line
Development	Postallantoic part of hindgut	Proctodeum
Blood supply	Superior rectal vessels	Middle and inferior rectal vessels
Lymphatics	Drain into internal iliac Group of lymph nodes	Drain into superficial inguinal Group of lymph nodes
Nerve supply	Autonomic nerves	Somatic nerve
Epithelium	Simple columnar	Stratified squamous

Q51. An ischioanal/ischiorectal abscess is extremely painful?

Ans. The ischioanal fossa is bounded by strong fascia and there is rich nerve supply, viz:
- Gluteal branch of posterior cutaneous nerve of thigh
- Perineal branch of sacral nerve
- Inferior rectal nerve.

So, in ischioanal abscess, there is distension of that area with pus and it is extremely painful.

Q52. Imperforate anus.

- It is a clinical condition in which the anal canal does not open to the exterior
- It is a developmental anal anomaly
- The anal canal develops from dual source:
  - The part above the pectinate line develops from endoderm—posterior allantoic hindgut
  - The part below the pectinate line develops from ectoderm
- Pectinate line is the demarcation between ectoderm and endoderm origin of anal canal and here lies the attachment of cloacal membrane
- This cloacal membrane ruptures at the 7–8th week of intrauterine life

- If the cloacal membrane fails to rupture then it results in imperforate anus where the anal canal does not open to the exterior
- It is a major anomaly and immediate surgical intervention is needed to save the life of the baby.

SURFACE ANATOMY OF ABDOMEN WHICH IS IMPORTANT TO THE CLINICIAN AND SURGEON

PLANES

1. *Right and left lateral planes (Fig. 4.32)*: Plane passing through midclavicular point to midinguinal point
2. *Transpyloric plane (Fig. 4.32)*: Cuts the lower border of L1 vertebra. One other hand, breadth below the xiphisternal joint of the individual on which the surface marking is done
   - Pylorus of stomach, hila of kidneys, duodenojejunal flexure and neck of pancreas lie in this plane
3. *Transtubercular plane (Fig. 4.32)*: Line joining the iliac tubercles represents this plane (5 cm behind the anterior-superior iliac spine). This plane lies at the level of L4 vertebra. It lies slightly below the umbilicus.

POINTS

1. *Origin of celiac artery*: Point 1.5 cm above transpyloric plane in the midline
2. *Origin of superior mesenteric artery*: A point just above the transpyloric plane in the midline
3. *Cardiac orifice*: Put a mark 2.5 cm left of the median plane on the seventh costal cartilage. Draw two short parallel lines 2 cm apart directed downwards and to the left
4. *Pyloric orifice of stomach (Fig. 4.32)*: At the transpyloric plane 1.25 cm to the right of the midline
5. *Tip of ninth costal cartilage (Fig. 4.32)*: At the junction of transpyloric planes and lateral border of rectus abdominis (it is prominent in muscular body)
6. *Fundus of gallbladder (Fig. 4.32)*: Tip of right ninth costal cartilage. It corresponds with an angle between right costal margin and linea semilunaris (lateral border of rectus muscle)

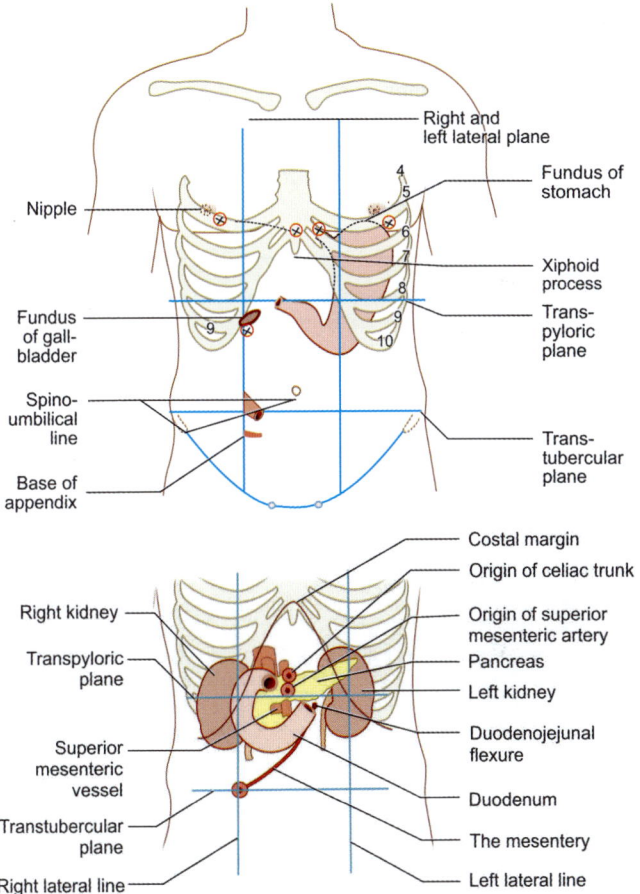

Fig. 4.32: Surface marking of abdomen

7. *Base of the appendix (Fig. 4.32)*: Lies 2 cm below junction between right lateral and the transtubercular planes
8. *McBurney's point*: At the junction between medial two-thirds and lateral one-third of spinoumbilical line (line joining

umbilicus and anterior-superior iliac spine). This point corresponds to maximum tenderness felt during appendicitis. The surface marking of appendicular orifice does not coincide with this point

9. *Duodenojejunal flexure*: 1 cm below the transpyloric plane and 2.5 cm to the left of midline
10. *Tip of fourth lumbar spine*: It corresponds with the highest point on the iliac crest.

> **Points to Remember**
>
> - Four pair of muscle (external oblique, internal oblique and rectus abdominis) forming the anterolateral wall are layered like plywood
> - Surface area of peritoneum is 2 m^2—equal to the surface area of skin, it has property of bidirectional transfer of substances. This property is used in peritoneal dialysis
> - Vertical midline incision is used for emergency laparotomy (opening up the abdomen) (Fig. 4.33)
> - The superficial veins of anterior abdominal wall are not prominent normally. In some conditions like portal hypertension, inferior vena caval obstruction, they become prominent
> - Sometimes a small inguinal hernia may be confused as femoral hernia. But, if the swelling is lateral to pubic tubercle, it is femoral hernia and medial to pubic tubercle it is inguinal hernia
> - Embryologically, gut is a midline structure. Because of these, the visceral pain arising from gut is first felt over the midline
> - Pain arising from stomach and duodenum is referred at epigastrium. Pain from the rest of the small intestine and ascending colon is referred to the area around umbilicus. From rest of the gut pain is referred to the hypogastrium
> - Spleen may be ruptured as a result of trauma and surgical removal (splenectomy) is needed
> - Normal renal mobility is 3 cm
> - The pelvic diaphragm may be greatly stretched during childbirth and may be weakened leading to prolapse of uterus or prolapse of rectum
> - Examination of interior of rectum and anal canal is called proctoscopy
> - The ureteric orifices appear as an oblique slit in cystoscopic (an instrument, which can pass through urethra) examination. However, in TB kidney, it is circular in shape due to shortening of urethra. This condition is known as golf hole urethra
> - Bilateral ligation of vas in the upper part of scrotum is done in male for permanent sterilization and this process is called vasectomy
> - One of the most important symptoms of prostatic enlargement is repeated and frequent desire to pass urine, but there is difficulty in doing so

Contd...

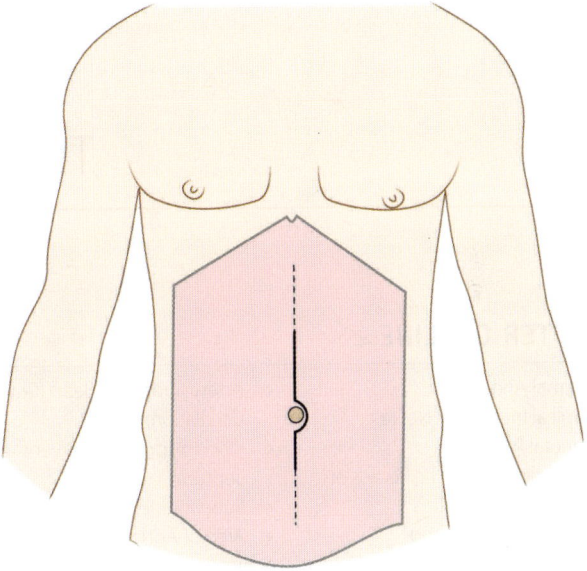

Fig. 4.33: Vertical midline incision is used for emergency laparotomy in peritonitis. Lengthy incision with wide exposure of the peritoneal cavity is advisable

Contd...

- Operation of choice is transurethral resection of prostate (TURP) in which the verumontanum (colliculus seminalis) serves as a guide to identify the urethral sphincter
- The ovary occupies the ovarian fossa only up to the time of first pregnancy. After pregnancy, the broad ligament becomes lax and ovaries may descend and may even lie in the rectouterine pouch.

5
CHAPTER

Thorax

CHAPTER OUTLINE

- Sternal Angle
- Typical Intercostal Nerve
- Parietal Pleura
- Costodiaphragmatic Recess of Pleura
- Azygos Lobe of Lung
- Mediastinal Surface of the Lungs
- Root of the Lung
- Bronchopulmonary Segments
- Azygos Vein
- Accessory Hemiazygos Vein or Inferior Hemiazygos Vein
- Artery Supply to Heart (Coronary Circulation))
- Blood Supply of Interventricular Septum
- Superior Mediastinum
- Arch of Aorta
- Tetralogy of Fallot
- Pericardial Cavity
- Coronary Sinus
- Constrictions of Esophagus with Clinical Importance
- Thoracic Duct

SHORT NOTES

STERNAL ANGLE (FIG. 5.1)

It is the junction between lower parts of manubrium with the upper end of the body of sternum. It is represented by a thin line, which can be visible in thin individual and palpable in obese person. It is an important landmark for the following:

- Junction between superior mediastinum and inferior mediastinum
- It corresponds with second costal cartilage. So, counting of ribs and intercostal space (ICS) is done from here which is important for surgeon and clinician
- Bifurcation of trachea occurs in this level
- Beginning and end of arch of aorta at this point.

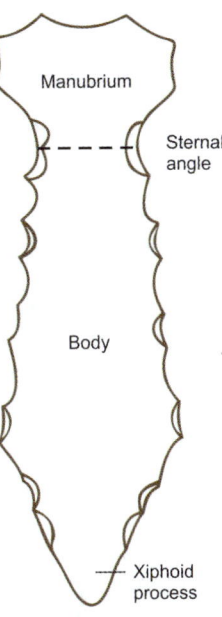

Fig. 5.1: Sternum anterior view

TYPICAL INTERCOSTAL NERVE

Anterior primary rami of third to sixth thoracic spinal nerves are called typical intercostal nerves. They are confined only to thoracic wall (Fig. 5.2).

Course

- The nerve passes through the respective intervertebral foramen and appears in the posterior part of ICS, medial to the superior costotransverse ligament
- It passes upward and laterally behind the sympathetic trunk and then intervenes in the endothoracic fascia between costal pleura and posterior intercostal membrane
- On reaching the angle of the upper rib, the nerve gives off a collateral and a lateral cutaneous branch

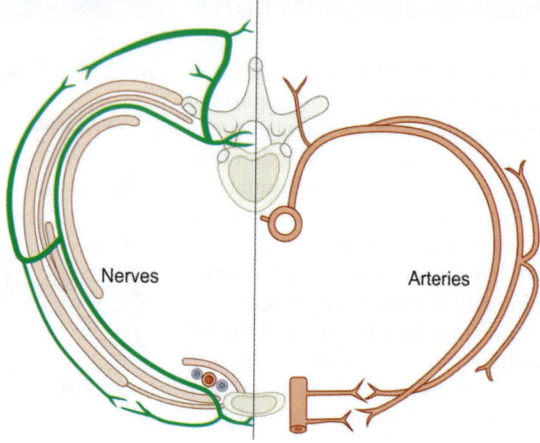

Fig. 5.2: Scheme showing the course and branches of typical intercostal nerve and intercostal arteries

- The trunk of the nerve passes forwards along the costal groove between intercostalis internus and intimus muscles
- In the costal groove arrangements of structures from above downwards are vein, artery and nerve
- In the anterior part of the space, the nerve passes in front of sternocostalis muscle, crosses internal intercostal and anterior intercostal membrane.

Applied Anatomy

In herpes zoster (viral infection) bulla is situated along the distribution of intercostal nerve.

PARIETAL PLEURA

Parietal pleura is thicker than the pulmonary pleura, and is subdivided into four parts. It develops from somatopleura layer of lateral plate mesoderm (Fig. 5.3).

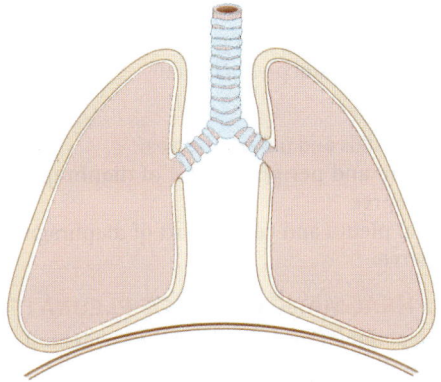

Fig. 5.3: Pleura

The divisions are:
1. Costal
2. Diaphragmatic
3. Mediastinal
4. Cervical.

Costal pleura: Lines the thoracic wall, which comprises of ribs and intercostal space to which it is loosely attached by a layer of areolar tissue called the endothoracic fascia.

Mediastinal pleura: Lines the corresponding surface of the mediastinum. It is reflected over the root of the lung and becomes continuous with the pulmonary pleura around the hilum.

Cervical pleura: It extends into the neck, nearly 5 cm above the 1st costal cartilage and 2.5 cm above the medial one-third of the cervical and covers the apex of the lung. It is covered by the suprapleural membrane of Sibso's fascia. Cervical pleura is related:
- *Anteriorly*—subclavian artery, scalenus medius
- *Posteriorly*—neck of the first rib and structures lying over it
- *Laterally*—scalenus medius
- *Medially*—large vessels of the neck.

Diaphragmatic pleura: It lines the superior aspect of diaphragm and below the base of the lung and gets continuous with mediastinal pleura medially and costal pleura laterally.

Nerve Supply

These are intercostals and phrenic nerves:
- Costal pleura and peripheral part of diaphragmatic pleura—intercostal nerve
- Mediastinal pleura and central part of diaphragmatic pleura—phrenic nerve.

COSTODIAPHRAGMATIC RECESS OF PLEURA (FIG. 5.4)

It is a cleft-like potential space between the lower limit of the pleural sac and the lower border of the corresponding lung. The costal and diaphragmatic pleura are in appositions in quit respiration, only separated by capillary layer of fluid. The lower limit of the pleura and lower border of the lung correspond with eighth, tenth and twelfth ribs in midclavicular, midaxillary and scapular lines, respectively.

Relations of the recess below the diaphragm:

Right Side
- Right lobe and caudate lobe of liver
- Upper part of the posterior surface of the right kidney.

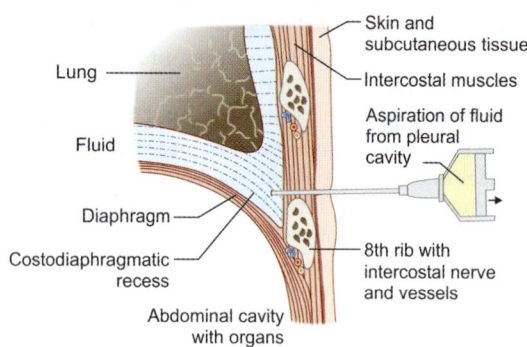

Fig. 5.4: Pleural reflection, costodiaphragmatic recess and pleural tap

Left Side
- Fundus of stomach
- Spleen
- Upper part of the posterior surface of left kidney.

Applied Anatomy
- It is a potential space, which allow expansion of the lung in full inspiration
- It is the most dependent part of the pleural sac so if fluid appears in the pleural sac it is connected first in this space, appears as haziness in X-ray.

Peculiarities
- Viewed is lateral aspect, the recess is widest in the midaxillary line where the lower border of the lung lies about 5 cm above the lower limit of pleura
- Right costodiaphragmatic recess crosses right costoexiphoid and costovertebra angles, whereas the left recess crossed the left costovertebral angle only.

AZYGOS LOBE OF LUNG

It is an accessory lobe of lung. They are of three types:
1. Upper azygos lobe
2. Lower azygos lobe
3. Lobe of azygos vein.

The former two types are of little clinical importance. The lobe of azygos vein is present in 1% of the population. It affects the upper portion of right lung, where the apex of the lungs splits into two; (1) medial and (2) lateral by a fissure formed by the arch of azygos vein the medial part of the split apex forms the lobe of the azygos vein.

Clinical Anatomy
It is one of the differential diagnoses of enlarged lymph node in the chest.

MEDIASTINAL SURFACE OF THE LUNGS (TABLE 5.1 AND FIGS 5.5A AND B)

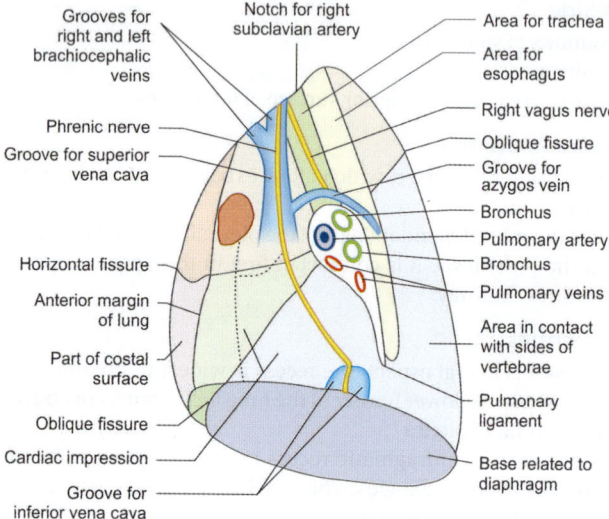

Fig. 5.5A: Right lung viewed from the medial side showing areas related to various structures

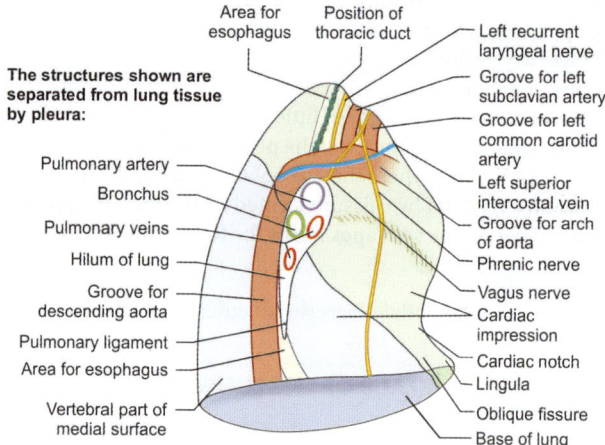

Fig. 5.5B: Left lung viewed from the medial side showing areas related to different structures

Table 5.1: Mediastinal surface of the lungs

Right lung (venous)	Left lung (arterial)
Right atrium and auricle in cardiac impression	Left ventricle, left auricle infundibulum and adjoining part of the right ventricle in cardiac impression
Small part of the right ventricle	Pulmonary trunk
Superior vena cava above cardiac impression	Arch of aorta—above the root of lung
Inferior vena cava below cardiac impression	Descending aorta—behind the root of left lung
Lower part of right brachiocephalic veins above cardiac impression	Left brachiocephalic vein esophagus
Esophagus behind the root of lung	Thoracic duct
Trachea above and behind the root of lung	Left vagus nerve
Right vagus nerve	Left phrenic nerve
Right phrenic nerve	Left subclavian artery
Azygos vein—arching over the root of lung	Left recurrent laryngeal nerve

ROOT OF THE LUNG

Root of the lung is a short and broad pedal, which connects the medial surface of the lung to the mediastinum. It is formed by the structures, which either enters or comes out of the lung through the hilum. The roots of the lung lie opposite the bodies of fifth, sixth and seventh vertebra (Fig. 5.6).

Arrangement of Structures in the Root (Table 5.2)

Table 5.2: Branches in the root of right and left lung

Right lung	Left lung
• Eparterial bronchus • Pulmonary artery • Hyparterial bronchus • Pulmonary vein	• Pulmonary artery • Bronchus • Pulmonary vein

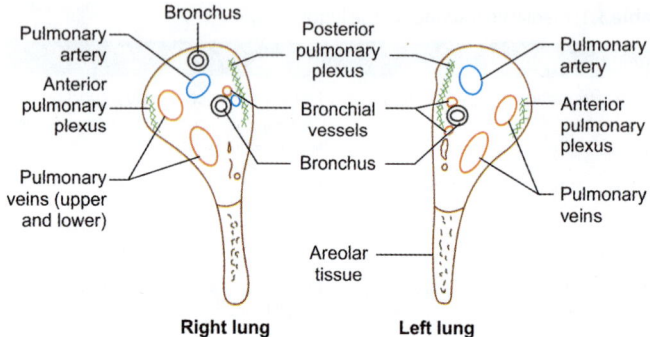

Fig. 5.6: Enlarged view of root of two lungs with its contents

Relations (Table 5.3)

Table 5.3: Relations between the right and left side of different lobes of lung

	Common of two sides	Right side	Left side
Anterior	Phrenic nerve Pericardiacophrenic vessels Anterior pulmonary plexus	Superior vena cava A part of right atrium	—
Posterior	Vagus nerve Posterior pulmonary plexus	—	Descending aorta
Superior	—	Terminal part of azygos vein	Arch of aorta
Inferior	Pulmonary ligament		

BRONCHOPULMONARY SEGMENTS (FIGS 5.7A TO D AND TABLE 5.4)

These are well-defined anatomical, functional and surgical segments of the lung, each one being aerated by a tertiary or segmental bronchus. Each segment is pyramidal in shape with its apex directed toward the root of the lung.

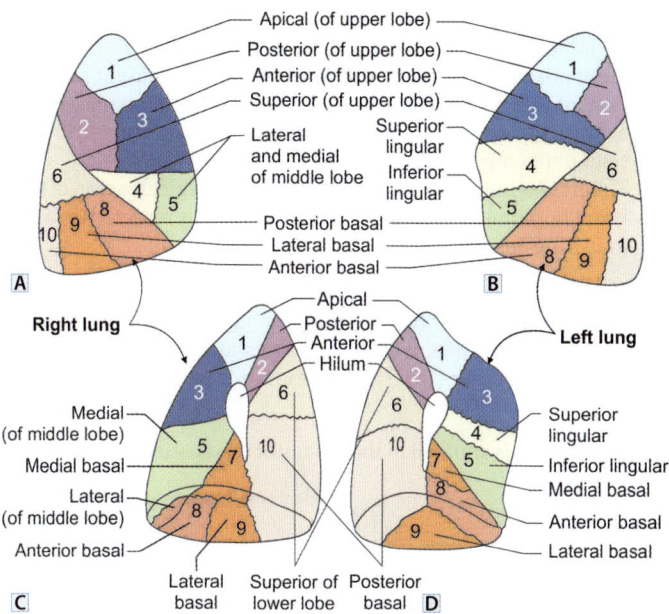

Figs 5.7A to D: Bronchopulmonary segments of the right and left lungs

Table 5.4: Bronchopulmonary segments of lung

	Lobes	Segment
Right lung	Upper	Apical, posterior, anterior
	Middle	Lateral, medial
	Lower	Apical, anterior basal, medial basal, lateral basal, posterior basal
Left lung	Upper	Apical, posterior, anterior, superior lingular, inferior lingular
	Lower	Superior, medial basal, anterior basal, lateral basal, posterior basal

Clinical Anatomy

- Knowledge of bronchopulmonary segment is important for postural drainage

- *Bronchoscopy*: It is the study of bronchopulmonary segment radiologically by installation of radiopaque dye
- Lung abscess is more common in posterior segment of upper lobe and apical region of lower lobe. Bronchopulmonary segment acts as an independent unit, hence infection is restricted in each segment except foreign body
- Tubercular lesion commonly affected in the apical region of lung
- Bronchopulmonary segment may be surgically resected in tumor or in lung abscess.

AZYGOS VEIN

It drains the right-sided thoracic wall upper-lumbar region, mediastinal structure and bronchus. It forms an important channel connecting the superior vena cava (SVC) and inferior vena cava (IVC) (Fig. 5.8).

Situation

Major part of it, is situated in the posterior mediastinum.

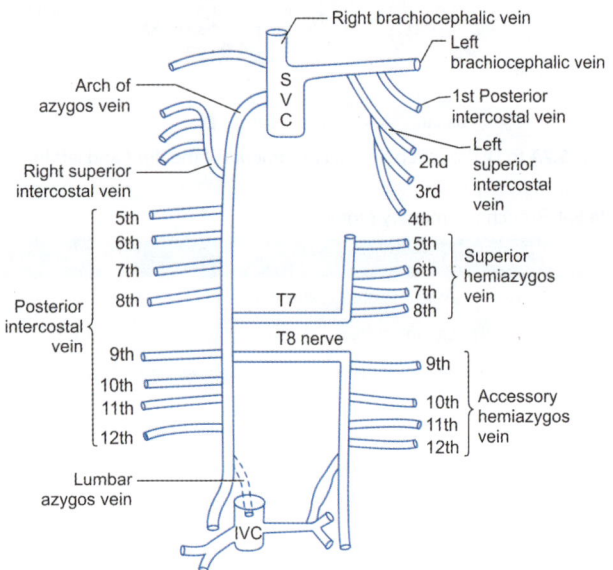

Fig. 5.8: Azygos system of veins
Abbreviations: SVC, superior vena cava; IVC, inferior vena cava

Formation

Arises in abdomen as lumbar azygos vein or may from union of right subcostal and right ascending lumbar veins.

Course

- The azygos vein enters the thorax by passing through the aortic opening of the diaphragm
- It ascends up to T4 vertebra, where it arches forward over the root of the right lung ends by joining the SVC just before the latter pierces the pericardium.

Relation

- *Anteriorly*: Esophagus
- *Posteriorly*:
  - Lower eight thoracic vertebra
  - Right posterior intercostal arteries
- *To the right*:
  - Right lung and pleura
  - Greater splanchnic nerve
- *To the left*:
  - Thoracic duct and descending aorta in lower part
  - Esophagus (right edge), trachea and right vagus in the upper part.

Tributaries

- Right superior intercostal vein
- Fifth to eleventh right posterior intercostal veins
- Hemiazygos veins at the level of T7 vertebra
- Accessory hemiazygos vein at the level of T8 vertebra
- Right brachial vein, near the terminal end of the azygos vein
- Several esophageal, mediastinal pericardial veins.

Applied Anatomy

In obstruction of SVC or IVC, the azygos vein acts as an important channel to establish collateral circulation.

ACCESSORY HEMIAZYGOS VEIN OR INFERIOR HEMIAZYGOS VEIN (FIG. 5.8)

Formation

Formed by the union of left ascending lumbar vein and left subcostal vein.

Termination

At azygos vein at about T8 level.

Tributaries

- Left lower three posterior intercostal veins
- Common trunk formed by ascending lumbar and subcostal, esophageal and mediastinal veins.

Area of Drainage

Lower parietes of thorax and structures of mediastinum.

ARTERY SUPPLY TO HEART (CORONARY CIRCULATION) (TABLE 5.5)

Table 5.5: Specification and supply to heart of left and right coronary artery

Name	Beginning	Course	Branches	Area supplied
1. Right coronary artery (smaller than left coronary artery) (Fig. 5.9) P.G.E.	It arises from ascending aorta from the anterior aortic sinus	1. It passes downwards in between the root of pulmonary trunk and the right auricle, it winds round the inferior border, passes in the posterior part of atrioventricular groove and terminates by anastomosis with left coronary artery	• Marginal • Posterior inter-ventricular • Nodal (60% case) • Anterior inter-ventricular • Branch to diaphragmatic surface of left ventricle	It supplies all the right ventricle, the variable part of diaphragmatic surface of left ventricle, post-one-third of interventricular septum, the right atrium part of left atrium and nodal tissue
2. Left coronary artery (Fig. 5.9) P.G.E.	It arises from ascending aorta from left posterior aortic sinus	2. It passes behind and then to the left of pulmonary artery. Between it and left auricle, it divides into circumflex and anterior interventricular branch		It supplies most of left ventricle, small area of right ventricle, anterior two-thirds of interventricular septum, most of left atrium

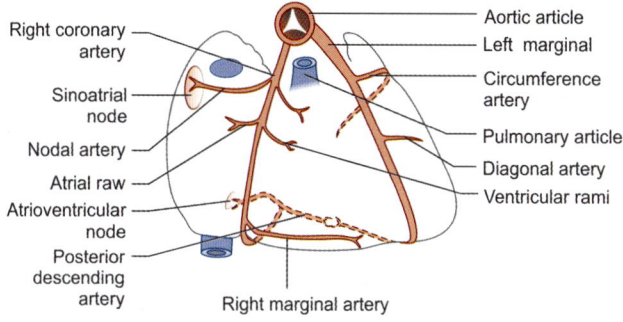

Fig. 5.9: Coronary circulation

BLOOD SUPPLY OF INTERVENTRICULAR SEPTUM

Interventricular septum separates the right ventricle from the left ventricle. It has got anterior inferior muscular part and small posterosuperior membranous part. Normally, right coronary artery supplies the posterior one-third of interventricular septum and left coronary artery supplies the anterior two-thirds and it is known as left dominance. When posterior two-thirds is supplied by right coronary artery, it is known as right dominance (Fig. 5.10).

Clinical anatomy—This is important for cardio thoracic surgery.

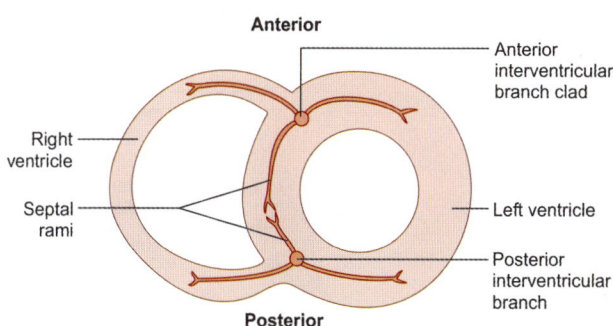

Fig. 5.10: Arterial supply of interventricular septum (in transverse section)

SUPERIOR MEDIASTINUM

Boundaries (Fig. 5.11)
- *Anterior:* Manubrium sterni
- *Posterior:* Upper four thoracic vertebra
- *Superior:* Pleura of the thoracic inlet
- *Inferior:* An imaginary plane passing through the sternal angle in front and the lower border of the body of fourth thoracic vertebra behind
- *On both side:* Mediastinal pleura.

Contents
- *Organs:*
  - Trachea and esophagus
  - *Muscles:* Origins of sternohyoid, sternothyroid and lower ends of longus colli
  - *Arteries:* Arch of aorta, brachiocephalic artery, left common carotid artery, left subclavicular artery
  - *Veins:* Right and left brachiocephalic veins, upper half of superior vena cava (SVC), left superior intercostal vein

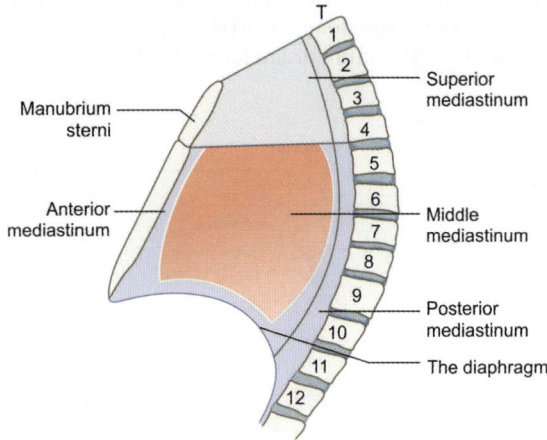

Fig. 5.11: Median section of thorax showing divisions of mediastinum

- *Nerves*: Vagus phrenic, cardiac nerves of both sides, left recurrent laryngeal nerve
- Thymus
- Thoracic duct
- *Lymph nodes*: Paratracheal, brachiocephalic and tracheobronchial.

ARCH OF AORTA (FIG. 5.12)

Arch of aorta is the continuation of the ascending aorta. It is an anteroposterior arch begins at sternal angle and arches over the root of the left lung and connects the ascending with descending aorta at the level of T4 vertebra. It is situated in the superior mediastinum and upper end of arch extends up to middle of manubrium sterni.

Development

It is developed from three sources:
- *Left side of the aortic sac*: Truncus arteriosus—forms the part between the brachiocephalic trunk and left common carotid artery

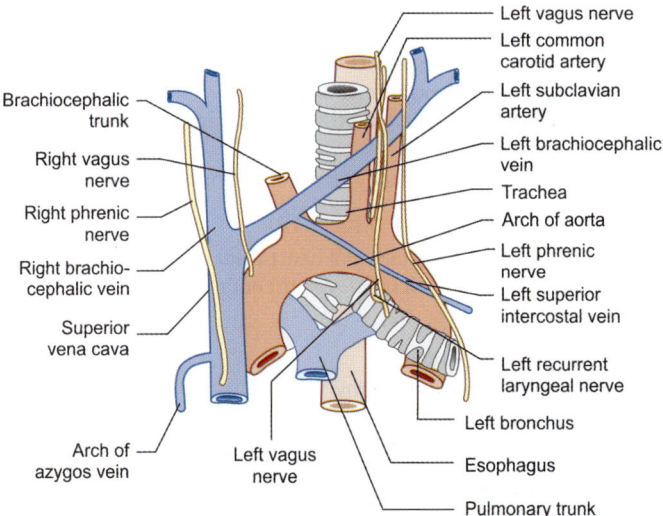

Fig. 5.12: Arch of aorta

- *Left-fourth aortic arch*: It forms the part between left common carotid artery and ductus arteriosus
- *Left dorsal aorta*: It forms the rest of arch up to descending aorta.

Relations

Anteriorly, it is related with left phrenic, cervical cardiac branch of left vagus, cardiac branch of left sympathetic, left vagus left superior intercostals vein, remains of thymus and all these are covered by left lung and pleura.

Posteriorly, it is related to deep cardiac plexus, trachea, left recurrent laryngeal nerve, esophagus and thoracic duct.

Branches

There are three branches in the area, i.e. brachiocephalic, left common carotid and left subclavian. All these are crossed by left brachiocephalic veins.

Abnormal Branches

Arteria thyroid ima, internal thoracic artery, left vertebral artery, bronchial artery and inferior thyroid artery. Arches may be of one side.

Clinical Anatomy

- Patent ductus arteriosus (PDA). In this case, blood is passing from arch of aorta to left pulmonary artery.
- *Clinical features:* Deficient growth, left ventricular hypertrophy and congestion of lung.
- *Coarctation of aorta:* It may be preductal or postductal.

TETRALOGY OF FALLOT (FIG. 5.13)

It is the most common congenital heart disease. On exertion, child develops breathlessness. It is a developmental defect.

Defects

- Pulmonary artery stenosis
- Right ventricular hypertrophy
- Over-riding of aorta
- Ventricular septal defects.

Clinical Anatomy

- Corrected by surgery.

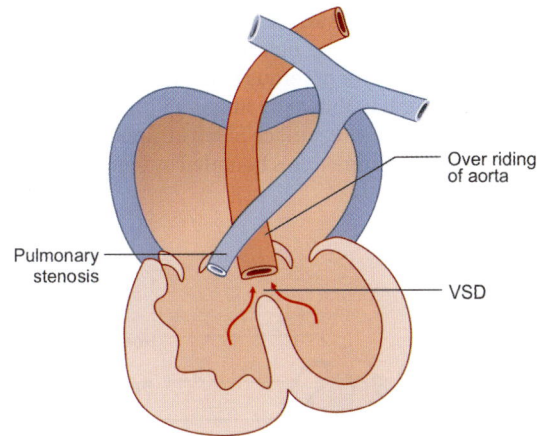

Fig. 5.13: Tetralogy of Fallot
Abbreviation: VSD, ventricular septal defect

PERICARDIAL CAVITY (FIG. 5.14A)

Heart lies within the pericardial cavity in middle mediastinum. The pericardium provides for heart a friction-free surface to accommodate its sliding movement. Parts of pericardium are:
- *Fibrous pericardium*: It consists of collagenous fibers and fused with the central tendon of diaphragm because they develop from same source
- *Serous pericardium*: The serous pericardium lines the inner wall of fibrous pericardium and visceral layer is reflected over the heart and it is known as epicardium. The pericardial cavity is the space between parietal and visceral layers. Two regions of pericardial cavities have special name.

Transverse Pericardial Sinus P.G.E. (Fig. 5.14B)

It is a space behind the ascending aorta and pulmonary trunk in front and posteriorly by upper border of left atrium and veins. It is an intervisceral space and one can pass a forceps behind the ascending aorta and pulmonary trunk to demonstrate it.

Oblique Pericardial Sinus P.G.E. (Fig. 5.14B)

It is the parietovisceral space behind the posterior surface of left atrium where parietal layer of serous pericardium reflected over the fibrous pericardium. It is shown by lifting up the apex of heart and behind the base or posterior surface of left atrium. It is a cul-de-sac, which opens inferiorly. The sinus is bounded by four pulmonary veins and IVC (five veins).

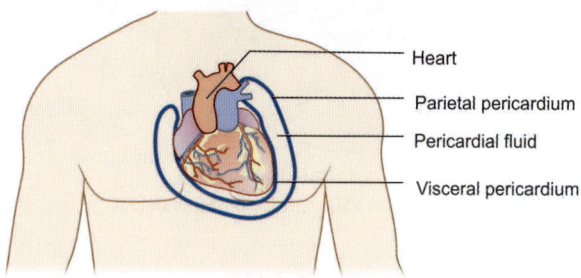

Fig. 5.14A: Pericardial cavity

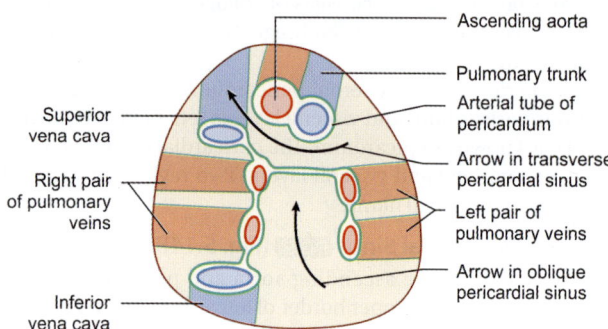

Fig. 5.14B: Oblique and transverse pericardial sinus

CORONARY SINUS (TABLE 5.6)

Cardiac Veins (Venous Drainage of Heart) (Fig. 5.15)

Table 5.6: Coronary sinus

Name	Formation	Termination	Tributaries	Area of drainage
Coronary sinus	It is formed behind the left atrium and left ventricle; 2–3 cm long	Open in the right atrium between the opening of inferior vena cava and right atrio-ventricular orifice	• Great cardiac vein (begins at cardiac apex, ascends in anterior inter-ventricular sulcus) • Small cardiac vein • Middle cardiac vein (begins at cardiac apex ascends in posterior interventricular groove) • Posterior vein of the left ventricle, oblique vein of left atrium	Whole heart

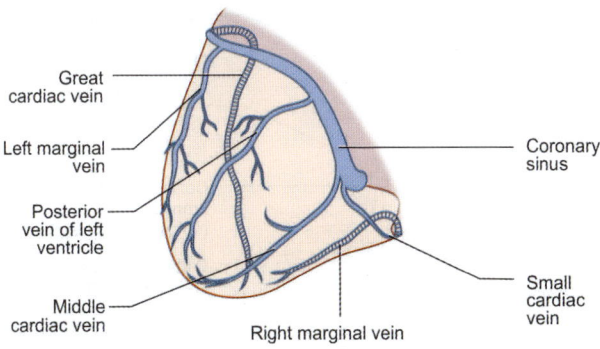

Fig. 5.15: Cardiac veins and coronary sinus

CONSTRICTIONS OF ESOPHAGUS WITH CLINICAL IMPORTANCE (FIG. 5.16)

Esophagus presents four constrictions from above downwards:
- At its commencement, opposite C6, about 6 inches from incision teeth
- Where it is crossed by the arch of aorta, opposite T4, about 9 inches from the incision teeth
- Where it is crossed by the left bronchus opposite T6, about 11 inches from the incision teeth
- At the esophageal opening of the diaphragm, opposite T10, about 15 or 16 inches from incision teeth.

Clinical Importance
- Swallowed foreign bodies can lodge in these sites
- These sites can cause difficulty in passing the esophagoscope or Ryle's tube.

Medical person should aware of this constriction because in intake of corrosive (acid) for suicidal attempt produces harm in constriction of esophagus.

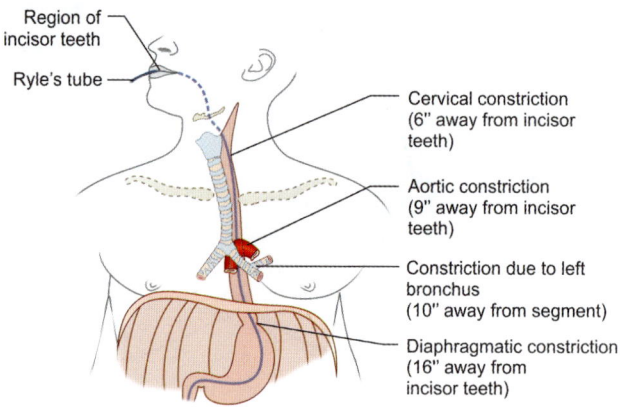

Fig. 5.16: Constrictions of esophagus

THORACIC DUCT (FIG. 5.17)

It is in elongated common lymphatic trunk, which conveys chyle and most of the lymph of the body. It drains the lymphatics from the whole body except the right side of head and neck, right upper limb, right half of the heart and convex surface of the liver.

Characteristics

It is flexible in character, beaded in appearance and is provided with numerous valves; valves are situated on those sites, which are exposed to pressure.

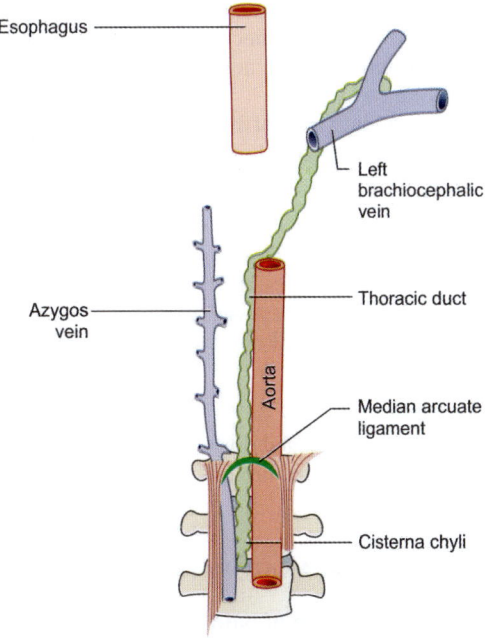

Fig. 5.17: Thoracic duct

Measurement
- Length—38-45 cm
- Breadth—0.5 cm.

Extent
Lower border of T12 vertebra upwards up to C7 vertebra.

Course
- The thoracic duct begins as a continuation of the upper end of the cysterna chyli near the lower border of the T12 vertebra and enters the thorax through the aortic opening of the diaphragm
- It then ascends through the posterior mediastinum crossing from the right side to the left and the level of T5 vertebra. It then runs through the superior mediastinum along the edge of the esophagus and reaches the neck
- In the neck, it arches laterally at the level of the transverse process of C7 vertebra
- Finally, it descends in front of the first subclavian artery and ends by opening into the angle of junction between the left subclavian and left internal jugular vein.

Tributaries
- In the thorax, it receives lymph vessels from posterior mediastinal nodes and from small interstitial lymph nodes
- At the root of neck, efferent vessels of the nodes in the neck form the left jugular lymph trunk and those from nodes in axilla form left subclavian trunk.

Clinical Anatomy
Thoracic duct may be damaged during the operation at the root of neck, the lymph usually flow through other channels, but if it fails chylous fistula may occur.

EXPLANATORY NOTES

Q1. A person complaining of pain radiating along the typical intercostal space.

Ans. Third to sixth intercostal nerves are typical intercostal nerves. They supply the typical intercostal space. When there is irritation of this nerve due to viral (herpes) or bacterial infection, this pain is radiates along the distribution of those nerves.

Q2. Coronary disease in old age is less fatal than in young age. Explain.

Ans. Anastomoses do exist between branches of coronary arteries at the precapillary level. Blockage of coronary arteries in old age is less fatal than in young age because anastomoses increase and collateral channels develop with the advancement of age.

Q3. Entry of foreign body is common to the right bronchus due to following reasons.

Ans.

- The right bronchus is shorter, wider and more vertical than left bronchus
- The keel-like median ridge at the bifurcation of the trachea between the orifices of two main bronchi (the carina) is slightly deviated to the left side.

Q4. T3 to T6 intercostal nerves are called typical intercostal nerve. Why?

Ans. These are anterior ramus of typical thoracic nerve. Those intercostal nerves, who are limited only, in the thorax are called typical intercostal nerve. These are T3 to T6 nerves.

- T1 to T2 distributed to both superior extremity and thorax
- T7 to T11 are distributed to both thorax and abdomen.

Q5. Transposition of great vessels. Explain.

Ans. This is one of the acyanotic diseases of heart due to transposition of great vessels. It is due to failure of aortic pulmonary septum to follow the normal spiral course.

Q6. Child with atrial septal defect presents foramen ovale. Explain.

Ans. Atrial septal defect (ASD) is one of the most common congenital anomalies of heart. There are many variables of ASD. The intra-atrial septum are formed from three sources—(1) septum primum, (2) septum secundum and (3) septum intermedium. The foramen ovale is a valvular gap between septum primum and septum secundum. It closes after birth when there is rapid increase in pressure of blood in left atrium due to beginning of lung circulation. But, when excessive reabsorption of septum primum or inadequate development of septum secundum or persistent ostium primum then there is persistent foramen ovale in ASD.

Q7. Explain tracheoesophageal fistula.

Ans. Fistula is an abnormal communication between two structures. Trachea is embryologically developed from the laryngeal bud that arises from the ventral part of foregut, which will form the esophagus. Later, the trachea and esophagus are separated by tracheoesophageal septum. If somehow the septum is not developed completely or absent, there is a communication between trachea and the esophagus. This is known as tracheoesophageal fistula.

Q8. In a chest X-ray, the left thoracic cavity is found to contain abdominal viscera/a child presents with peristaltic sounds in the chest. Explain.

Ans. Child may present with peristaltic sounds in the chest when there is herniation of abdominal viscera in the thorax.

This takes place through the diaphragm and can be considered as a case of diaphragmatic hernia.

The stomach and part of small intestine can enter thorax through the foramen of Morgagni or through the *Bochdalek triangle*.

The junction of the esophagus and stomach may herniate (rolling type of hernia) or the fundus of the stomach may herniate (sliding type of hernia).

Q9. Chest X-ray shows arching of ribs in coarctation of aorta. Explain.

Ans. Coarctation of aorta means narrowing of the lumen of the aorta. It may be preductal and postductal. Postductal coarctation is more common. Here, there is more flow of blood through posterior intercostal artery. In X-ray, there is rib notching due to erosion of lower border of ribs.

In case of postductal coarctation, there is swelling of posterior intercostal artery. Radiological sign of rib notching due to more pressure on the lower part of the ribs.

Q10. How intercostal nerve block is accomplished?

Ans. Intercostal nerve block is accomplished by injecting an anesthetic immediately beneath the inferior edge of a rib in the back. This is very effective way of relieving pain caused by a fractured rib.

- Local irritation of an intercostal nerve by a disease of thoracic vertebrae gives rise to pain in front of the chest
- Pus from the region of thoracic vertebra gives rise to pain in course of intercostal nerve around the chest wall and points outward at the sides of exist of cutaneous branches.

Q11. Following tumor of apical lobe of lung there is enlargement of neck vein and Horner's syndrome. Explain.

Ans. Behind the apical lobe of lung lies first posterior intercostal vein, which drains into corresponding brachiocephalic vein and also T1 sympathetic thoracic ganglion. Tumor mass presses on these structures and there will be enlargement of neck vein and Horner's syndrome (characterized by ptosis).

Q12. Central tendon of the thoracoabdominal diaphragm is blended with the basal part of the fibrous pericardium. Explain.

Ans. Central tendon of thoracoabdominal diaphragm and fibrous pericardium are developed from same source that is septum transversum. So, both of them are fused together.

Q13. Explain pericardial effusion.

Ans. When excess fluid is accumulated (more than 300 cc), it is known as pericardial effusion. There is compression symptom (cardiac tamponade). The cardiac output is reduced and heart beats in abnormal rhythm; and eventually cardiac arrest.

Clinical anatomy: To relieve pain, a tapping is done through left costoxiphoid angle as the lungs here are apart from pericardial cavity and heart.

Q14. Why in adult the respiration is thoracoabdominal and in child that is abdominal?

Ans. The thorax up to 2 years after birth is circular in cross-section. Therefore, the diameter of thorax cannot be increased within the circumference, the length of which remains constant. Therefore, in children up to the 2 years of age, the respiration is almost entirely abdominal.

Q15. Collection of pus in posterior mediastinum may come from pharynx. Explain.

Ans. The posterior portion of pretracheal fascia is covering the posterior pharynx and esophagus. Infection (pus) in this vertical space may pass inferiorly into the posterior mediastinum of thorax.

Q16. Anterior interventricular branch of left coronary artery is known as the artery of sudden death. Explain.

Ans.
- The anterior interventricular branch [or left anterior descending artery (LAD)] arises at the branching point of left main coronary artery (the trunk or LMCA) and descends along anterior interventricular groove and terminates by meeting the end of posterior interventricular artery—either at the apex or winding around the apex at the posterior interventricular groove
- The anterior septal branches supply the anterior two-thirds of the interventricular septum
- It is evident that the LAD supplies a large area of the left ventricle and the interventricular septum
- Neuropsychological studies and recent angiographic studies have demonstrated that this artery is very much prone to atherosclerosis and narrowing, particularly in men. Blockage of this artery causes massive and fatal infarction. On account of this, the artery is termed as the *"Artery of sudden death"* or *"Widow maker".*

SURFACE ANATOMY OF THORAX WHICH IS HELPFUL TO CLINICIAN AND SURGEON

- *Bifurcation of trachea (Fig. 5.18)*: It is a point, located to the slightly right of midpoint of sternal angle
- *Sternal angle (Fig. 5.19)*: Junction of manubrium with the body of sternum.
  Importance of sternal angle:
  - Counting of ribs
  - Junction of superior and inferior mediastinum
- *Apex of the heart (Fig. 5.20)*: In the left fifth ICS 9 cm away from midline (i.e. below and medial to left nipple)
- *Right border of heart (Fig. 5.20)*:
  - Point at the upper border of right third costal cartilage 1.25 cm from the lateral border of sternum
  - Point on the lower border of right sixth costal cartilage at the level of xiphisternal joint

Thorax

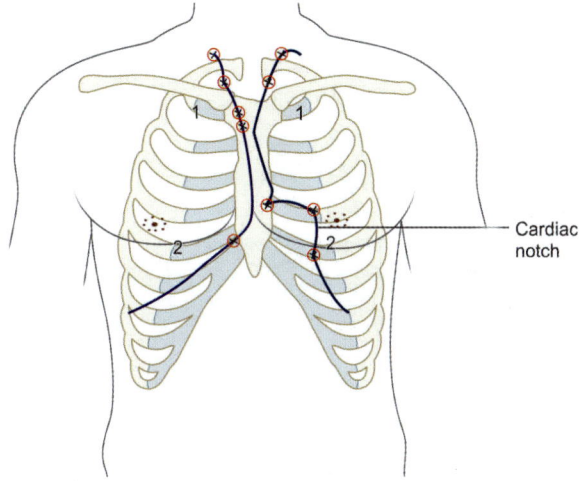

Fig. 5.18: Surface marking of: (A) Anterior border; (B) Lower border of both lungs

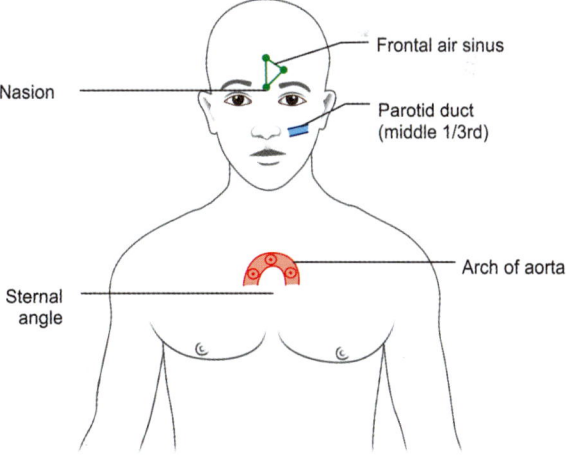

Fig. 5.19: Sternal angle, arch of aorta, frontal air sinus and parotid duct

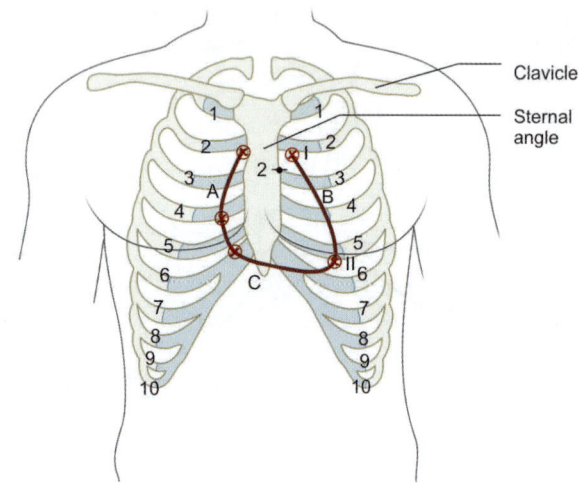

Fig. 5.20: Surface marking of heart (only give the linear diagram) (A) Right border; (B) Left border; and (C) Inferior border

- Point on the right fourth space 3.8 cm from midline convex line. Joining the above three points represents right border of heart.
- *Left border of heart (Fig. 5.20):*
  - Point on lower border of left second costal cartilage 1.2 cm from lateral margin of sternum
  - Point in the left fifth ICS 9 cm away from the midline (where apex beat is felt)
  - Join the above points with convexity toward the left.

CLINICAL ANATOMY (HEART AND PERICARDIUM)

- *Angina pectoris*: It is an intermittent, transient and central chest pain. It is due to coronary artery insufficiency and always manifests after exertion

- *Valvular disease*: It is commonly seen in rheumatic fever, produces valvular incompetence (incapability to hold blood), seen most commonly in mitral and aortic valves
- *Heart failure*: When diastolic pressure of ventricle increases (normal pressure 0)—there is gradual heart failure. Any one of the four chambers of heart can fail separately, which increases back pressure. There is edema (accumulation of fluid) in feet and breathlessness on exertion
- *Arterial aneurysm*: Abnormal dilation of a segment of main artery is known as aneurysm
- *Atherosclerosis*: It is characterized by irregular lipid deposit (fat) in the inner wall of large- and medium-sized artery. Common in middle- and old-aged group; produces partial ischemia, (less blood supply) of the region supplied and required bypass surgery
- *Coronary bypass (Fig. 5.21)*: It is a surgical procedure to direct blood from root of aorta to coronary vessels by putting a saphenous vein graft or internal mammary artery graft for coronary artery obstruction.

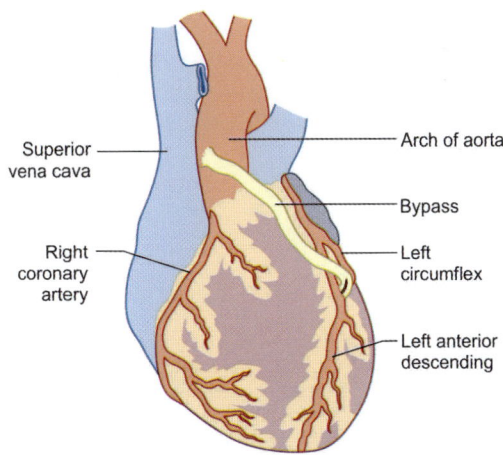

Fig. 5.21: Coronary bypass

- *Myocardial infarction or heart attack*: As coronary arteries are functionally end arteries blockage of main branches by atherosclerosis produces damage of large amount of heart tissue and patient died immediately
- Narrowing of valve orifice due to fusion of cusps is known as stenosis, e.g. mitral stenosis, etc.
- Dilatation of valve orifice due to stiffening of cusps is known as incompetence or regurgitation. It is due to imperfect closure of valve, e.g. aortic incompetence.

> **Points to Remember**
> - Collection of pus within the pleural cavity is known as empyema
> - Tracheostomy is of two types—(1) emergency tracheostomy and (2) elective tracheostomy
> - Cryosurgery—it is the destruction of tissues by controlled cooling, e.g. wart removal.

6
CHAPTER

Head, Neck and Brain

CHAPTER OUTLINE

- Sutural Joint
- Scalp
- Lacrimal Apparatus
- Posterior Cricoarytenoid Muscle
- Palatine Tonsil
- Waldeyer's Ring
- Little's Area of Epistaxis
- Cornea
- Taste Buds
- Temporalis Muscle
- Hypoglossal Nerve
- Movement of Temporomandibular Joint
- Parotid Gland
- Thyroid Gland
- Orbital Fissure
- Nasal Cavity

Brain and Eyeball
- Filum Terminale
- Types of Sulci
- Neural Crest Cells
- Paracentral Lobule
- Blood–Brain Barrier
- Ciliary Body
- Iris
- Corpus Callosum
- Third Ventricle
- Aqueous Humor
- Arachnoid Granulations
- Rhomboid Fossa
- Circle of Willis
- Midbrain

SHORT NOTES

SUTURAL JOINT

Introduction
Sutural joints are formed when bones are united by fibrous tissue; therefore, these are examples of fibrous joints.

Location
Most of the joints of the skull, where bones ossify in membrane.

Types (Fig. 6.1)
- *Serrate suture*: Edges of articulating bones present saw-tooth appearance, e.g. sagittal suture.

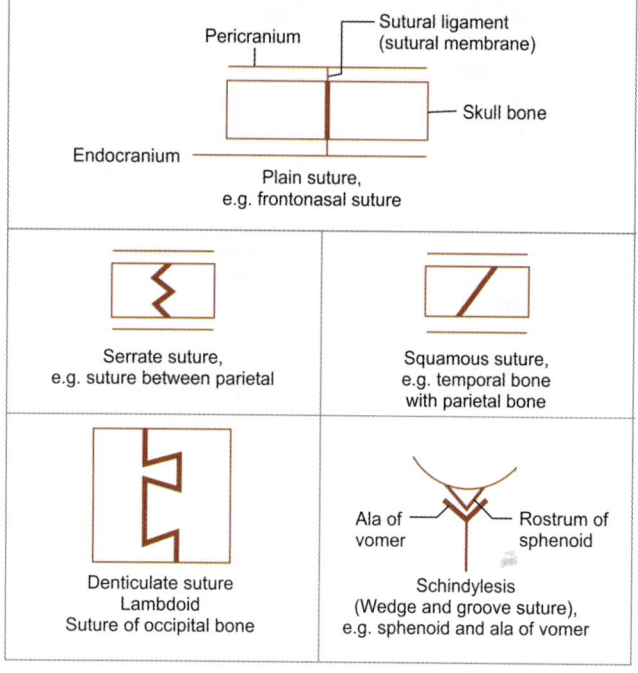

Fig. 6.1: Types of sutures

- *Denticulate suture*: Edges of articulating bones present teeth-like appearance, e.g. lambdoid suture
- *Squamous suture*: Edges of articulating bones united by overlapping, e.g. between parietal and squamous part of the temporal bone
- *Plane suture*: Edges of articulating bones being plane united by sutural ligament, e.g. between palatine process of two maxillae
- *Wedge-and-groove suture*: (Schindylesis) edges of one bone fit into the groove of other, e.g. between the rostrum of sphenoid with the upper margin of vomer.

SCALP

- *Five word*—it consists of five layers (Fig. 6.2), from outside inwards they are:
    - *Skin*—skin is hairy and contains plenty of sebaceous glands. It is adherent to the epicranial aponeurosis through the dense superficial fascia, as in the palms and soles
    - *Connective tissue (superficial fascia)*: It is very dense and contains plenty of blood vessels and nerves. The cut vessels are not able to retract due to adherence of their wall with the dense connective tissue
    - *Aponeurosis (galea aponeurosis or epicranial aponeurosis)*: This contains occipitofrontalis muscle. It has occipital and frontal belly. The occipital belly arises from external occipital protuberance and highest nuchal lines. The frontal belly arises

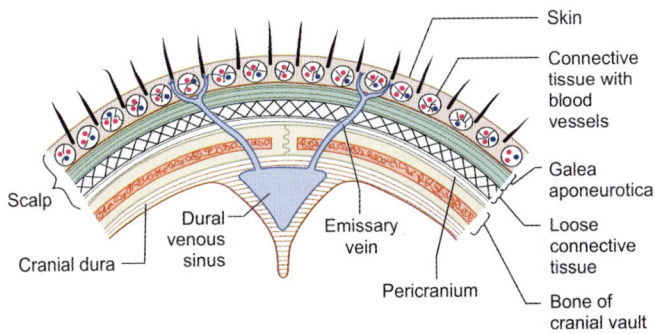

Fig. 6.2: A coronal section through the scalp showing the different layers

from epicranial aponeurosis and merges with the procerus, corrugator supercilii and orbicularis oculi. The direction of the fibers is anteroposteriorly
- *Loose areolar tissue*: It extends:
  - Posteriorly up to highest and superior nuchal lines
  - Laterally up to superior temporal lines
  - Anteriorly into the eyelids
- The fourth layer, i.e. loose areolar tissue is called dangerous area of the scalp. The infection of this layer reaches dural venous sinuses through emissary veins. The bleeding in this layer results into black eye as frontalis muscle is not attached to bone
- *Pericranium*—periosteal layer—adherent to suture line
- **Arterial supply**—in front of auricle—supratrochlear, supraorbital, superficial temporal behind auricle—posterior auricular, occipital
- **Nerve supply**—motor—temporal branch of facial nerve—frontal belly
- Posterior auriclater branch of VII—occipital belly
- Sensory supply of scalp
- **In front of ear**—four branches, behind ear—four branches. They are: supratrochlear, supraorbital, greater auricular C2, C3, lesser occipital C2.

Clinical Anatomy

- *First layer*—common site of sebaceous cyst
- *Second layer*—bleeding in second layer is profuse due to:
  - Rich blood supply
  - *The torn vessels are prevented from constriction because the walls of the vessels are adherent to the dense connective tissue*
- *Third layer*—the injury in anteroposterior direction heals fast. There is delay in the healing of the transverse injury
- *Fourth layer*:
  - *This is the dangerous area of scalp.* The infection from this layer spread to the brain through emissary vein
  - Accumulation of blood and pus in this layer result in black eye
  - *Caput succedaneum*—collection of fluid/blood in loose areolar tissue in newborn due to forceps delivery produces swelling, which is diffuse
- *Fifth layer*—cephalhematoma—collection of blood below periosteal layer of scalp due to injury.

Head, Neck and Brain

LACRIMAL APPARATUS (FIG. 6.3)
It consists of following:

Lacrimal Gland
- *Shape*: Almond-shaped
- *Position*: It is situated at the anterolateral surface of the orbit, medial to the zygomatic process of the frontal bone in lacrimal fossa
- *Description*: It is divided by levator palpebrae superioris into two parts: (1) gland proper and (2) palpebral part
    - Gland proper is producing the secretion and the secretion enters the conjunctiva by the lacrimal ducts.

Lacrimal Ducts
- Six to twelve in number. The gland proper contains four to six ducts and rests are connected with the palpebral part. Thus ducts are opening into the conjunctival sac in the upper conjunctival fornix.

Conjunctival Sac
- Part next to the lacrimal duct. It has two parts: (1) palpebral part and (2) ocular or orbital part:
    - Palpebral part overlaps the upper and lower eyelids
    - Orbital part is lying behind the palpebral part up to the corneoscleral junction.

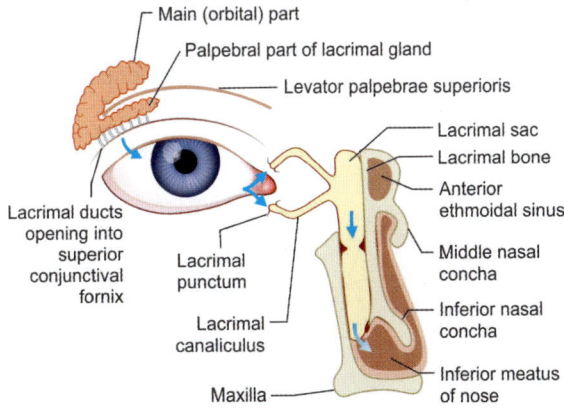

Fig. 6.3: Lacrimal apparatus

Lacrimal Canaliculi
- It is situated at the medial part of the orbital cavity. It consists of the two parts: (1) superior canaliculi and inferior canaliculi
    - *Superior canaliculi*—starting from the puncta lacrimalis—ascends 1–1.2 cm and then descends forming dilated ampulla—ends in the lateral border of the lacrimal sac
    - *Inferior canaliculi*—starting from puncta lacrimalis—descend 1–1.2 cm and then go horizontally to end in the lateral border of the lacrimal sac.

Lacrimal Sac
- It is a dilated sac at the medial part on the lacrimal bone guarded by the medial palpebral ligament. From this, a duct arises called the nasolacrimal duct
    - *Nasolacrimal duct*: It is a duct starting from the lacrimal sac enclosed in a lacrimal bone and the frontal process of maxilla to end in the inferior meatus of the lateral wall of nose.

Arterial Supply
- Middle palpebral artery
- Lateral palpebral artery
- Lacrimal artery.

POSTERIOR CRICOARYTENOID MUSCLE (FIG. 6.4)
- *Origin*: External surface of posterior lamina of cricoids cartilage
- *Insertion*: Muscular process of arytenoid cartilage
- *Fibers*: It consists two types of fibers: (1) horizontal fibers and (2) vertical fibers

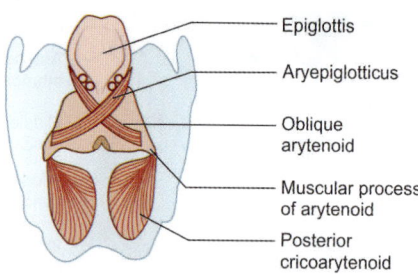

Fig. 6.4: Intrinsic muscles of larynx showing posterior cricoarytenoid

- *Functions*: Horizontal fibers help in rotator movement of vocal folds
- Vertical fibers help in the gliding movement of the vocal folds
- As a whole, this muscle helps in abduction of vocal folds
- *Nerve supply*—recurrent laryngeal nerve

Clinical Anatomy

In normal breathing, this muscle helps in abduction of the vocal cords and maintains the pentagonal shape of the rima glottidis. Thus, posterior cricoarytenoid acts as the safety muscle of the larynx.

PALATINE TONSIL

Introduction

Palatine tonsils are collection of lymphoid tissue situated on either side of oropharynx in-between palatoglossal arch in front and palatopharyngeal arch behind. It lies within tonsillar fossa (bed) (Fig. 6.5).

Function

Protection of body by formation of lymphocytes, antibodies and localization of infection.

Measurements and Brief Discussions

It is 2.5 cm long, 1.9 cm wide and has:
- Anterior border (overlapped partially by palatoglossal arch)
- Posterior border (overlapped by palatopharyngeal arch)
- Upper pole (marked by intratonsillar cleft)

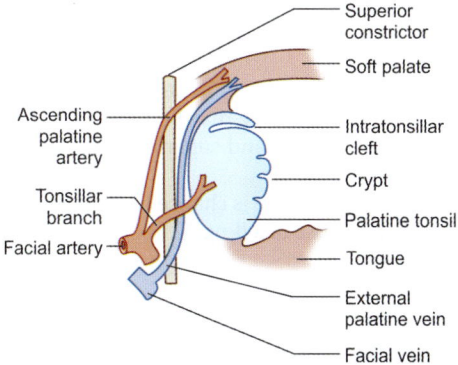

Fig. 6.5: Coronal section through the palatine tonsil

- Lower pole (rest on dorsum of tongue)
- *Medial surface (facing oropharynx)*: It shows 10–15 small orifices (crypts), which leads inside the substance of tonsil
- *Lateral surface or tonsillar bed related to*: (1) capsule, (2) subcapsular tissue containing paratonsillar vein, (3) pharyngobasilar fascia, (4) superior constrictor muscle, (5) buccopharyngeal fascia, (6) facial artery branch of carotid artery:
    - Superior tonsillar
    - Inferior tonsillar
    - Anterior tonsillar
    - Posterior tonsillar arteries.

All arteries are the subbranch of external carotid artery.

- *Tonsillar venous plexus*® drain into pharyngeal venous plexus® then internal jugular vein
- Few vein drain into paratonsillar vein® then internal jugular vein
    - Into jugulodigastric group of deep cervical nodes.
    - Glossopharyngeal nerve
    - In tonsil, partial capsule is present, whereas in LN complete capsule is present
    - No system of sinuses like lymph node within tonsil, so blood filter occurs directly through the follicle.

Lymphoid tissue, including palatine tonsil attains their maximum size in early childhood. After puberty they gradually atrophy.

Clinical Anatomy

- *Tonsillitis*: Inflammation of tonsil is known as tonsillitis. The pain may refer to ear as glossopharyngeal nerve may supply the middle ear
- *Peritonsillar abscess (Quinsy)*: Repeated attack from tonsillitis and in untreated case, there may be formation of peritonsillar abscess between capsule and superior constrictor muscle also known as quinsy
- During tonsillectomy, there is chance of damage of paratonsillar vein producing profuse bleeding.

WALDEYER'S RING

- There is a ring of tonsillar tissue around the entrance into oropharynx—known as Waldeyer's ring or tonsillar ring. The ring is formed (Fig. 6.6):

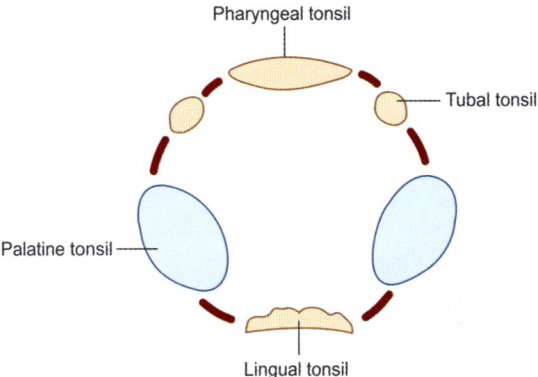

Fig. 6.6: Waldeyer's ring or tonsillar ring

- *Superiorly*: By nasopharyngeal tonsil (enlarged to form adenoid—it produces mouth breathing in children)
- *Inferiorly*—by lingual tonsil
- *Superolaterally*—by tubal tonsil
- *Laterally*—by palatine tonsil.

They form a strong defense system to prevent the spread of infection from oral and nasal mucosa to larynx and lower respiratory tract.

LITTLE'S AREA OF EPISTAXIS

The nasal septum is formed anteriorly by hyaline cartilage (the septal cartilage) and posteriorly by perpendicular plate of ethmoid and vomer. Minor contribution by nasal spine of frontal bone and nasal crest of maxilla and palatine bones. The anteroinferior part of nasal septum is highly vascular where septal branch of facial artery, a branch from long sphenopalatine, and greater palatine artery anastomoses (Fig. 6.7). It is known as "little's area of epistaxis" which produce bleeding in children (commonly due to pricking of nose).

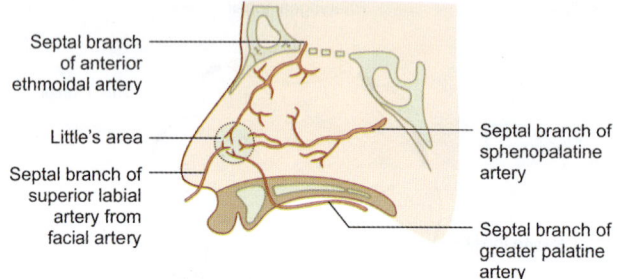

Fig. 6.7: Blood supply of nasal septum P.G.E.

CORNEA

- The cornea is a thin, clear and transparent avascular tissue projecting forward like a dome from the sclera (Fig. 6.8)
- It is convex anteriorly
- Radius of curvature:
  Anterior surface—7.8 mm
  Posterior surface—6.5 mm.

From before backward, cornea is made up of five layers:

1. *Corneal epithelium*: Nonkeratinized stratified squamous epithelium usually five cells thick, continuous with the conjunctival epithelium at the sclera corneal junction it becomes 10 cells thick.
2. *Bowman's (anterior limiting) membrane*: Basel cells of corneal epithelium rests on a lamina of substantia propria, which is a

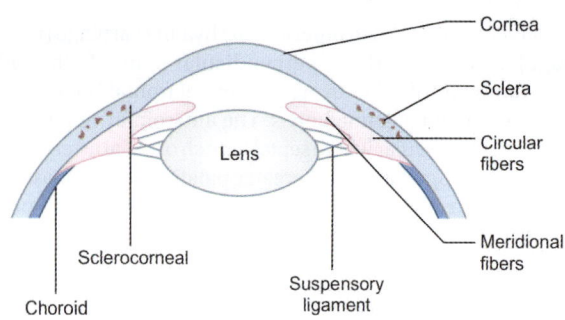

Fig. 6.8: Cornea and associate structure

cellular and densely packed layer of fine collagen fibers called Bowman's membrane. Once eroded, it does not regenerate and leaves a superficial scar tissue behind.

3. *Substantia propria (stroma)*: This layer forms about 90% of corneal thickness, composed of flattened lamellae of fine collagen fibrils and fibroblasts ensheathed by acid, mucopolysaccharides and set in a ground substance of chondroitin sulfate and keratan sulfate. These fine fibers are of regular diameter, spaced equidistally as a lattice with interfibrillar spacing of less than a wavelength of light, but directed in different angles to each other in successive lamellae, maintaining the transparency of cornea.

4. *Descemet's membrane*: A thin acellular homogeneous and elastic layer made of collagen fibers on which corneal endothelial cells rest. At the periphery, the fibers spread posteriorly to form trabecular network forming the inner wall of sinus venosus sclera.

5. *Endothelium*: Single-layer cuboidal cells, which maintain hydration of corneal stroma. It covers the posterior surface. This layer is identified by specular microscope (×500).

   Intermediate layers (two to three cells deep) are polyhedral wing cells with flat nuclei.

   Surface epithelial cells (about two cells deep)—flat with microvilli and microplicae, which retain the tear fluid.

Nerve Supply

- Long and short ciliary nerves from ophthalmic division of trigeminal nerve. Cornea has no proprioceptive senses. No end organs, no Schwann cells
- *It is devoid of blood supply or veins or lymphatics.* Capillary arcades from sclera and conjunctiva supply at sclera–corneal limbus. Tear fluid and aqueous humor provide its nutrition (also oxygen from the air).

Clinical Anatomy

- Abnormal curvature of the refractive surfaces of cornea:
  - If flatter—curvature hypermetropia
  - If steeper—curvature myopia
- Irregular or unequal curvature in different meridian gives rise to astigmatism

- Inflammation of corneal tissue, which may or may not form an ulcer:
  - Bacterial
  - Viral
  - Fungal
  - Neuropathic
- Resultant opacity of the cornea is known as nebula, macula glaucoma
- Gray-green or golden-brown coloring in cornea—due to deposition of copper in the Descemet's membrane—seen in hepatolenticular degeneration or Wilson's disease
- *Keratoplasty*—replacement of diseased cornea by a graft of homogeneous tissue. It is improved today due to increased eye donations
- Excimer laser is nowadays extensively used for phototherapeutic keratectomy.

TASTE BUDS

Taste buds are present in relation to circumvallate papillae, fungiform papillae and to leaf-like folds of mucosa (folia linguae) present on the posterolateral aspect of the tongue (Fig. 6.9).

Taste buds are also present on the epiglottis, soft palate, the palatoglossal arches and posterior wall of the oropharynx.

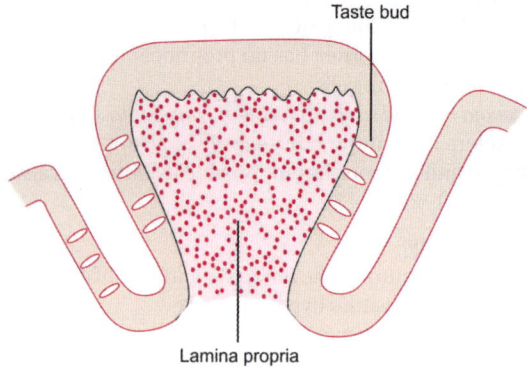

Fig. 6.9: Papillae, circumvallate

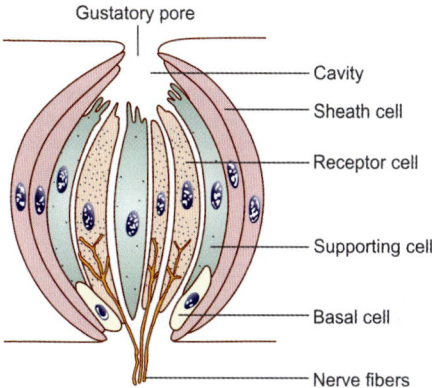

Fig. 6.10: Arrangement of cells in a taste bud (schematic representation)

Each taste bud is pyriform structure made up of modified epithelial cells. The taste bud has small cavity that opens to the surface through a gustatory pore. There are two types of cells in taste buds—(1) elongated receptor cells or gustatory cells and (2) supporting cells. Gustatory cells are related with afferent nerve ends. Different modalities of taste sensation, e.g. sweet—felt in the tip of tongue; sour—on the sides; bitter—at the vallate papillae and epiglottis by the same types of taste bud (Fig. 6.10).

TEMPORALIS MUSCLE (TABLE 6.1)

Table 6.1: Temporalis muscle

Muscle	Origin	Insertion	Description	Nerve supply	Action
Temporalis	Mandibular fossa of temporal bone	Coronoid process (its tip and anterior border)	Fan-shaped muscle. Its contraction is easily felt during clenching of teeth	Branch of mandibular nerve	Elevates mandible and clenches teeth

HYPOGLOSSAL NERVE (TABLE 6.2) (FIG. 6.11)

Table 6.2: Hypoglossal nerve—It is puraly motor nerve

Name and components	Origin and course	Function	Clinical testing	Clinical anatomy
Hypoglossal nerve (XII cranial nerve). It consists of only somatic efferent component. Nucleus is elongated 2 cm in length. Subependymal position. Situated in the floor of 4th ventricle	Fibers arise by a series of rootlets from medulla between olive and pyramid and exit from skull via hypoglossal canal and supplies tongue muscles (both extrinsic and intrinsic except palatoglossus)	It supplies all muscles of tongue (except palatoglossus) and controls its shape and movement	Person is asked to protrude tongue. Any deviation can be noted	In lesion of hypoglossal nerve, protruded tongue deviates toward affected side. It causes difficulty of speech (moderate dysarthria)

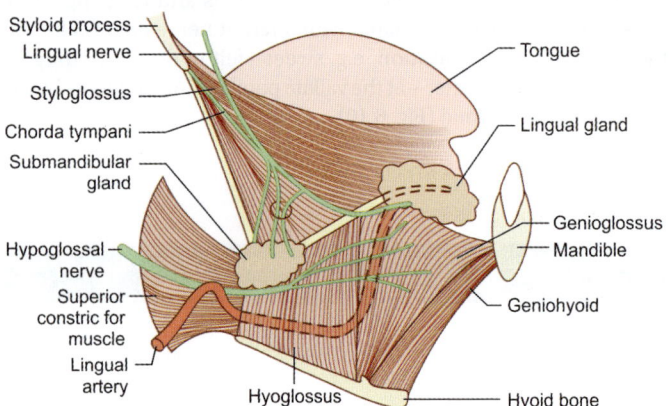

Fig. 6.11: Submandibular region and hypoglossal nerve

MOVEMENT OF TEMPOROMANDIBULAR JOINT (TABLE 6.3 AND FIG. 6.12)

Table 6.3: Movement of temporomandibular joint

Name and bones concerned	Ligaments	Movements	Muscles concerned	Nerve supply
Temporo-mandibular (TM) joint Bones concerned: • Articular area of head of mandible • Articular area of mandibular fossa of temporal bone and its articular tubercle • Articular cartilage (fibrocartilage) in nature	• Capsular ligament • Lateral temporo-mandibular ligament • Stylo-mandibular ligament	• Protrusion • Retraction • Elevation • Depression • Side-to-side chewing movement	• Lateral and medial pterygoid muscle • Temporalis (posterior fiber), assisted by—masseter, digastric, geniohyoid • Temporalis masseter • Medial pterygoid Lateral pterygoid Digastric geniohyoid	Auriculo-temporal—from posterior division of mandibular Masseteric branch—from anterior division of mandibular

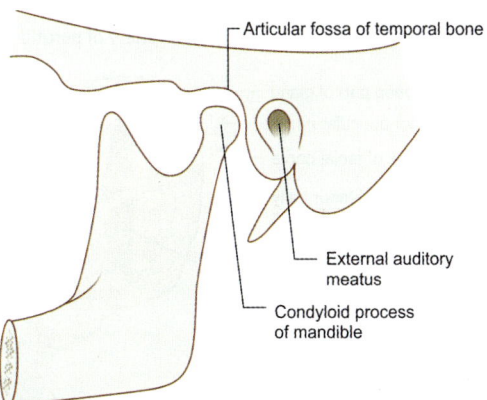

Fig. 6.12: Bones forming the temporomandibular joint

PAROTID GLAND (FIGS 6.13 AND 6.14)

It is one of the salivary glands. Others are submandibular and sublingual. The large triangular parotid gland lies in parotid mold (fossa), between masseter muscle and skin. The fossa is bounded anteriorly by mandible, behind by mastoid process, medially by styloid process and above by zygomatic arch. The gland is covered on lateral aspect by thick parotidomasseteric fascia (part of deep-cervical fascia).

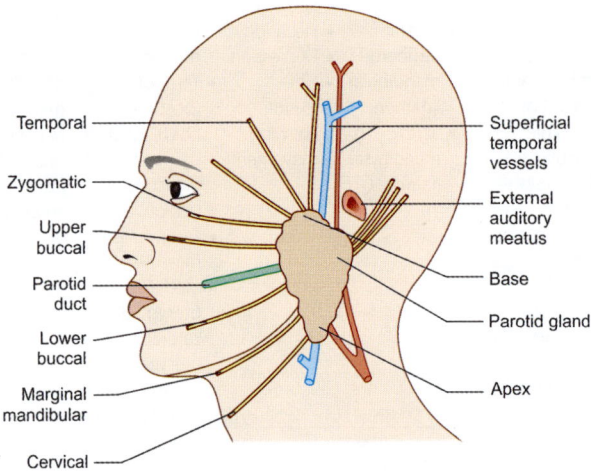

Fig. 6.13: Structures emerging at the periphery of parotid gland

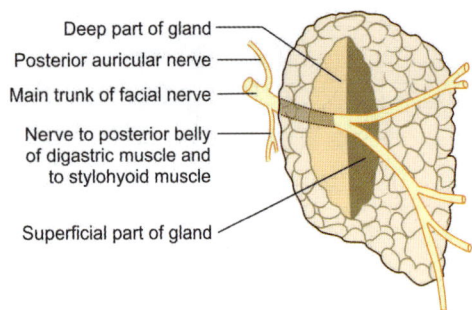

Fig. 6.14: Superficial and deep part of parotid gland

Presenting Parts

The gland presents a tapering apex (placed downwards), a concave broad base (placed below the external acoustic meatus) and three surfaces—(1) superficial (related to skin and subcutaneous tissue), (2) anteromedial surface (deeply grooved by ramus of mandible) and (3) posteromedial surfaces (large and related to mastoid process, styloid process, transverse process of atlas, facial nerve and external carotid artery). Facial nerve and its five branches (the pes anserinus) divide the gland into superficial and deep parts.

Parotid Duct

By parotid duct, the gland pours its secretion in the vestibule of mouth opposite the crown of upper second molar tooth. Length is 5 cm and can be palpable when teeth are clenched.

Arterial Supply

By external carotid artery and its branches.

Nerve Supply

By autonomic nervous system. Parasympathetic secretomotor fiber passes through auriculotemporal nerve.

Clinical Anatomy

- Viral infection of parotid gland is known as mumps; common in children
- Inflammatory swelling of gland is very painful due to tough fascial covering
- *Mixed parotid tumor*—it is slow growing, benign, painless tumor and of huge size.

Anatomical Position

- Placed concave broad base, above (often external auditory meatus attached with it)
- Tapering apex below
- Anterior border (identified by the presence of parotid duct) and it should be hold by other hand anteriorly
- Lateral surface is smooth and placed outside
- Medial surface (identified by fossa and ridges) should be placed inside.

THYROID GLAND (FIGS 6.15 AND 6.16)

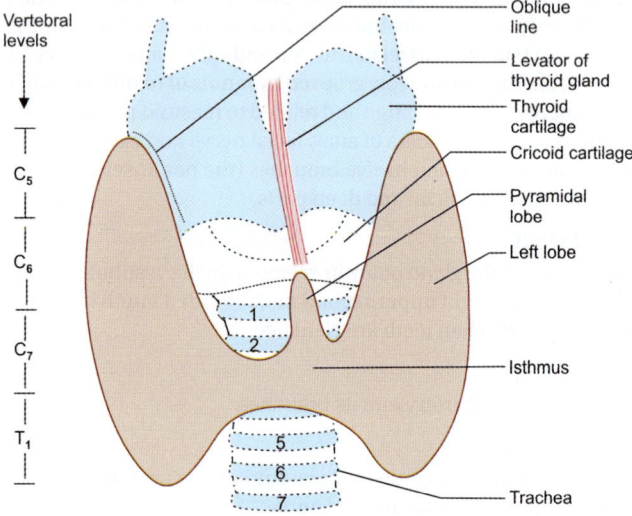

Fig. 6.15: Outline of the thyroid gland as seen from the front and its relationship to the larynx and trachea

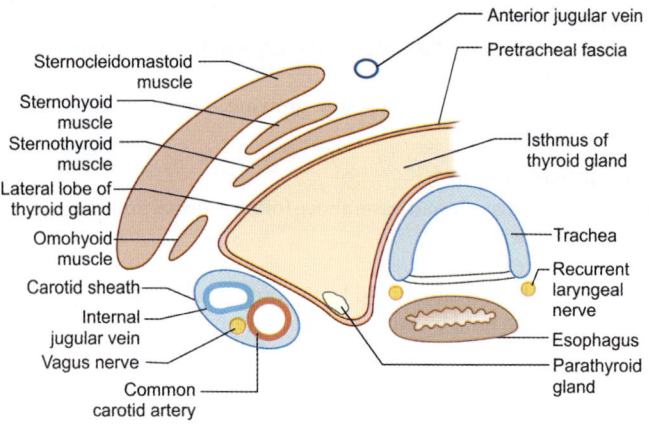

Fig. 6.16: Transverse section across the thyroid gland and related structures

Parts

Butterfly-shaped largest endocrine gland situated in front of neck over trachea.

It has two lobes connected by median tissue mass called isthmus. The lateral lobe presents upper pole (extends up to oblique line of thyroid cartilage), external LN is close to apex. Lower pole (extends up to sixth tracheal ring); recurrent LN is close to it. Three surfaces—superficial (muscular surface), posterior (vascular surface) and medial (tubal surface) and three borders.

Muscular Surface

It is related to sternothyroid muscle and thyrohyoid muscle.

Vascular Surface

It is related to carotid sheath with common carotid artery and internal jugular vein.

Tubal Surface

- It is related to two tubes; two nerves and two muscles.
    - Lower part of larynx and upper part of trachea
    - Lower part of pharynx and upper part of esophagus
    - *Nerves*—external laryngeal and recurrent LNs
    - *Muscles*—inferior constrictor and cricothyroid.

Arterial Supply

Highly vascular thyroid gland is supplied by superior thyroid (branch of external carotid) and inferior thyroid (branch of thyrocervical trunk) arteries; occasionally by arteria thyroidea ima. During thyroid operation, inferior thyroid artery should be tied away from lower pole otherwise recurrent LN will be damaged (which supplies all the muscles of larynx except cricothyroid) producing hoarseness of voice.

Clinical Anatomy

- Slight enlargement of thyroid gland during puberty is known as pubertal goiter
- Noninflammatory; nonneoplastic growth of thyroid gland is known as goiter
- Cancer of thyroid is also common

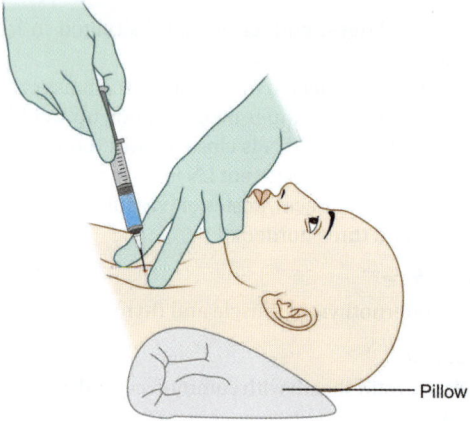

Fig. 6.17: Fine-needle aspiration cytology of thyroid

- Fine-needle aspiration cytology (FNAC)—study of tumor cells whether benign or malignant (Fig. 6.17)
- Diagnosis of cancer can be done by FNAC.

Anatomical Position
- Hold the butterfly-shaped gland in such a way that tapering upper pole should above
- Flat superficial surface laterally.

ORBITAL FISSURE (FIG. 6.18)

Structures passing through Superior Orbital Fissure
- 22 cm long
- Separates lesser wing of sphenoid from greater wing
- Transmits IIIrd, IVth and VIth cranial nerve and sympathetic plexus, superior ophthalmic veins.

Structures passing through Inferior Orbital Fissure
- Located between lateral orbital wall and the orbital floor
- Transmit maxillary division of trigeminal nerve and pterygoid nerve

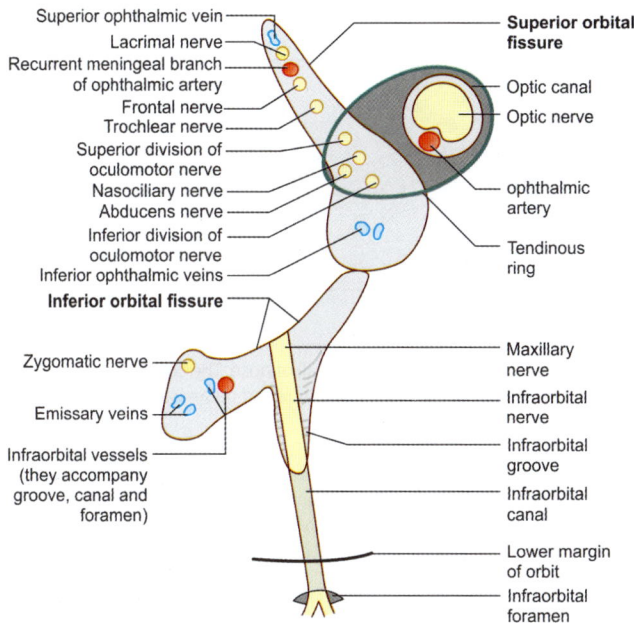

Fig. 6.18: Structures passing through the optic canal, the superior orbital fissure, and the inferior orbital fissure

- Infraorbital nerve (a branch of trigeminal enters the infraorbital canal for sensation of lower eyelid, cheek, upper lid, upper teeth)
- Inferior ophthalmic vein.

NASAL CAVITY (FIG. 6.19)

The nasal cavity lies posterior to external nose. Air enters the nasal cavity through nostrils. The cavity is divided into two by a midline nasal septum. The nasal cavity is continuous behind with the nasopharynx by choanae (posterior nares). The roof is bounded by ethmoid and sphenoid bone; floor is formed by palate (which separates it from oral cavity), the lateral wall is formed by medial wall of maxilla, the ethmoid, the palatine bone, etc.

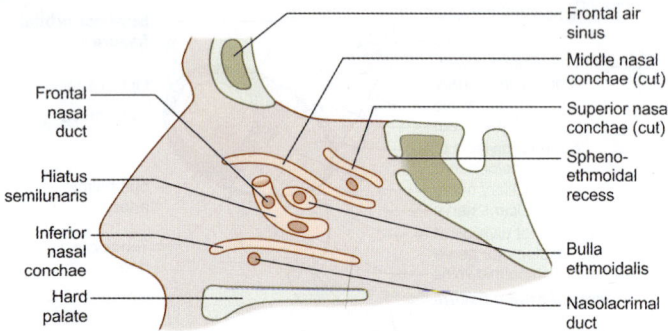

Fig. 6.19: Openings in the lateral wall of nose. The conchae have been partially removed to show the different paranasal air sinuses

Nasal septum Major contribution P.G.E.	The septum is formed anteriorly by hyaline cartilage (the septal cartilage) and posteriorly by perpendicular plate of ethmoid and vomer. Minor contribution by nasal spine of frontal bone and nasal crest of maxilla and palatine bones. The antero-inferior part of nasal septum is highly vascular where septal branch of facial artery, a branch from long sphenopalatine, and greater palatine artery anastomoses. It is known as 'Little's area of epistaxis' which produce bleeding in children (commonly due to pricking of nose) P.G.E.
Parts of nasal cavity	The portion of nasal cavity superior to the nostril is called vestibule, is lined by skin. Hair is present for filtering of dust and bacteria from inspired air. Small slit-like area at the roof is covered with olfactory mucosa (contains receptor for sense of smell). The rest of the area is covered with respiratory mucosa (lined by pseudostratified ciliated columnar epithelium). The paranasal air sinuses open into the respiratory region.
Nasal conchae	Protruding medially from lateral wall of nasal cavity are three mucous-covered projection known as conchae or turbinates. The superior and middle conchae are part of ethmoid bone and inferior nasal conchae is a separate piece of bone. The space under the conchae are named superior, middle and inferior meatus respectively. Openings that are situated on the lateral wall of nasal cavity:

Contd...

Contd...

	A. Superior meatus—Opening of posterior ethmoidal sinus. B. Middle meatus contains—1. Ethmoidal bulla (elevation) which contains middle group of ethmoidal air cells and it opens on it. 2. Hiatus semilunaris where maxillary sinus, frontonasal duct and anterior group of ethmoidal air cells open. C. Inferior meatus—Nasolacrimal duct opens here P.G.E.
Clinical anatomy	• Inflammation of nasal cavity is known as rhinitis. • The nasal septum is not truly median. Excessive deviation of nasal septum is known clinically as deflected nasal septum (DNS). Patients with DNS frequently suffer from common cold and often, respiratory difficulty. • Benign growth in the nasal cavity is commonly known as polyps. • Lesion of olfactory nerve due to breakage of cribriform place (usually in motor car accident) and CSF may dribble (drop by drop) through the breakage.
Paranasal air sinuses (Figs 6.20A and B)	The nasal cavity is surrounded by a group of air sinuses known as paranasal air sinuses (PNS). It makes the bone lighter and add moisture to the inspired air. Each sinus is lined by ciliated columnar epithelium. The sinuses are located in frontal, ethmoid, sphenoid and maxillary bones. The sinuses possess a sensory nerve supply and the mouth (ostium) of the sinus is more sensitive and other parts are relatively insensitive. **Maxillary sinus**—Largest paired sinus whose floor is 1 cm deeper to floor of nasal cavity. It is bounded by: • Apex (laterally situated)—Zygomatic process of maxilla • Base (directed medially)—Medial surface of maxilla; an opening called maxillary hiatus is present here • Roof (above)—Orbital surface of maxilla • Floor (below)—Alveolar process of maxilla • Anterior wall—Anterolateral surface of maxilla • Posterior wall—Posterolateral surface of maxilla Its opening to the nasal cavity is minimized by lacrimal (in front), palatine (from behind) uncinate process of ethmoid from above and a process of inferior nasal concha from below **Ethmoidal air sinus (cells):** It lies within labyrinth of ethmoid bone. They are grouped into anterior, middle and posterior groups.

Contd...

Contd...

	Frontal air sinuses: It is paired, unequal size, more prominent in male. In section triangular shape. It produces more prominent glabella and superciliary arch, in male and it is absent at birth. **Sphenoidal air sinus:** Unpaired, situated in middle, lies within the body of sphenoid. It is related to pituitary above and cavernus sinus on both sides. It opens in sphenoethmoidal recesses.
Clinical anatomy	• Inflammation of sinus due to common cold virus is known as sinusitis. It produces pain • Accumulation of infected material in maxillary sinus produces much pain due to poor natural drainage (as the floor of the sinus is deep). Surgical drainage is done by breaking the lateral wall of inferior meatus and middle meatus • Paranasal air sinuses are well-visualized in X-ray skull (in occipitomental view) • As the frontal air sinus is nearer to frontal lobe of brain repeated, infection may give rise to frontal lobe abscess

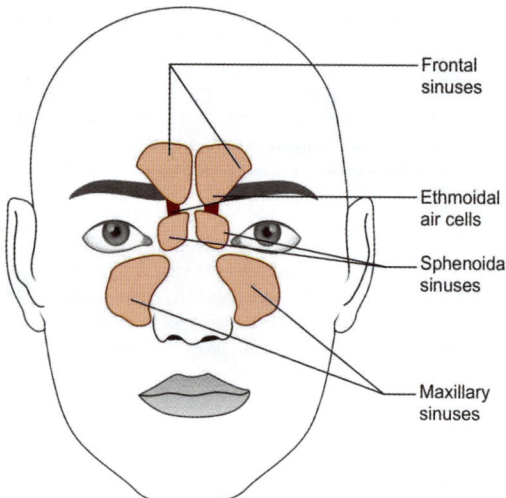

Fig. 6.20A: Relative position of air sinuses in face

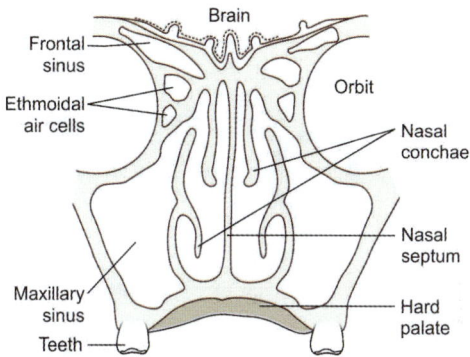

Fig. 6.20B: Paranasal air sinuses (coronal section)

BRAIN AND EYEBALL

FILUM TERMINALE

Introduction
- Filum terminale is a non-nervous filamentous thread-like pial modification
- Length—about 20 cm.

Attachment
- *Above*—tip of conus medullaris
- *Below*—blending with periosteum of dorsal surface of first coccygeal vertebra.

Parts
- *Proximal*: 15 cm within dural sheath, called *filum terminale internum*
- *Distal*: 5 cm resting outside dural sheath called *filum terminale externum.*

Other features: Central canal of spinal cord may extend up to upper 5–6 mm of filum terminale as terminal ventricle (Fig. 6.21).

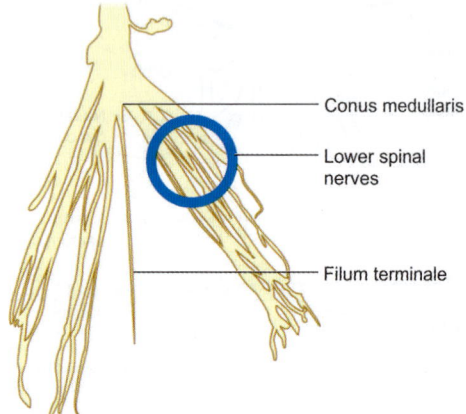

Fig. 6.21: Cauda equina and filum terminale

TYPES OF SULCI (TABLE 6.4)

Table 6.4: Types of sulci

Sl. No.	Name	Description	Examples
1.	Limiting sulcus	Separates to functionally and structurally different areas	Central sulcus
2.	Axial sulcus	Sulcus develops in the long axis of a rapidly growing cortical (functional) area	Posterior part of calcarine sulcus
3.	Operculated sulcus	Separates two areas by its lips and contents a third area in the walls and floor of the sulcus	Lunate sulcus
4.	Complete sulcus	Very deep sulcus, so as to produce elevation on the walls of lateral ventricles	Collateral sulcus
5.	Secondary sulcus	They appear secondary due to growth of the brain	Lateral sulcus

NEURAL CREST CELLS

During formation of neural tube, a group of cells are formed on either side of neural tube. The cells get detached from the surface and migrate laterally, from the neural crest cells. These cells extend from forebrain up to the level of caudal somites.

Derivatives of neural crest cells are as follows:
- Primitive cranial ganglia
- Primitive spinal ganglia.

Derivatives of primitive cranial ganglia:
- Sensory ganglia of fifth, seventh, eighth, ninth, tenth cranial nerve
- Parasympathetic ganglia
- Ciliary, otic, submandibular and pterygopalatine ganglia
- Pia mater and arachnoid mater.

Derivatives from primitive spinal ganglia:
- Dorsal root ganglia of spinal nerves
- Adrenal medulla
- Sympathetic ganglion.

Derivatives from both the cranial end and spinal ganglia:
- Pharyngeal cartilage cells
- Pigment cells
- Satellite cells
- Mesenchyma of head region
- Chromaffin cells
- Odontoblast
- Schwann cells.

PARACENTRAL LOBULE

The paracentral lobule is present in the medial surface of cerebral hemisphere.

Boundary

- *Above*—Superomedial border of cerebral hemisphere
- *Below*—Cingulate sulcus
- *Behind*—Upturned end of cingulated sulcus
- *In front*—A ramus from cingulated sulcus.

Histological Importance
Central sulcus from the superolateral surface end in paracentral lobule dividing into it agranular cortex in front and a granular cortex behind.

Functions
- Sensory regulation of the trunk and limb below knee
- Motor regulation of trunk and limb below knee
- It is center of micturition and defecation reflex.

Lesion
Lesion in paracentral lobule leads to:
- Sensory loss of the trunk and limb below knee
- Involuntary micturition and defecation.

BLOOD–BRAIN BARRIER
- It is a barrier formed by structures between blood and nerve cells of brain. The barrier at capillary level is formed by mere capillary endothelium with neuroglia and ground substance
- It permits a selective transport of blood content to nervous tissue. So, it prevents normally the passage of toxic and harmful substances to the brain and protects it.

CILIARY BODY
- This is the thick part of the uveal tract. It is continuous with iris in front and choroid behind
- Its anterior part forms ciliary process. Its posterior part is smooth and broad
- It is attached to lens by suspensory ligament of lens. There are smooth ciliary muscles with longitudinal, radial and circular fibers
- The muscle arises from scleral spur, which is a projection from sclera from sclerocorneal junction
- All the three fibers relax the suspensory ligament of the lens and thus the lens becomes more convex. It helps in accommodation
- The muscles are supplied by parasympathetic nerve fiber component of occulomotor nerve.

IRIS
It is a muscular diaphragm of eyeball formed by a middle coat of eyeball. Literally, "iris" means rainbow because the color of the iris

varies from blue to dark-brown. The iris is placed between the lens behind and the cornea in front. Peripheral margin is attached to the middle of the choroid. In the center, there is an aperture known as pupil. The main function of the iris is to regulate the amount of light that reaches the lens. The iris divides the space behind cornea and in front of lens into two chambers—(1) anterior chamber and (2) posterior chamber.

Muscles of Iris

- *Sphincter pupillae*: It encircles the pupil. When the muscles contract, the pupil gets narrowed (myosis). It is supplied by parasympathetic through ciliary ganglion
- *Dilator pupillae*: It is a smooth, thin muscle and radially arranged fibers. Merge with those of the sphincter pupillae at the margin. On contraction, it produces dilatation of the pupil (mydriasis). It is supplied by the sympathetic T1-T2 segment.

Arterial Supply

By long posterior ciliary and anterior ciliary artery.

Clinical Anatomy

- Parasympatholytic drugs like Atropin relax the sphincter pupillae muscles, thereby causing dilatation of the pupil. It is required for ophthalmoscopic examination of retina
- Injury to the sympathetic (T1-T2) produces Horner's syndrome in which the pupil is constricted.

CORPUS CALLOSUM

It is the largest commissure, 10 cm in length. Anterior end is 4 cm behind the frontal pole and posterior end is 6 cm in front of the occipital pole. It is divided into four parts from anterior to posterior aspect (Fig. 6.22) they are: (1) rostrum, (2) genu, (3) body and (4) splenium. As the corpus callosum is shorter than cerebral hemisphere, the callosal fibers linking the frontal and occipital poles curve forwards and backwards, and form forceps minor and major, respectively. As the splenium interconnects the occipital cortex, it is concerned with visual functions. Fibers arising from posterior part of body is not crossed by corona radiata fiber is known as tapetum (Fig. 6.23).

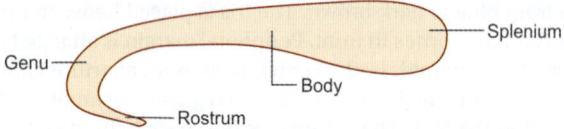

Fig. 6.22: Parts of corpus callosum (sagittal section)

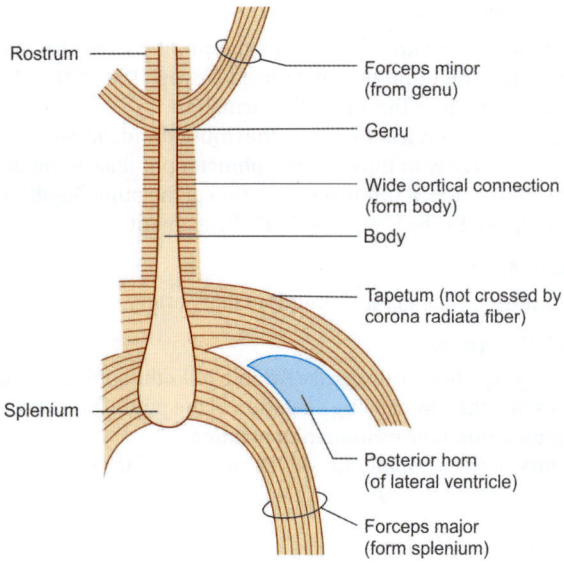

Fig. 6.23: Corpus callosum (laid out flat) showing fibers

Arterial Supply

By anterior and posterior cerebral arteries and artery of Heubner.

Clinical Anatomy

Destruction of splenium of corpus callosum by stroke or tumor leads to posterior disconnection syndrome. Such individuals can speak and write but cannot understand written material. Chronic epilepsy (fit)

patients may be treated by section of corpus callosum to control the fit. But the drawback is that the person cannot name objects.

These fibers connect between the cerebral cortex and various subcortical areas. These fibers pass through corona radiata and internal capsule. Fibers may be centripetal (toward the cortex) and centrifugal (away from the cortex).

Internal Capsule (Fig. 6.24)

It is the important neocortical projection fiber. Corona radiata fibers become condensed in a narrow area, and form internal capsule between thalamus and caudate nucleus medially and the lentiform nucleus laterally. The internal capsule is angulated like boomerang and has got anterior limb, genu, posterior limb, retrolentiform and sublentiform part. Through anterior limb pass fibers from thalamus to prefrontal cortex, also fibers from frontal cortex to pontine nucleus (pons). Through genu passes corticonuclear fibers. The posterior limb contains corticobulbar and corticospinal motor fibers and thalamocortical fibers to somatosensory cortex. Through retrolentiform part passes optic radiation fiber to visual cortex. Through sublentiform part passes auditory radiation fiber.

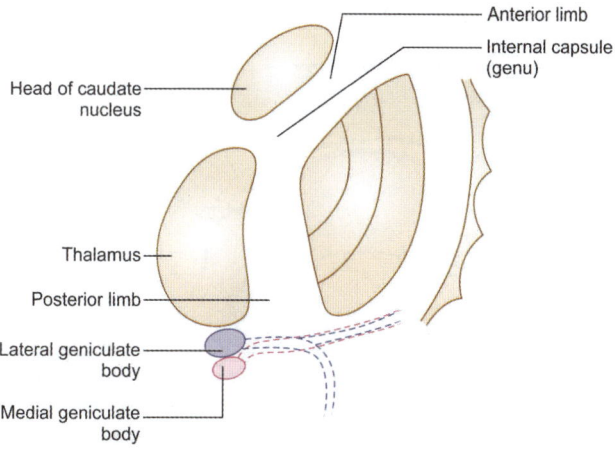

Fig. 6.24: Basal nuclei and internal capsule

Surgical Anatomy

Clinical Importance

As the important pathways are closely packed together in internal capsule, a small lesion may produce widespread disability.

Arterial Supply

- *Supplied by lenticulostriate arteries*: Branch of anterior and middle cerebral artery. One of them is large, known as Charcot's artery, supplies the lower limb region and is frequently ruptured. It is known as artery of cerebral hemorrhage.

THIRD VENTRICLE (FIG. 6.25)

It is a midline ventricular cleft extending from lamina terminalis in front (thin sheet of gray matter extended from optic chiasma to rostrum of corpus callosum) to pineal body behind. It is deep in front.

Boundary

- *Lateral wall*: By thalamus and hypothalamus
- *Floor*: By hypothalamus (from before backwards tubular cinereum with infundibulum, mammillary body, posterior perforated substance, upper surface of cerebral peduncle)

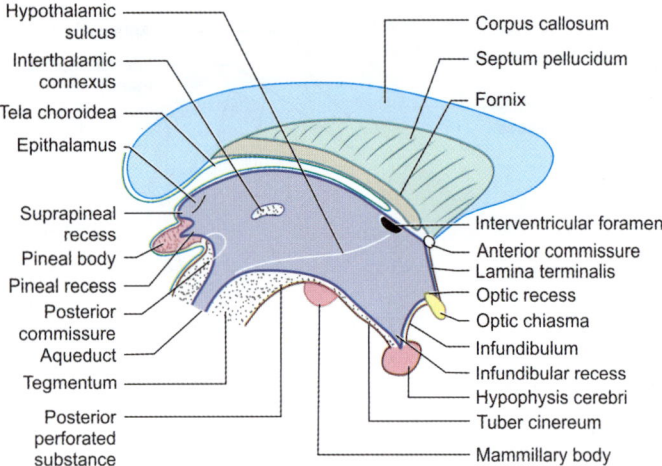

Fig. 6.25: Boundaries and recesses of the third ventricle. Note the mode of formation of the tela choroidea that lies in the roof of the ventricle

- *Anterior wall*:
    - By lamina terminalis
    - Anterior commissure running transversely
    - Anterior pillar of fornix.
- *Posterior wall*:
    - Upper end of cerebral aqueduct
    - Stalk of pineal body with pineal recess
- *Roof*:
    - Ependyma of third ventricle
    - Tela choroidea of third ventricle
    - Body of fornix
    - Body of corpus callosum.

Communication

With two lateral ventricles through the interventricular foramen and with the fourth ventricle through aqueduct of Sylvius.

AQUEOUS HUMOR

It is one of the refractive media of the eyeball.

Formation

It is formed by active transport and diffusion from capillaries of ciliary processes.

Situation

It is situated in the space between cornea in front and the lens behind. The space is divided by iris into anterior chamber and posterior chamber, which communicates freely with each other through pupil.

Composition

It is a clear fluid, rich in glucose, amino acid and vitamin C.

Circulation

After formation from posterior chamber, it passes to anterior chamber through pupil. From anterior chamber, it is drained into anterior ciliary veins through the spaces of iridocorneal angle, which is an angle of anterior chamber.

Function

Nutrition to cornea and lens maintains the intraocular pressure.

Clinical Anatomy

Any interference with the drainage of aqueous humor into canal of Schlemm leads to increased intraocular pressure known as glaucoma. If not treated, may cause blindness.

ARACHNOID GRANULATIONS

Arachnoid granulations are known Pacchionian bodies. These are rounded, pink, fleshy protrusion of arachnoid tissue into the cavity of venous sinuses particularly along the superior sagittal sinus. It is more prominent in old age and produce deep marking in the bone.

Function

Cerebrospinal fluid (CSF) drains through the arachnoid granulation to the bloodstream by filtration.

RHOMBOID FOSSA (FIG. 6.26)

The floor of 4th ventricle is known as rhomboid fossa. It is bounded:
- *Superiorly*—by two superior cerebellar peduncles
- *Inferiorly*—by two inferior cerebellar peduncles and gracile and cuneate nuclei.

The median sulcus extends into the fossa and divides it into left and right halves. The medullary striae divide the fossa into upper and lower halves of hindbrain. In the floor of fourth ventricle, the following nerve nuclei are present:

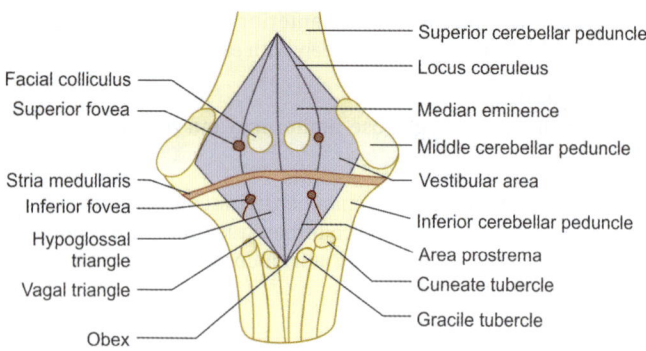

Fig. 6.26: Floor of the fourth ventricle (rhomboid fossa—diagrammatic)

Head, Neck and Brain

- Hypoglossal trigone placed medially formed by hypoglossal nuclei
- Vestibular area formed by vestibular nuclei is laterally placed
- Vagal trigone (formed by dorsal nucleus of vagus) is placed in intermediate position
- Facial colliculus (an elevation formed by curving facial nerve fiber around the abducens nucleus) is placed in intermediate position
- Apneustic center is situated in central part of floor of fourth ventricle
- A small area in the inferior angle of floor of fourth ventricle is known as area postrema. No blood–brain barrier lies in this site.

Clinical Anatomy
- The most common malignant (invasive) tumor in the children is medulloblastoma. It presses the vital center located beneath the floor of fourth ventricle producing cardiac irregularities, irregular respiration and vasomotor disturbance
- If the opening of the roof of the fourth ventricle is blocked by adhesion during meningitis or by tumor—the CSF cannot escape from ventricular system and accumulation of it is known as hydrocephalus
- Clinically area postrema is important and become true vomiting center. So, drugs or circulatory toxins may stimulate this center to produce vomiting.

CIRCLE OF WILLIS

It is polygonal rather than circular. It is bounded anteriorly by anterior cerebral arteries (from internal carotid) which are joined by anterior communicating artery. Posteriorly, the basilar artery divides into two posterior cerebral arteries, each joined to the same-sided internal carotid by a posterior communicating artery. Small aneurysm (Berry aneurysm) is common here due to congenital weakness of arterial wall. The circle of Willis equalizes the pressure of either side and also helps in establishing collateral circulation immediately (Figs 6.27 and 6.28).

Clinical Anatomy
- *Angiogram*: Visualization of arterial tree by radio-opaque dye is known as angiogram. At the upper limb brachial artery (just above the cubital fossa) and radial artery (region where radial pulse is felt) are the common site, common carotid artery in neck (near

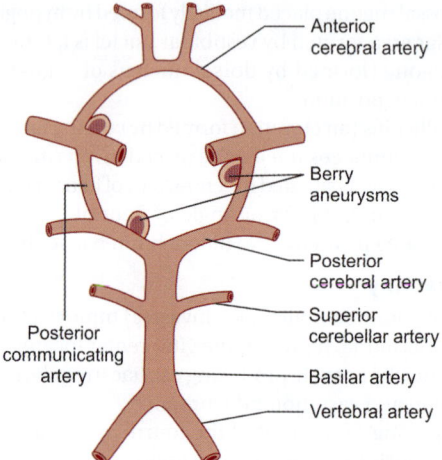

Fig. 6.27: Berry aneurysm in circle of Willis

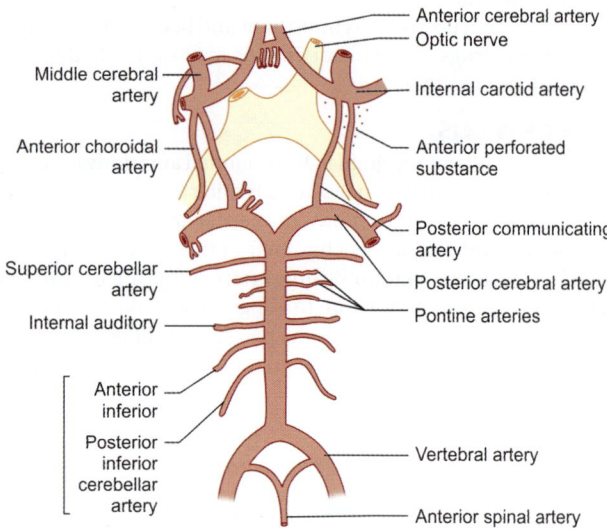

Fig. 6.28: Circle of Willis

its bifurcation) and femoral artery in lower limb (just below the inguinal ligament) in the site of choice for angiography
- Atheroma is the accumulation of cholesterol and other lipid compound developed in the tunica intima of arteries. Arteries mostly affected are coronary arteries, arteries of brain, small intestine, kidneys, etc.
- *Arteriosclerosis*: Progressive degeneration of arterial walls with aging and accompanied by high-blood pressure
- *Aneurysm*: It is the dilatation of blood vessels where part of the artery inflates like a balloon. The wall is weak, and there is chance of rupture.

MIDBRAIN (FIGS 6.29 AND 6.30)

It lies between diencephalons and pons. A hollow tunnel (cerebral aqueduct) passes through it. An imaginary line passes through the aqueduct, divides the midbrain into ventral cerebral peduncle (stalk) and dorsal tectum (roof).

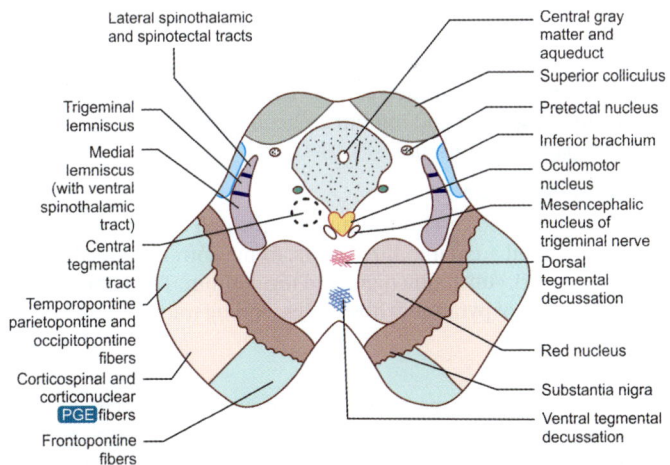

Fig. 6.29: Transverse section of midbrain—level of the superior colliculus and the red nucleus

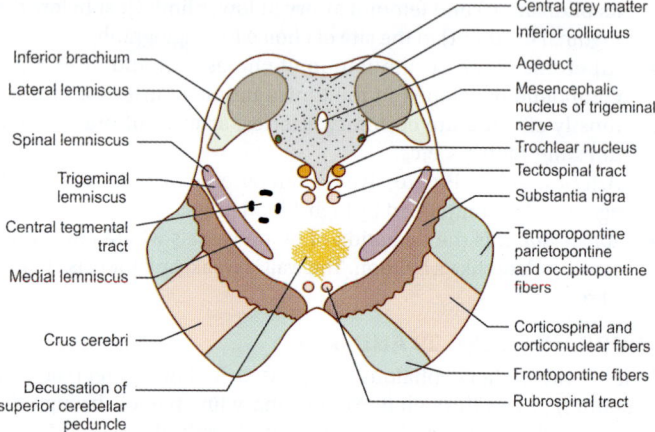

Fig. 6.30: Transverse section of midbrain—level of the inferior colliculus and the decussation of the superior cerebellar peduncle

Tectum

Tectum consists of two pairs of elevated masses, superior and inferior colliculi. They are the reflex center. The superior colliculi receive fibers from optic tract and inferior colliculi receive fibers of auditory pathway (lateral lemniscus).

Cerebral Peduncle

The ventraly placed cerebral peduncle is divided by substantia nigra (dark pigmented area) into three parts; from ventral to dorsal aspect lies crus cerebri, substantia nigra and tegmentum. The middle-third of crus consists of pyramidal fibers (descending tract).

Substantia Nigra

It is a dark pigmented area visible in naked eyes (section of midbrain). The substantia nigra has both afferent and efferent connections with basal nuclei (corpus striatum). It is associated with extrapyramidal system.

Head, Neck and Brain

Tegmentum

It consists of ascending fibers (medial and lateral lemnisci) and discrete gray matter. Third nerve nucleus lies in gray matter (ventral to aqueduct) at the level of superior colliculi. At this level lies iron containing red nucleus (important motor nucleus of extrapyramidal system) and fourth nerve nucleus lies ventral to aqueduct at the level of inferior colliculi. All through the tegmentum lie scattered masses of gray matter known as reticular formation. Decussation of tract to Gall and Burdach, trigeminal lemniscus, lateral lemniscus carrying auditory fiber and spinal lemniscus present here.

Clinical Anatomy

Benedict's Syndrome

In this lesion, tegmentum of midbrain is destroyed resulting in destruction of red nucleus, medial lemniscus, fibers of oculomotor nerve and superior cerebellar peduncle. The characteristics features are loss of tactile, muscle, joint, vibratory, pain and temperature sensation in the opposite half of body lateral squint, tremor and irregular twitching of opposite arm and leg.

Weber Syndrome

It is due to vascular lesion of midbrain, which destroys third cranial nerve nuclei and the corticospinal tract, resulting features are lateral squint, contralateral hemiplegia.

EXPLANATORY NOTES

Q1. Why circle of Willis is important for blood supply of brain?

Ans.

- Circle of Willis is an arterial anastomotic channel formed by basilar artery and internal carotid artery and situated in base of brain. It is the major supply of brain. It is polygonal in shape
- Situated in the interpeduncular fossa in interpeduncular subarachnoid cistern
- It is formed anteriorly by anterior cerebral artery and anterior intercommunicating artery, posteriorly by two posterior cerebral arteries and laterally by posterior communicating artery
- Through anterior, middle and posterior cerebral artery, most of the brain gets its blood supply

- By the circle, there is mixing of blood of vertebrobasilar system with carotid system. So, it maintains equilibrium of blood pressure.

Applied: Small berry aneurysm is common in this circle of Willis. Rupture of this may lead to formation of subarachnoid hemorrhage.

Q2. Safety muscles of tongue. Explain.

Ans. Genioglossus is the extrinsic muscle of the tongue and it is called safety muscle. It prevents the tongue from falling back behind the oral cavity as it arises from upper genial tubercle and inserted in fan-shaped manner into the base of tongue. Genioglossus places the tongue on the floor of the mouth.

Clinical importance: In unconscious patients, genioglossus muscle prevents the tongue from falling back inside and prevents the blocking of the air passage thus preventing the person from choking to death.

Q3. Hyaline cartilage is present in trachea and bronchi. Explain.

Ans. For proper functioning of trachea-bronchi, they should be kept patent, because during the period of respiration there is chance of collapse of these structures. Due to presence of hyaline cartilage, the hyaline cartilage is U-shaped and elastic in character; it prevents the collapse. If in place of cartilage if bone present, was extra-blood supply of bone would have been required. But cartilage does not need extra-blood supply.

Q4. Why optic nerve cannot regenerate after injury?

Ans. Optic nerve is devoid of neurolemma sheath (obtain from Schwann cells in case of a peripheral nerve, but optic nerve is an extension of white fibers of diencephalon). It is only supported by neuroglial cells. Myelination of the nerve is derived from the oligodendroglia. Due to the absence of neurolemma sheath and endoneurium, the optic nerve cannot regenerate, if damaged.

Q5. Blow to the root of the nose causes loss of olfaction, dribbling of CSF (meninges torn both dura and arachnoid).

Ans. Fracture of nasal and cribriform plate of the ethmoid as 16–20 nerve rootless carrying the sense of smell passes through cribriform plate, there is loss of olfaction and flow of CSF through the nose— known as CSF rhinorrhea. There is tearing of dura and arachnoid mater.

Q6. Careless removal of foreign body from pyriform fossa may be a cause of death. Explain.

Ans. During the removal of the foreign body like fish bone, which is deeply stuck in pyriform fossa, the internal LN, which is a branch of vagus, is severely irritated. As stimulation of vagus produces bradycardia and if the bradycardia is severe, it may cause death.

Q7. The depth of focus on the retina is so diminished in people aged over 50 that they are often required to wear convex eye glasses for reading a book. Explain.

Ans. During accommodation reflex, the ciliary body contracts, as a result in which the anterior curvature of the lens becomes negatively more convex and thus the image of near distance is focused on retina but during the presbyopic ages (usually from 36–40 years of age) the plasticity of the lens is lost, so the image of the near object falls behind the retina. So, to accommodate the image on the retina convex lens is used.

Q8. A child suffering from repeated throat infection presents discharge of pus through ear. Explain.

Ans. Throat means the region of nasopharynx. It is connected to middle ear cavity by auditory tube or Eustachian tube.

So, repeated throat infection produces spread of infection to the middle ear. There is formation of pus, which gives pressure over tympanic membrane. The membrane ruptures and pus discharges through ear.

Q9. A man develops "black eye" within 48 hours of lacerated injury to scalp. Explain.

Ans. Scalp consists of 5 layers, out of which 4th layer is known as layer of loose areolar tissue and it lies below the epicranial aponeurosis. Behind the epicranial aponeurosis connected with occipitalis muscle and they are attached to superior nuchal line. Laterally, the epicranial is tightly attached to zygomatic arch. In front, the galea is attached with frontalis muscle, which has no bony attachment but merges with skin and subcutaneous tissue of the eyebrows. So, in a lacerated injury of scalp or a blow on the head develops "black eye" within 48 hours of injury.

Q10. Vocal folds are the watershed line of larynx. Explain.

Ans. Watershed line means from where water separates into two directions, that means the part above the vocal folds have different arterial supply, venous drainage, lymphatic drainage and nerve supply.

- Above the vocal fold—vascular supply—superior laryngeal vessels
- Below the vocal fold—vascular supply—inferior laryngeal vessels
- Above the vocal fold—nerve supply (sensory)—internal lymphnode
- Below the vocal fold—nerve supply (sensory)—recurrent lymphnode.

So, vocal folds are called the watershed lines of larynx.

Q11. The superficial temporal and facial arteries are sometimes termed as "anesthetic arteries". Explain.

Ans. The superficial temporal and facial arteries are termed as anesthetic arteries, because the anesthetics being at the head end of operating table, it is convenient for them to measure the superficial temporal pulse at the root of the zygomatic process and facial arterial pulse against the lower border of mandible at the anteroinferior angle of zygomatic process.

Q12. A newborn suffers from acute respiratory distress and cyanosis while suckling milk. Explain.

Ans. This is because there is presence of cleft palate. During sucking, milk enters the nasal cavity as there is partial or total absence of hard and soft palate. That is why a newborn suffers from acute respiratory distress and cyanosis while suckling milk.

Q13. Two bellies of digastric muscle are supplied by two different nerves. Explain.

Ans. Anterior belly of digastric muscle is developed from first branchial arch (also named as mandibular arch) and the nerve of the first branchial arch is mandibular nerve. So, it is supplied by the same. Precisely, it is supplied by the mylohyoid branch of the inferior alveolar nerve of mandibular division of the trigeminal nerve.

Posterior belly of the digastric muscle is developed from the second branchial arch, also known as hyoid arch and the nerve, which innervates the hyoid on posterior mandibular arch, is facial nerve. Hence, it is supplied by the facial nerve.

Q14. Explain parotid abscess is drained by a horizontal incision.

Ans. As the facial nerve comes out and branches close to its anterior aspect horizontally and also the duct horizontal incision is preferred to drain the parotid abscess otherwise there will be more damage to the nerve and facial muscles paralysis.

Q15. The voice of a baby change at puberty. Explain.

Ans. At puberty due to androgen hormone, this is increased angulation of thyroid cartilage, which produces elongation and tension of vocal fold. Due to increased angulation, the voice of the body changes at puberty.

Q16. Water passes to nose during crying. Explain.

Ans.
- Because—nasolacrimal duct opens into the inferior meatus of nose
- Through this, duct tear enters into inferior meatus and then passes down the nose during crying.

Q17. Facial nerve palsy in the facial canal causes hyperacusis. Explain.

- Stapedius is a very small muscle, which has got dampening effect over sound
- Lesion of facial nerve in facial canal (which is situated in the middle ear segment) causes damage to nerve to stapedius and there is paralysis of stapedius muscle
- So, dampening of the sound is lost and there will be hyperacusis.

Q18. Syringing of external auditory meatus may cause cardiac arrest. Explain.

Ans. Syringing of ear sometimes cause irritation of auricular branch of vagus nerve. This may cause sudden cardiac arrest and death due to vagal stimulation.

Q19. Removal of palpebral part of lacrimal gland is equivalent to functional removal of whole gland?

Ans. Because the duct of orbital part also passes through palpebral part. So, when the palpebral part is removed, secretion of orbital plate cannot be drained.

Q20. Posteroinferior quadrant of tympanic membrane is chosen for myringotomy. Explain.

Ans. The tympanic membrane is a fibrous sheet, which separates external ear from middle ear. Oblique in position and it makes an angle of 55° with the floor. Clinically, the membrane is divided into four quadrants by means of two imaginary lines passing through umbo. Myringotomy is done in posteroinferior quadrant due to following reason:
- To avoid injury to the chorda tympani nerve
- To avoid injury to blood vessels
- Heals quickly
- It is the most dependent part.

Q21. Why is the facial artery tortuous?

Ans. Facial artery is a branch of the external carotid artery, which enters the face after crossing the base of mandible near the anteroinferior branch of masseter muscle. This artery undergoes tortuous course in face because:
- It accommodates with the movement of the mandible. If the artery was straight then the movement of the mandible will lead to tearing of the artery
- The tortuosity prevents the tearing of the artery during movements of mandible
- The facial artery is away from fulcrum of mandibular movement, so more stretching is needed, whereas the vein is close to fulcrum, so less stretching occurs.

Q22. Hyperacusis due to lesion of intrapetrous part of facial nerve.

Ans. From the intrapetrous part of facial nerve, nerve to stapedius arises. This muscle has got dampening effect on movement of ossicular chain. So, in lesion of intrapetrous part, there is hyperacusis.

Q23. Facial nerve injury in babies. Explain.

Ans. As the facial nerve is rudimentary in birth, the facial nerve is more easily damaged in babies. Birth injury can therefore cause an ipsilateral facial palsy, and it affects the suckling reflex.

Q24. The tongue and its muscles are supplied by the facial nerve, whereas the vallate papillae are supplied by the glossopharyngeal nerve. Explain.

Ans. Tongue and tongue muscles are developed from second pharyngeal arch. So, they are supplied by second pharyngeal arch nerve, i.e. facial nerve. But vallate papillae develop from third arch and gets position on the tongue in the anterior two-third. But, as it developed from third arch, it is supplied by glossopharyngeal nerve.

Q25. Repeated throat infection may lead to mastoiditis, if neglected. Explain.

Ans.
- Bacteria from the infected throat pass nasopharynx where there is opening of pharyngotympanic tube (auditory tube)
- The other end of auditory tube is connected with middle ear cavity
- So, middle ear cavity is infected and gives rise to otitis media
- This infection then spread to mastoid air cells and results in mastoiditis.

Q26. Explain lingual thyroid.

Ans.
- The thyroid tissue may lie anywhere along the line of descent of thyroglossal duct
- The thyroglossal duct starts behind the foramen cecum and descends up to trachea
- Lingual thyroid is commonly found in base of tongue, just behind the foramen cecum
- This is due to failure and descent of thyroglossal duct. The lingual thyroid lies either under the mucosa of the dorsum of the tongue or may be embedded within the musculature of tongue. It may form a swelling that may cause difficulty in swallowing.

Q27. Explain pituitary tumor patient suffers bitemporal hemianopia.

Ans. Pituitary tumor presses upon the nasal fibers of the optic chiasma. It causes loss of temporal fields of both sides called bitemporal hemianopia.

Q28. Why layers of loose areolar tissue is called dangerous layer of scalp?

Ans. The scalp consists five layers of soft tissue. The fourth layer is loose areolar.
- Infection from this layer may spread directly to the dural venous sinuses via valveless emissary veins
- Pus or blood can easily spread through this layer because of looseness of tissue
- As there is no nerve endings in this layer, infection may spread without giving rise to any pain sensation.

Q29. Occlusion of posterior cerebral artery causes contralateral homonymous hemianopia with macular sparing. Explain.

Ans. Contralateral homonymous hemianopia with macular sparing happens when lesion occurs in visual cortex with some degree of macular sparing. The macular vision is spared because it is represented in occipital pole, which has dual blood supply, from posterior cerebral as well as from middle cerebral artery. Anastomosis exists between the branches of middle and posterior cerebral artery in the occipital pole.

Q30. A patient with scalp injury presents black cyc. Explain.

Ans. The scalp consists of five layers. From when outside inwards skin, subcutaneous tissue, epicranial aponeurosis, loose areolar tissue and pericranium. If loose areolar tissue of scalp is injured, blood is collected in this layer and the whole scalp will be swollen. Blood may trickle down due to gravity and under the origin of frontalis in the upper eyelid, causing black eye.

There is fracture in middle cranial fossa because it is the weakest part of base of skull. The weakness is due to:

- Presence of numerous foramina
- Presence of middle ear cavity within the petrous part of temporal bone.

As there is damage to the middle ear cavity the blood and CSF pushes the tympanic membrane and there is rupture of the membrane and blood comes out through ear.

Q31. Explain Argyll Robertson pupil.

Ans. In neurosyphilis, there is destruction of the pretectal region of midbrain. Light reflex cannot be elicited though accommodation reaction will be present. The condition is called Argyll Robertson pupil, where the pupils are small and with irregular margins. In this case, the accommodation reflex is present but light reflex is lost. It is seen in tabes dorsalis.

Q32. Explain ectopic thyroid.

Ans. It is a very rare anomaly. The thyroid gland grows into the posterior triangle. It may be dragged behind the sternum called retrosternal thyroid.

Q33. A pimple in danger area of face may cause cavernous thrombosis. Explain.

Ans. The danger area of the face includes the upper lip, nasal septum, ala of nose and the adjoining area. These areas are drained by the veins from the ala and superior labial vein, which drain into the anterior facial vein.

Infections from these areas reach the cavernous sinus through two routes:
- Superior ophthalmic vein to cavernous sinus
- Deep facial vein—pterygoid venous plexus emissary vein—cavernous sinus.

Reasons:
- Vein has no valves
- Wall of the vein is thick and does not collapse when cut
- No barrier to the spread of infection due to absence of the deep fascia in face.

Q34. Parotid gland enlargement in mumps is very painful. Why?.

Ans. Swelling of the parotid gland in (mumps) viral infection is painful as it is limited laterally by the strong facial capsule derived from investing layer of deep cervical fascia. So, slight enlargement produces pain.

Q35. Explain wounds of scalp bleed profusely.

Ans. The scalp consists of five layers of soft tissue that cover the skull cap. From superficial to deep they are:
1. Skin
2. Dense connective tissue
3. Epicranial aponeurosis
4. Loose areolar tissue
5. Pericranium.

Scalp laceration is most common type of head injuries. The wound of scalp bleed profusely due to following reasons:
- The scalp is richly supplied by arteries (5 on each side of midline), which anastomose with each other
- These vessels are present in dense connective tissue where fibers are attached to the outer coat of arteries. Therefore, the cut vessels are not able to contract leading to profuse bleeding.

Q36. Superior parathyroids are inferior in position. Explain.

Ans. The superior parathyroid develops from fourth pharyngeal pouch. The inferior parathyroid develops from third pouch along with thymus. Inferior parathyroid is dragged down by thymus and become inferior in position. But superior parathyroid loses its connection with the developing pharynx and is attached to superior part of developing thyroid. So, during early development, it is inferior in position.

Q37. Thyroglossal duct when present, extends up to foramen cecum.

Ans. An endodermal diverticulum grows from floor of the first pharyngeal pouch caudal to the tuberculum impar. This is called median thyroid diverticulum.

It starts from foramen cecum. It grows ventral to the arches up to the level of fourth pouch.

Part from foramen cecum, up to the thyroid—disappears.

When whole of it persists, it is called thyroglossal duct, and it extends up to foramen cecum.

Q38. Types of articulation found in occipital bone. Explain.

Ans. The articulations are as following:
- *Atlanto-occipital joint*—between condylar process of occipital with superior kidney-shaped articular process of atlas
- Articulates along its lambdoid border with posterior border of two parietal bones forming lambdoid suture
- Articulates with mastoid border of two temporal bones forming occipitomastoid sutures.

Q39. Explain optic nerve is not a peripheral nerve.

Ans. Optic nerve develops from the neuroectoderm of the forebrain vesicles. Optic groove appears in the cranial end of forebrain. They grow and evaginate to form hollow optic vesicle and proximal part from (optic stalk) form optic nerve. So, this is not a peripheral nerve.

Q40. In tonsillitis, pain is referred to the middle ear. Explain.

Ans. The tonsil is supplied by glossopharyngeal nerve as branch from this nerve also forms tympanic plexus and supplies middle ear so in tonsillitis pain may be referred to the middle ear.

Q41. Optic disc in the eye is called the blind spot. Explain.

Ans. A circular depressed white to pink area is present in retina, called optic disc. From here, optic nerve fibers arise.

The optic disc does not contain photoreceptor cells and hence does not respond to light. So, it is called blind spot of eye.

Q42. Surgeon thoroughly clears the blood clots in the tonsillar fossa after performing tonsillectomy.

Ans. This is done to prevent postoperative hemorrhage because the clots in the tonsillar fossa interfere with the retraction of the vessels walls or preventing the contraction of the surrounding muscles, i.e. the muscles forming the boundaries of the tonsillar fossa.

Q43. Following operation of the thyroid gland patient develops hoarseness of voice.

Ans. The external lymph node (LN) stays behind thyroid gland. In operation of thyroid gland, it may be damaged. The external LN is important for the pitch of voice because it supplies cricothyroid muscle, which is a tensor of the vocal cord.

So, damage to this nerve may cause loss of phonation that develops hoarseness of voice.

Q44. An intracranial tumor causes papilledema of optic disc.

Ans. The optic nerve is surrounded by all the meninges of brain, that is dura mater, arachnoid mater and pia mater. There is extension of subarachnoid space containing CSF around the optic disc. An intracranial tumor raises the presence of CSF and produces congestion of retinal veins and bulging forward of optic disc and its edema. This condition is known as papilledema.

Q45. Paralysis of soft palate causes nasal regurgitation of fluid.

Ans. While deglutingfood, nasopharyngeal isthmus closes. It prevents the food from entering in the nasopharynx. It is done by levator palatini, which elevates the soft palate. When soft palate is paralyzed this does not occur. It leads to nasal regurgitation of fluid/food.

Q46. Horner's syndrome and its manifestation.

Ans. Its symptoms are:
- Apparent enophthalmos
- Slight drooping of upper eyelid
- Pupillary constriction
- Redness of conjunctiva
- Anhidrosis
- Abolition of ciliospinal reflex.

During sympathectomy of upper limb, Horner's syndrome results due to:
- Paralysis of the cervical sympathetic fibers
- Removal of stellate ganglion
- Damage to T1 segment of spinal cord.

Q47. What sympathetic disorders are like to arise from injury of T1 segment of spinal cord?

Ans. Injury to the T1 segment of spinal cord results from an interruption of the sympathetic nerve supply to the head and neck. This is known as Horner's syndrome. The effected person exhibits constriction of pupil, slight drooping of eyelid, vasodilation of skin, arterioles and loss of sweating.

Q48. Pain in the ear in dental caries.

Ans. In dental caries, inferior dental branch of mandibular nerve is affected and produce pain in the teeth. As auriculotemporal nerve is another branch of mandibular nerve; sometimes, pain is referred to the ear and temporal region, because the said nerve supplies these regions.

Q49. Upper half of the face escapes in supranuclear lesion of facial nerve.

Ans. The part of motor nucleus, which supplies the muscles of forehead and eye (orbicularis oculi) is controlled by corticonuclear fibers (pyramidal tract) of both the side but muscles of lower half of face are controlled by opposite-sided corticonuclear fiber. So, in supranuclear lesion upper half of the face escapes from paralysis.

Q50. Thyroid gland moves with deglutition.

Ans. The thyroid is enclosed in the pretracheal layer of the deep cervical fascia, it is attached to hyoid bone, thyroid cartilage and cricoids cartilage of larynx. A fibrous band known as ligament of Berry is derived from pretracheal fascia. It connects the lobe of thyroid gland with cricoids cartilage.

The thyroid gland also moves up and down with the larynx being fixed to its cartilages by the pretracheal fascia.

Q51. Why left recurrent laryngeal nerve is longer than right?

Ans. Fused cranial end of endocardial heart tubes form aortic sac and its right and left horn. Six arterial arches appear stagewise. Major part of the first and second arch disappears. But the remnant of first arch is maxillary artery and second is stapedial artery. Next, there is disappearance of fifth arch. Recurrent LN lies under the sixth arch. Part of the sixth arch artery between lung bud and dorsal aorta is known as ductus arteriosus on left side. On the left side, the ductus arteriosus persists as ligamentum arteriosum. Due to disappearance of ductus arteriosus on the right side and disappearance of fifth arch the right recurrent LN goes to the neck and hooks the right subclavian artery. So, the right remains in the neck and left recurrent LN comes down in the thorax. So, left is longer than the right.

Q52. Inflammation of parotid gland is very painful.

Ans. The superficial or lateral surface of the gland is covered by the strong parotidomasseteric fascia.

The facial layer covering the parotid gland merges with the fascia covering the masseter leading to formation of this strong sheath, which remains closely adhered to the gland.

Hence, due to the unyielding or inelastic nature of this sheath, inflammation of the parotid is painful.

Q53. Motor aphasia after injury over pterion. Explain.

Ans. Pterion of the parietal bone lies over motor area of speech or Broca's area (area 44 and 45) of the brain.

Hence, its injury can lead to severe damage of the Broca's area and its consequent loss of function.

Thus, it will lead to motor aphasia in which, although the words can be understood, the person is unable to speak as the muscular movements are not permitted.

Q54. Fourth layer is the dangerous layer of scalp, explain why?

Ans. Fourth layer/loose areolar layer—potential space traversed by valveless emissary veins connecting extracranial scalp veins with intracranial venous sinus. So, any scalp infection passes through valveless communication to intracranial sinuses.

Q55. Lesion of pretectal nucleus causes Argyll Robertson pupil.

Ans. Argyll Robertson pupil light reflex absent but accommodation reflex present. Light reflex afferent limb optic nerve, optic chiasma, optic tract pretectal nucleus of midbrain fibers of pretectal nucleus, occulomotor nucleus of both side efferent limb third nerves. So lesion in pretectal nucleus—efferent pathway disrupts no light reflex.

Accommodation reflex afferent limb optic nerve, optic chiasma, optic tract-LGB-optic radiation—visual cortex long association fiber frontal eye field (area 8)—projection fiber through internal capsule third nerve nucleus efferent limb third nerve. So, it is retained.

Q56. Boy presents with discharge of pus through ear following recurrent throat infection.

Ans. Throat infection spread to middle ear in children as auditory tube is shorter 18 mm, wider and horizontal. In adult it is longer 36 mm, narrower and directed downward forward medially.

Q57. In tonsillitis pain referred to middle ear.

Ans. Tonsil supplied by glossopharyngeal nerve irritated in tonsillitis pain referred to middle ear along tympanic border of glossopharyngeal nerves, which form tympanic plexus over promontory of middle ear and supply mucous membrane of ear.

 ## SURFACE ANATOMY OF HEAD AND NECK WHICH IS HELPFUL FOR CLINICIAN

1. *Isthmus of thyroid gland*: Put a point at the center of the isthmus. *Upper border*: 1.2 cm below the lower border of cricoid cartilage. Lower border 2 cm below the upper border. Borders are 1.2 cm long. It lies over first, second and third tracheal ring.
   - Here tracheostomy is done by lifting the isthmus.
2. *Anterior arch of cricoid cartilage (Fig. 6.31)*: A point at the midline of anterior arch of cricoid, most prominent part below the thyroid.
3. *Tip of greater cornu of hyoid bone (Fig. 6.31)*: Uppermost and lateralmost bony point from the body of the hyoid, can be palpated between thumb and the index finger.

   In throttling greater cornu of hyoid is fractured.
4. *Thyroid eminence*: The most prominent eminence in the midline below the hyoid bone. More marked in male.
5. *Nasion (Fig. 6.31)*: It overlies the frontonasal suture, marked by the depression at the root of the nose.
6. *Bifurcation of common carotid artery*: A point at lower one-third opposite upper border of thyroid cartilage at the anterior margin of sternocleidomastoid.
7. *Tip of seventh cervical spine*: A point at lower end of nuchal furrow, a prominent bony elevation in the midline felt when the head is bowed down.

Head, Neck and Brain

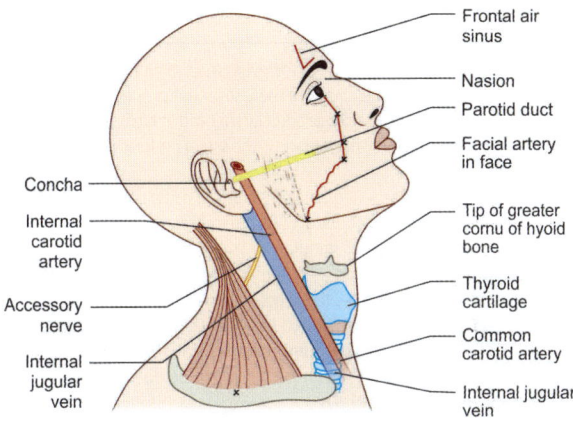

Fig. 6.31: Surface marking of head and neck

8. *Infraorbital foramen*: It lies vertically below the supraorbital notch and 1 cm below the infraorbital margin.

Points to Remember

- Anterior two-third and posterior one-third of dorsum of tongue differ in location, gross features, sensory innervation and development of mucosa
- The inspection of dorsum of the tongue helps the clinician in diagnosis of not only the disease of tongue but also systemic disease. The black hairy tongue is characteristic of AIDS. In inflammation, i.e. glossitis of the tongue looks red
- Congenital anomalies like lingual thyroid may present as a red and round swelling at the foramen cecum on the dorsum of tongue or inside the tongue
- Deviated nasal septum (DNS) is a common cause of nasal obstruction
- Frontal air sinus are absent at birth. They start developing 2–3 years after birth
- Due to anatomical proximity of sphenoidal sinus and pituitary gland the sinus is used as a route for surgery of pituitary gland (transsphenoidal hypophysectomy)
- The maxillary sinus is more prone to infections in chronic smokers because of loss of mucosal cilia. It is very often filled with pus due to poor natural drainage and due to its position favoring collection of pus due to frontal sinusitis
- Peritonsillar space is the plane along which tonsil is removed during tonsillectomy. The paratonsillar vein that passes through the space is often source of postoperative bleeding

Contd...

Surgical Anatomy

Contd...

- The internal LN is intimately related to the pyriform fossa. During removal of foreign body the internal LN may be injured, if the instrument pierces the mucosa
- Infant larynx is smaller (one-third of adult larynx) and at higher level
- The central part of tympanic membrane is the site of perforation because of poor blood supply here
- Fracture of roof of middle ear (tegmen tympani) may cause rupture of the tympanic membrane and escape of blood and CSF from the ear
- Otitis media (inflammation of middle ear) is common because bacteria easily reaches middle ear through auditory tube
- Mastoiditis is a complication of otitis media
- Presbycusis is the physiological hearing loss associated with aging process
- The spina bifida is usually found in lumbosacral region. This defect is due to failure of closure of posterior neuropore. It is believed to be due to deficiency of folic acid in mother
- The term "bulb" was earlier used for medulla oblongata. Hence, one come across the terms like corticobulbar fibers, bulbar palsy, etc.
- Lesion in the corpus striatum causes disturbances in the initiation and cessation of motor event. This results in various kinds of abnormal movements
- The spinal nerve roots (ventral and dorsal) are the filaments by which spinal nerve is attached. So, the spinal nerve is formed by the union of ventral and dorsal nerve roots.

7
CHAPTER

Histology

CHAPTER OUTLINE

- Transitional Epithelium
- Respiratory Epithelium
- Histology of Lung
- Histology of Duodenum
- Microanatomy of Appendix
- Histology of Ureter
- Histology of Parotid Gland
- Kupffer Cells
- Skin
- Classical Hepatic Lobule
- Histology of Esophagus
- Sructure of Lymph Node
- Suprarenal Gland
- White Pulp
- Histology of Fallopian Tube
- Histology of Spinal Cord (At T10 Segment)
- Dermatome
- Histology of Cerebellum
- Histology of Adrenal Cortex

SHORT NOTES

TRANSITIONAL EPITHELIUM P.G.E.

> *Shape*: Multilayered with superficial umbrella cells layer (3–4 cell layers).
> *Function*: Distension.
> *Situation*: Ureter and urinary bladder.

RESPIRATORY EPITHELIUM

The respiratory system provides oxygen to the body and eliminates carbon dioxide. It consists of two parts:
1. *Conducting part*: It includes nasal cavities, nasopharynx, larynx, trachea, bronchi and bronchioles. This conducting part is lined by pseudostratified columnar epithelium. Terminal bronchiole is lined by simple columnar cells. The number of goblet cells decreases from distal.
2. *Respiratory part*: It includes respiratory bronchioles, atria and alveoli. Respiratory bronchiole is lined by cuboidal epithelium, alveoli are lined by (i) simple squamous epithelium (type I cells), which is extremely thin and gaseous exchange takes place; (ii) small cuboidal secretory cells (type II)—they secrete a surfactant (phospholipid) that spreads over the epithelial surface. Apart from these cells, there are lung macrophages known as dust cells.

Clinical Anatomy
- Surfactant reduces surface tension and it prevents alveolar collapse. Premature infants suffer from respiratory distress syndrome due to insufficient surfactant.
- Under certain conditions, one type of epithelium may change into another type. For example, in heavy smokers, the ciliated columnar epithelium lining the respiratory tract may change into stratified squamous epithelium. This process is called metaplasia.
- Malignant tumor (cancer) arising from epithelial tissue accounts for 90% cancer in adults.

HISTOLOGY OF LUNG

The lungs are essential organ of respiration. It provides O_2 for body metabolism and helps to eliminate CO_2. It is conical in shape, covered

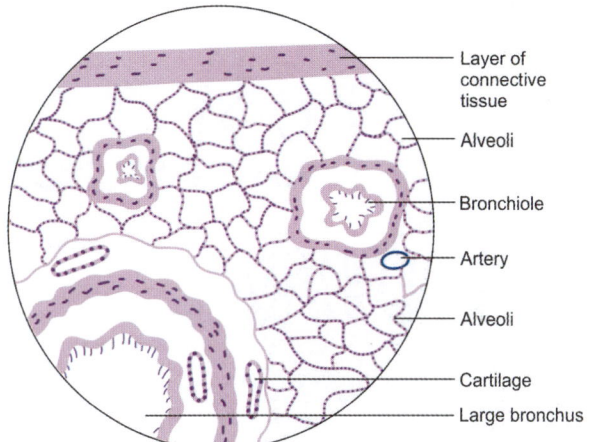

Fig. 7.1: Sectional view of lung (H & E stained)

by visceral pleura (pulmonary pleura). Each lung has conical apex directed above, concave semilumbar base directed below thin anterior border facing forward and thick rounded posterior border facing backward, costal surface (identified by impression of ribs) and medial surface (identified by hilum). It contains the terminal parts of bronchial tree that is intrapulmonary branches of bronchiole, respiratory bronchiole, alveolar ducts, and alveoli along with blood vessels (Fig. 7.1).

- Presence of innumerable alveoli lined by squamous epithelium.
- Presence of bronchus (identified by incomplete ring of hyaline cartilage).
- Presence of bronchiole (cartilage absent and flower-like appearance).

HISTOLOGY OF DUODENUM

It is the proximal fixed part of the intestine C-shaped. From inside outward (Fig. 7.2):

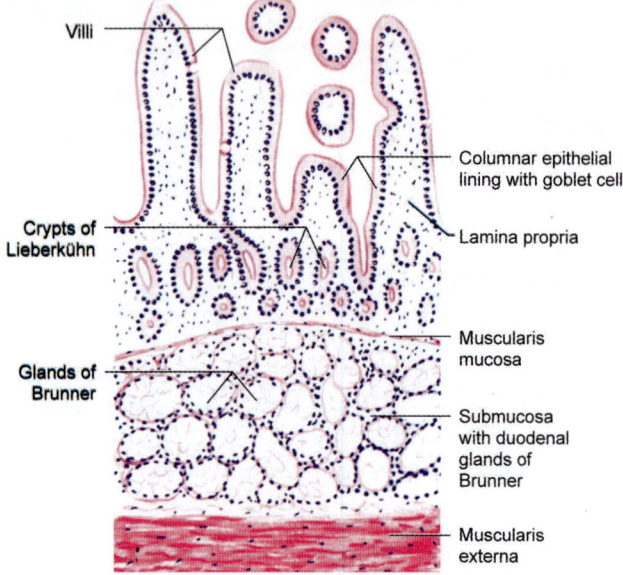

Fig. 7.2: Duodenum

1. The epithelium shows numerous broad villi lined by columnar cells with brush border and goblet cells. Lamina propria contains crypts, diffuse lymphocytes.
2. Muscularis mucosa is made up of two thin layers of muscle fiber.
3. The submucosa is characterized by the presence of compound racemose mucous gland known as gland of Brunner. These glands fill up most of submucosa.
4. Muscularis externa consists of two layers of smooth muscle fiber outer longitudinal and inner circular.
5. The outermost layer is serosa/adventitia.

MICROANATOMY OF APPENDIX

Worm-like organ 2–9 cm in length, attached to the posteromedial aspect of cecum. It has a very narrow lumen and a thick wall (Fig. 7.3).

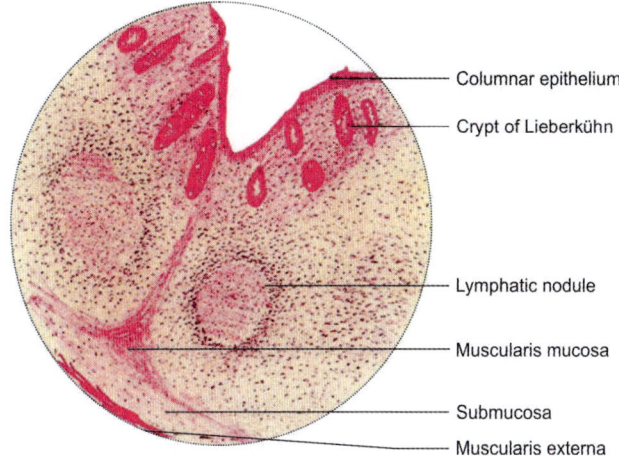

Fig. 7.3: Vermiform appendix

- Absence of intestinal villi.
- Columnar epithelium with goblet cells.
- Prominent lymphoid tissue in submucous coat.
- Presence of gap in the muscular coat (hiatus muscularis).

Clinical Anatomy

Due to hiatus muscularis, infection of appendix is common.

HISTOLOGY OF URETER

The ureters are two muscular tubes, each tube transmits urine from renal pelvis to urinary bladder by regular peristaltic movements. The ureter pierces the bladder wall very obliquely so that during contraction of bladder the opening is closed and backflow is prevented.

- From within outward lined by transitional epithelium (from which outward).
- Lamina propia present.
- Muscular coat: Inner longitudinal and outer circular.
- Outermost fibrous coat (Fig. 7.4).

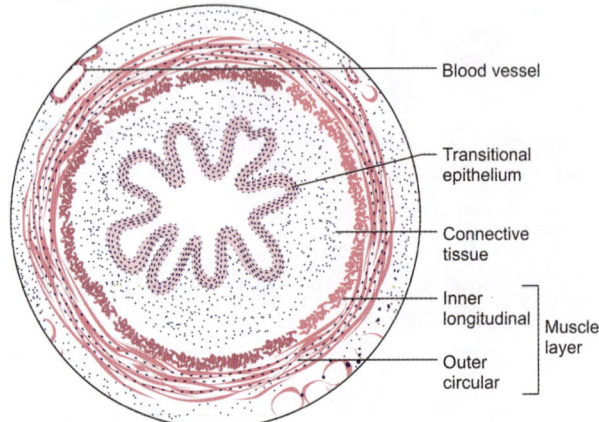

Fig. 7.4: Transverse section of ureter (H & E stained)

HISTOLOGY OF PAROTID GLAND

Largest among the three major salivary glands. Other major salivary glands are—submandibular and sublingual. The minor salivary glands are small labial, buccal, lingual, and palatine glands (Fig. 7.5).

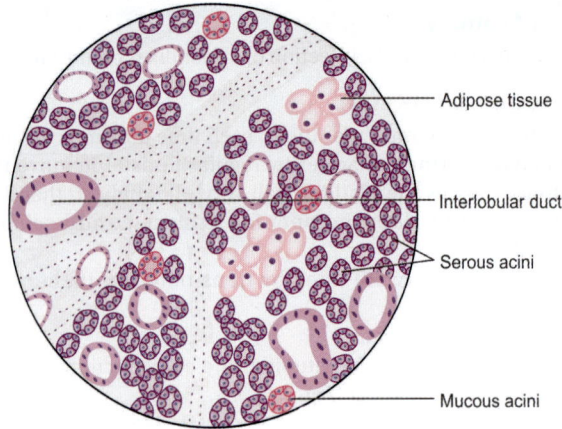

Fig. 7.5: Salivary gland parotid (H & E stained)

- Connective tissue septa divide it into a number of small lobules containing mainly serous and few mucous acini.
- No islets of Langerhans.
- Ducts are lined by pseudostratified columnar epithelium.

KUPFFER CELLS

- Total macrophages of body form the tissue macrophase system. It was previously known as reticuloendothelial system.
- The macrophages are known by different names in different places.
- In the liver, the macrophages are known as Kupffer cells. They protect against the invasion of microbes from gastrointestinal tract via portal circulation.

SKIN

It is the widest organ of the body covering the external surface. Its surface area is 2 m^2, like that of peritoneum.

Histology

- It has two parts—(1) epidermis (responsible for different coloration of skin) and (2) dermis (collagen fiber in it, is responsible for cleavage lines). The epidermis is a vascular. The dermis is tough, strong and very vascular. Here roots are situated in dermis or subcutaneous tissue.
- It has two types of glands—(1) sebaceous gland (secretes oily substance) and (2) sweat gland.
- It has two appendages—(1) nail and (2) hair follicle.
- It has two thickenings—(1) in palm and (2) sole.
- In the cadaver, the skin feels more thick due to preservative material.

Skin (Fig. 7.6): The skin has two main parts: (1) Epidermis, and (2) Dermis.

Underneath the dermis lies hypodermis or subcutaneous tissue containing blood vessels, nerves and fat. The color of the skin depends on the amount of melanin pigment and circulatory status of the dermis. In section through skin, the site of junction of epidermis and dermis is not straight. There is wavy projection known as dermal papillae. The skin is of two varieties: (1) thick skin—found over palm and sole, and hairless, (2) thin skin—found in other regions of body and contains hairs. The appendages of skin are—(a) hairs, (b) nails

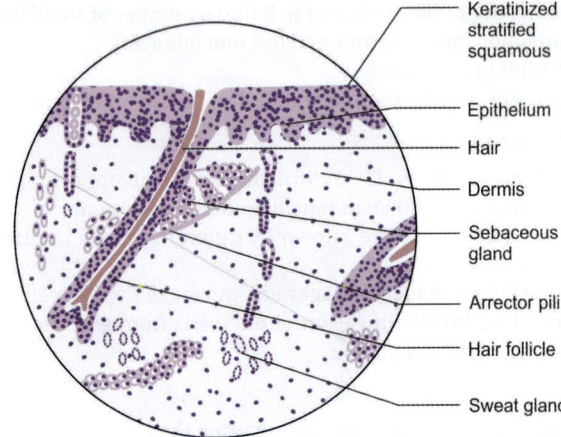

Fig. 7.6: Sectional view of skin

and (c) the glands (sebaceous and sweat glands). Functions of the skin are the following:

1. Protection against physical, chemical and biological agents
2. Thermoregulation
3. Largest sense organ with wavy receptor ending
4. Minor excretion through sweat
5. Produce vitamin D on exposure to sunlight
6. Absorbs certain lipid-soluble substance.

Epidermis has got five layers (from inside outward):

1. Stratum basale: Low columnar cells
2. Stratum spinosum: Several layers of polygonal cells with spinous processes on the surface
3. Stratum granulosum: Few layers of flat cells with keratohyalin granules
4. Stratum lucidum: Cells with no nuclei
5. Stratum corneum: Flat cells with no nuclei.
    - From superficial to deep presence of stratified squamous keratinized epithelium
    - Hair follicle present.

Clinical Anatomy
- Basal cell carcinoma arises from basal cells of epidermis. It begins in keratinocytes of stratum spinosum.
- The melanoma is the cancer of melanocytes. It is a highly metastatic cancer.
- Superficial fascia lies adjacent to dermis and contains variable amount of fat.
- Subcutaneous injection is preferred where slow absorption of drug is needed. For example, insulin and local anesthetic. Similarly low molecular weight heparin is given by this route (in anterior abdominal wall) after coronary bypass surgeries.

CLASSICAL HEPATIC LOBULE

Liver is the largest gland of the body and has got both endocrine and exocrine functions, endocrine function is glucose formation and exocrine function is bile formation. Classical hepatic lobule is hexagonal in shape, they form the units of liver. Polyhedral plates of hepatocytes radiate from central vein to periphery of lobule. In between two rows of hepatocytes lie sinusoids which are lined by Kupffer cells. Kupffer cells phagocytes bacteria (Fig. 7.7).

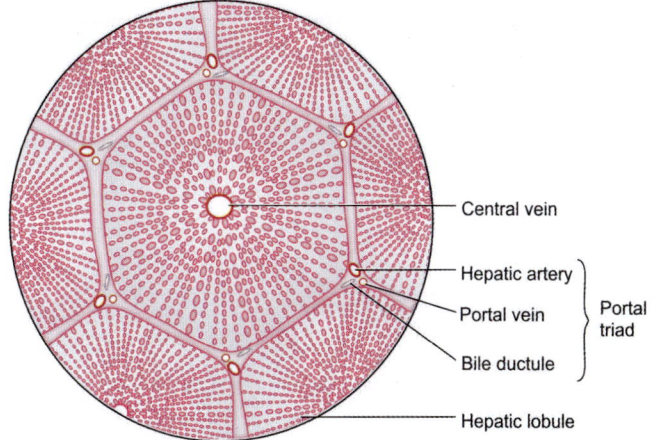

Fig. 7.7: Transverse section of liver (H & E stained)

Presence of portal triad (consists of branch of portal vein, a branch of hepatic artery and small bile channel) at different corners of the lobule.

Space is small between hepatocytes and portal triad, lymphatic channel originates from here.

Space of perisinusoidal space lies between liver sinusoids and hepatocyte.

Clinical Importance

Liver has got extraordinary power of regeneration. The loss of hepatic tissue initiates a mechanism by which hepatocytes begin to divide. In human being, the capacity is restricted.

Destruction of liver parenchyma and replacement by connective tissue is known as "cirrhosis of liver".

HISTOLOGY OF ESOPHAGUS

Esophagus: It is a muscular tube, lying between pharynx and the stomach. It begins at inferior border of cricoids cartilage, opposite C6 vertebra and ends at the cardiac opening of the stomach opposite T11 vertebra (Fig. 7.8).

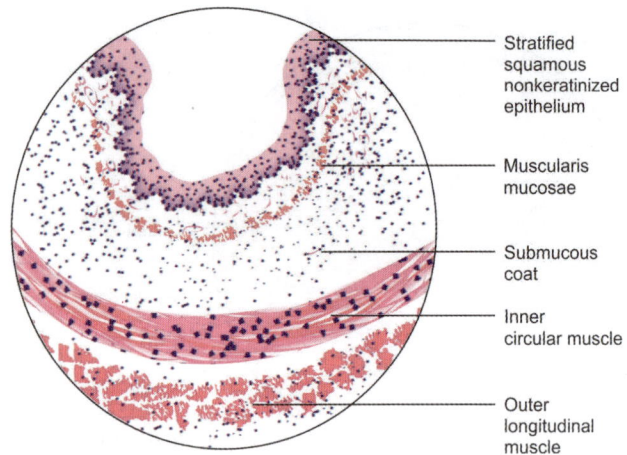

Fig. 7.8: Transverse section of upper esophageal wall (H & E stained)

Histology from within outward:
- Mucous membrane lined by stratified squamous epithelium with thin muscularis mucosa
- Muscularis externa
- Outer longitudinal
- Inner circular.

STRUCTURE OF LYMPH NODE (FIG. 7.9)

It is a bean-shaped structure situated along the course of lymphatic vessels. Each lymph node is covered by connective tissue capsule. The septa from the capsule extend to the gland known as trabecule. Peripheral motor part is where cortex where trabecule extends. The afferent lymphatic vessels are many in number and enter through hilum (indented portion) of lymph node may be one or two in number.

- Medullary cords and sinuses are present in medulla.
- The lymphatic nodules present in the cortex are B lymphocytes. The inner cortical zone which is poorly demarcated is known as paracortex. It contains T-lymphocytes.
- Medulla has two components: (1) darkly stained medullary cords with H&E-stained, and (2) lightly stained medullary sinuses.

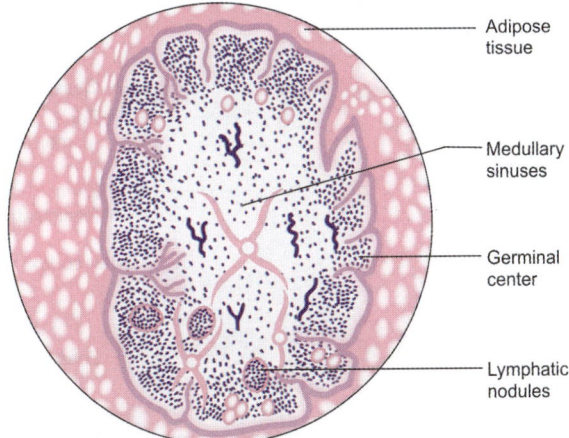

Fig. 7.9: Lymph node (panoramic view) (H & E stained)

Functional Importance
- It is an important part of the immune system.
- Phagocytosis and filtration of bacteria.
- Produce B lymphocytes which are important source of antibody.

SUPRARENAL GLAND (FIG. 7.10)

They are paired flattened glands located at upper pole of kidney. The glands are composed of two distinct parts: (1) cortex and (2) medulla that differ in origin, structure and functions. Under the microscope one can see the cortex surrounded by connective tissue capsule from which septa goes inside carrying blood vessels and lymphatics.

- *Zona glomerulosa*: Here the columnar cells are arranged in small clusters.
- *Zona fasciculata*: It consists of large polyhedral cells arranged in parallel columns, one or two cell thick separated by sinusoids.
- *Zona reticularis*: It has rounded cells with branching column.

Suprarenal medulla is composed of chromatin cells with connective tissue and many blood vessels and nerves.

Two cell types are seen:
1. Cells secreting epinephrine (stains quickly).
2. Cells secreting norepinephrine (stains well).

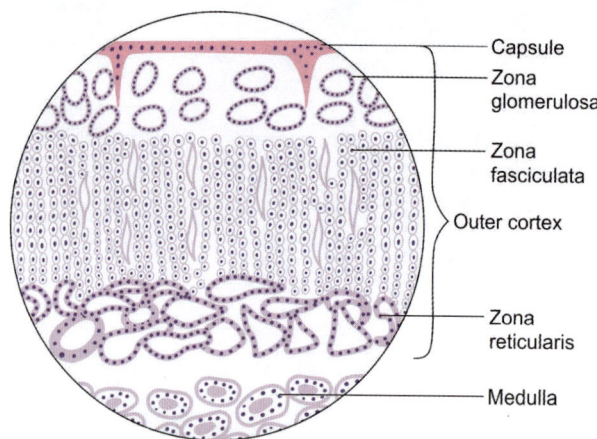

Fig. 7.10: Sectional view of suprarenal gland

Clinical Anatomy

- *Zona glomerulosa*: Secretes mineralocorticoids. Hypersecretion of this layer produces Cohn's syndrome.
- *Zona fasciculata*: Secretes glucocorticoids, increases secretion, produces Cushing's syndrome. Hyposecretion produces Addison's disease.
- *Zona reticularis*: Secretes sex steroids. Increased secretion produces hirsutism in females.
- *Adrenal medulla*: Increased secretion produces rise of blood sugar level. Tumor of adrenal medulla known as pheochromocytoma causes transient increase of blood pressure.

WHITE PULP

- White pulp present in the spleen which is the largest lymphoid organ.
- Microscopically, it is made up of aggregation of lymphoid tissue around a small artery or arteriole. It looks relatively pale area in hematoxylin and eosin stain. The artery is known as central artery with eccentric in position. It is a branch of trabecules artery that leaves the trabeculum and enters into white pulp (Fig. 7.11).

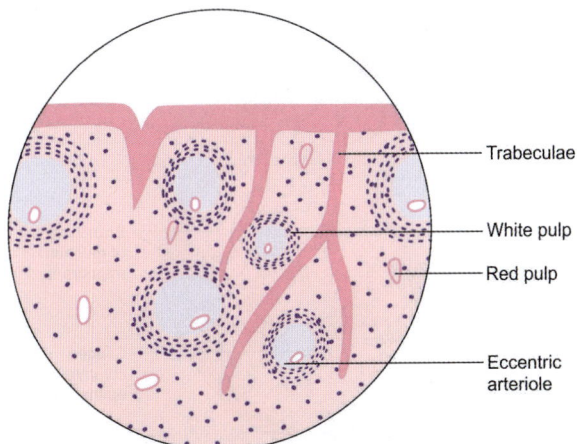

Fig. 7.11: Section of spleen (panoramic view) (H & E stained)

- On entering the white pulp, it is surrounded by lymphoid tissue populated by T-lymphocytes.
- Collection of B lymphocytes is seen along the germinal centers (white pulp).
- The white pulp is surrounded by an immunologically active zone containing many macrophages, few T-lymphocytes and blood sinuses. This functional zone between white and red pulp is known as marginal zone.
- The central artery leaves the white pulp and enters the red pulp and divides to form straight penicillar arterioles.

HISTOLOGY OF FALLOPIAN TUBE (FIG. 7.12)

- Fallopian tube is attached with the lateral angle of the uterus.
- It has four parts (from medial to lateral): (1) Intramural, (2) isthmus, (3) ampulla, and (4) infundibulum with fimbriae.
- Histologically, wall of fallopian tube has three layers from inside out:
    1. Mucous membrane
    2. Muscular layer
    3. Serosa (peritoneum).

Mucous Membrane

- It is composed of lining epithelium and lamina propria.

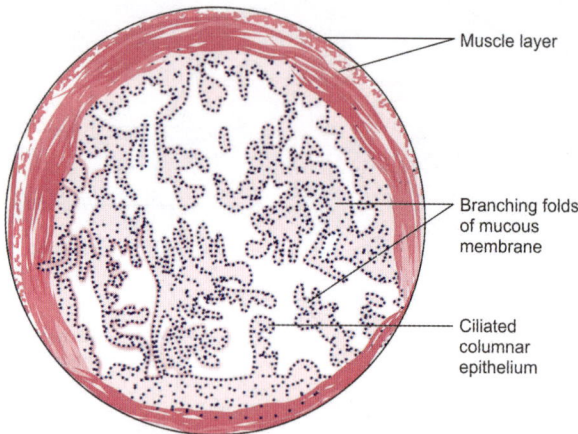

Fig. 7.12: Section of the uterine tube (H & E stained)

- Lining epithelium (mainly) is ciliated columnar and some secretory cells (peg cells).
- Lamina propria contains loose areolar tissue, blood vessels and nerves.
- Most important feature is folds of mucosa—folds are of primary, secondary and tertiary types and it is so dense in adult that the lumen is rarely seen.

Muscular Layer
- Inner circular and outer longitudinal
- Smooth muscles
- Muscular layer is thick in the intramural part and isthmus

Serous Layer
- It is covered on all sides by peritoneum.

Functional and Clinical Importance
- The fallopian tube helps in grabbing the ovum and carrying it toward the ampulla where fertilization takes place.
- Cilia is meant for beating movement for carrying the ovum. In any diseases of the fallopian tube, the cilia are destroyed and lead to infertility.
- Sometimes the lumen of tube is blocked by pus and leads to infertility.

The microscopic difference between jejunum and ileum are described in Table 7.1.

Table 7.1: Microscopic differences between jejunum and ileum

Jejunum	Ileum
• Presence of more circular mucous fold and long leaf-like villi	• Many short club-like villi
• No Peyer's patches or Brunner's gland	• Lamina propria contains many lymphatic nodules including Payer's patches
• Intermediate number of goblet cells	• No circular folds
• Walls are thicker and redder (because of mucous fold)	• Walls are thinner
• Feeding jejunostomy is done • In case of paralyzed patient	• In typhoid fever, the Peyer's patches are affected and produce perforation of gut if not treated
• Both jejunum and ileum are susceptible to trauma (external injury)	

HISTOLOGY OF SPINAL CORD (AT T10 SEGMENT) (FIG. 7.13)

The spinal cord is 45 cm in length, cylindrical in shape, lies within the vertebral canal and extends from upper border of 1st cervical vertebra up to 1st lumbar vertebra in adult. In children, it extends up to 3rd lumbar vertebra. The spinal cord consists of central core of gray matter containing cell bodies of neurons (Fig. 7.13).
- H-shaped gray matter inside (pink stain is more)
- Outer white matter
- Anterior median fissure and posterior median sulcus present
- Anterior horn is bulbous.

The anterior gray column large size multipolar motor neurons and cytoplasm contains dark-staining basophilic Nissl substance. The neurons of posterior gray column are much smaller than anterior horn cells. Within the gray matter, besides the sensory or motor nerve cells, there are neurons, neuroglial cells and blood vessels.

The white fibers are mainly myelinated fibers but also neuroglial cells and blood vessels.

Clinical Anatomy

Multiple sclerosis is the most common disorder of the nervous system affecting young adults. There is progressive damage of myelin sheath. This affects the sensation, movements, body functions and balance.

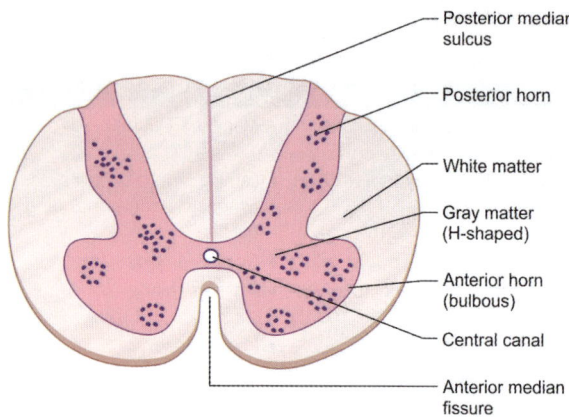

Fig. 7.13: Histology of spinal cord (at T10 segment)

DERMATOME

The area of skin supplied by the spinal nerve is known as dermatome. No area of skin of trunk is supplied by one spinal nerve as there is an overlapping in the distribution of spinal nerve to the skin. Loss of one dorsal root of a spinal nerve results in diminished sensation. At least three consecutive intercostal nerves to be divided. The important spinal segments are:
1. The T9 supplies the epigastrium.
2. The T10 supplies the umbilical region.
3. The T12 supplies the region midway between umbilicus and pelvis. The iliohypogastric (L1) supplies the hypogastrium.

HISTOLOGY OF CEREBELLUM

The cauliflower-like cerebellum is the largest part of hind brain. The cortex is highly folded. The folia (folds) are separated by closely placed parallel transverse fissures. Each folium consists of a core of white matter cover outside by gray matter (Fig. 7.14).

From outside inward, outer gray matter divided into three zones:
1. Outer molecular layer (lightly stained)
2. Intermediate Purkinje layer (flask-shaped)
3. Inner granular (dark bluish violet stained) well-defined layer

Inner white matter contains nerve fiber-stained pink.

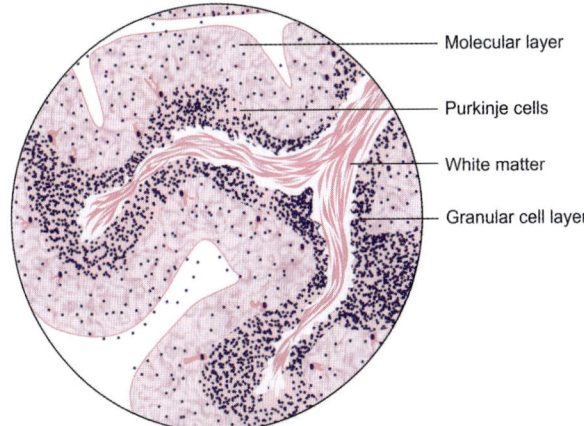

Fig. 7.14: Section of cerebellum

EXPLANATORY NOTE

PIMPLES OR ACNE IS COMMON IN PUBERTY

Pimples are small elevation on facial skin due to swelling of sebaceous gland due to accumulation of sebum. Under the influence of sex hormone, the sebaceous subsequent infection produces pimple or acne. It usually occurs in non-hairy region of skin-like face and back.

> **Points to Remember**
> - In Huntington's disease (autosomal dominant) striatal neurons are lost from cerebral cortex and putamen
> - Spleen does not possess subcapsular space like lymph nodes
> - Hassel's corpuscles are aggregation of flattened epithelial reticular cells, which later undergo degeneration.

8 CHAPTER

Genetics

CHAPTER OUTLINE

- Definition
- Chromosome
- Karyotyping
- Classification of Chromosomes
- Codominant Genes
- Down's Syndrome (Mongolism)
- Nondisjunction
- Turner Syndrome
- Klinefelter Syndrome
- Barr Body (Sex Chromatin) or X Chromosome Inactivation
- Sex Chromosome
- Allelic Gene
- Translocation
- Philadelphia Chromosome
- Albinism
- Abnormalities due to Alteration of Chromosomal Morphology

Surgical Anatomy

DEFINITION

Genetic is the study of heredity, a process by which children inherit certain character (traits) from family and from their parents.

These traits pass from parents to children by genetic code situated in the nucleus of the cell. The code is formed by deoxyribonucleic acid (DNA molecule). The functional unit of DNA is called gene. The total genetic information in a cell is known as genome. The human genome comprises 50,000–100,000 genes.

SHORT NOTES

CHROMOSOME (FIG. 8.1)

Human possess diploid number of chromosomes (46). They are best seen when they are maximally coiled. This takes place during the metaphase of mitosis and meiosis. Metaphase chromosomes are utilized for karyotyping. There are two types of chromosomes: (1) autosome, and (2) sex chromosomes. Parts of chromosome have been given in Box 8.1.

Box 8.1: Parts of chromosome

• Short upper limb	P arm
• Lower longer limb	Q arm
• Intervening nonstaining gap	Centromere
• End of chromosome	Telomere

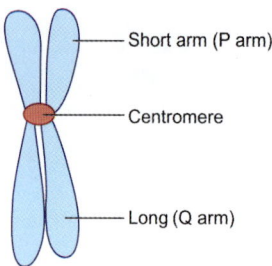

Fig. 8.1: Parts of chromosome

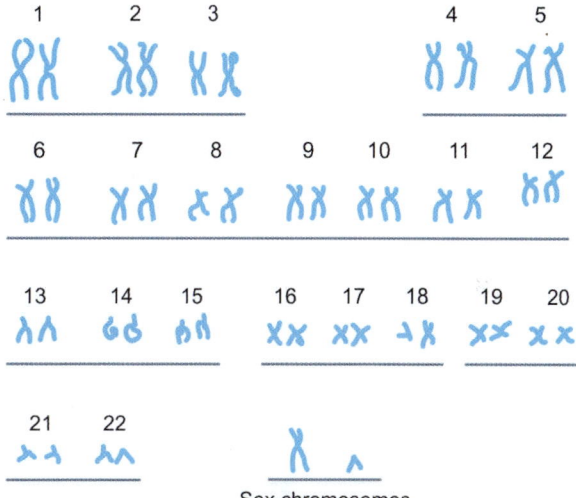

Fig. 8.2: Karyotyping chromosome

KARYOTYPING (FIG. 8.2)

It is a process by which chromosomes are classified and numbered on the basis of decreasing length and position of centromeres. Chromosomes are also present in mitochondria. Mitochondria DNA is inherited from mother.

Clinical Importance

A number of genetic abnormalities can be directly related to chromosomal pattern, the karyotyping is of considerable diagnostic importance.

CLASSIFICATION OF CHROMOSOMES (FIG. 8.3)

They are classified into four types depending on position of centromere. (1) Metacentric chromosomes, where the centromere is situated near the center of the chromosome, making the arm almost equal in length; (2) Submetacentric chromosome, here the centromere is situated somewhat between the midpoint and the

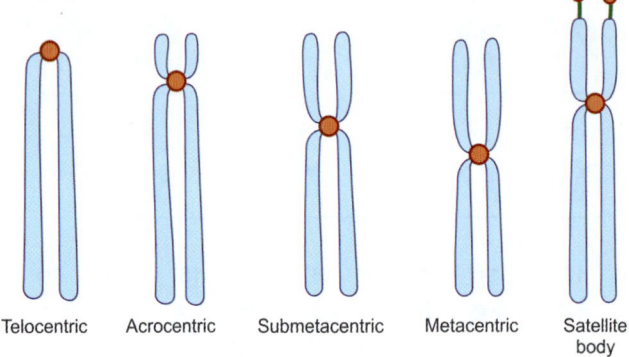

Fig. 8.3: Classification of chromosomes

Table 8.1: Chromosome classification

Group	Number	Feature
A	01–03	Largest metacentric
B	04–05	Largest submetacentric
C	06–12, X	Medium submetacentric
D	13–15	Largest acrocentric
E	16–18	Smallest submetacentric
F	19–20	Smallest metacentric
G	21–22, Y	Smallest acrocentric

end of chromosomes making one arm short and the other arm long; (3) Acrocentric centromere is situated near the end with a very short and very long arm; (4) Telocentric, chromosomes, here the centromere is situated at the end having only one arm (not present in human being). Classification of chromosome has been given in Table 8.1.

CODOMINANT GENES

When both the alleles of a pair are fully expressed in the heterozygote, the genes are known as codominant.

Examples of codominance are the various blood groups. A person having AB blood group has both A and B antigen, in his or her red blood cells, showing that allelic genes are fully expressed and therefore the genes are codominant genes.

DOWN'S SYNDROME (MONGOLISM) (FIGS 8.4A AND B)

This is a numerical chromosomal abnormality affecting the autosome. Here, there is trisomy 21. Down's syndrome occurs in every 700 births.

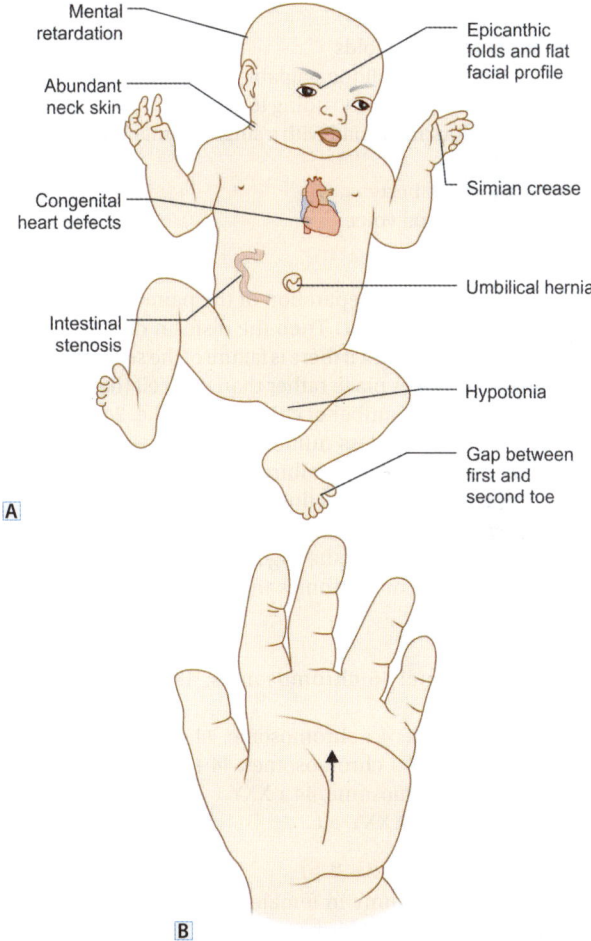

Figs 8.4A and B: An infant with Down's syndrome (mongolism)

The probability of Down's syndrome increases with the age of the mother.

Clinical Features
- Mental retardation
- Brachycephalic
- Presence of epicanthal folds
- Mongoloid face with oblique palpable fissure
- Open mouth with long-protruding tongue
- Hand is very short and broad with a single palmar crease (simian crease)
- There is delayed puberty
- Low-pitched guttural voice.

NONDISJUNCTION

In meiosis cell division, the separation of the paired chromosomes takes place during anaphase 1. Then the disform diploid cell (2n) becomes haploid cells (n). But if there is failure of the separation of the paired chromosome takes place rather than one cell (daughter cell) may contain one excess number of chromosome (i.e. 24 in number) and the other will contain less number of chromosome (i.e. 22 in number). This phenomenon of failure of separation of the paired chromosome is called nondisjunction.

So during fertilization, the gametes will unite with normal gamete (2n) will result in formation of the zygote which will contain either excess or less number of chromosomes and this phenomenon is called "aneuploidy".

Example:
1. Turner's syndrome: 45 chromosomes, 44 + X0 (only one X chromosome)
2. Klinefelter syndrome: 4 + chromosome, 44 + XXY
3. Triple X syndrome: 4 + chromosomes, 44 + XXX
4. Supermale: 4 + chromosome, 44 + XXY
5. Others: 48XXXY, 49XXXXY, etc.

TURNER SYNDROME (FIG. 8.5)

It is also called X monosomy in females. It was first described by Turner. Occurs in every 3,000 births.

Karyotype 45, X0. No Barr body.

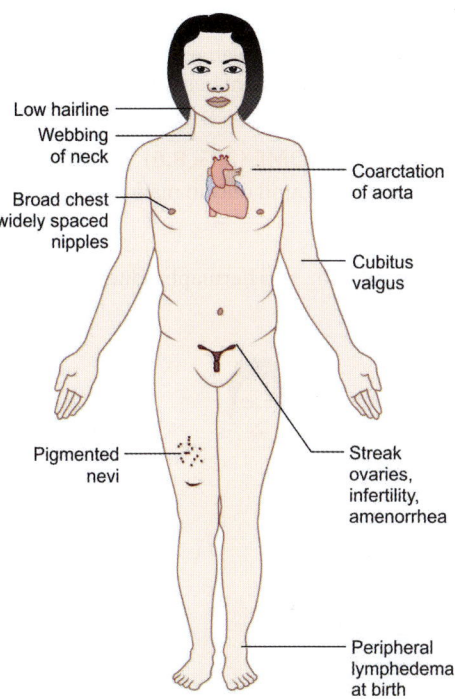

Fig. 8.5: A patient with Turner syndrome

Clinical Features
- Phenotypically female
- Short stature, webbing of neck
- Presence of cubitus valgus
- Broad chest with widely spaced nipple
- Coarctation of aorta or ventricular septal defect (VSD) may present
- Renal anomaly and streaks like gonad
- There is primary amenorrhea.

Treatment

Anabolic steroid administration about 10–12 years of age helps them to gain height. Estrogen treatment helps in development of secondary sexual characters.

KLINEFELTER SYNDROME (FIG. 8.6)
- Trisomic condition found only in male
- Karyotype 47, XXY
- Barr body present
- Patients are tall, thin, and hermaphrodite

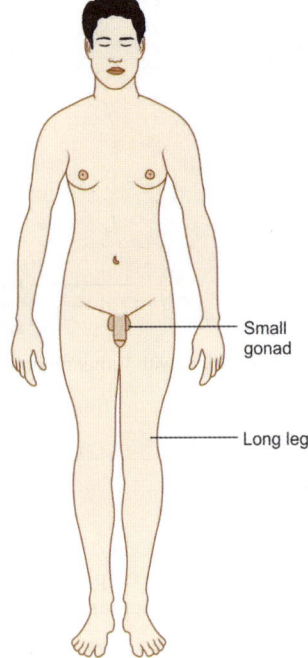

Fig. 8.6: A patient with Klinefelter syndrome

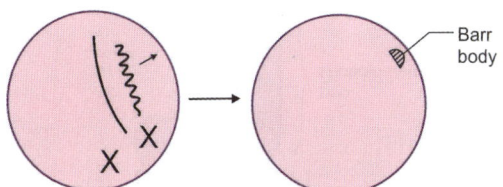

Fig. 8.7: Barr body (sex chromatin) or X chromosome inactivation

- Long legs, poorly develop secondary sexual character
- Normal intelligence
- Testis is small, scrotum, and penis show hypoplasia. Spermatogenesis is absent.

BARR BODY (SEX CHROMATIN) OR X CHROMOSOME INACTIVATION (FIG. 8.7)

Barr and Bertram discovered a small chromatin body in the nuclei of neuron of female cats. This is called Barr body. It is a characteristic feature of interphase nuclei of all female mammals and can be used for nuclear sex determination. It is studied in buccal smear, skin, leukocytes, etc. The study of sex chromatin is widely used in medicine. The Barr body is due to the result of inactivation of one X chromosome. The number of Barr body in a cell is equal to the total number of X chromosome minus one. In normal male and in Turner syndrome no Barr body is present. In normal female, Klinefelter syndrome one Barr body is present. In XXX syndrome (superfemale) double Barr body is present.

SEX CHROMOSOME (FIG. 8.8)

Sex chromosomes are pair of chromosomes that are responsible for sex determination. They differ in males and females. The two sex chromosomes of males are different from one another and are designated as XY. The two sex chromosomes in females are similar and designated as XX. The X of male is similar to X in female but Y is much smaller in size than X. Clinical syndromes due to numerical chromosomal abnormalities involving sex chromosome are Turner syndrome, Klinefelter syndrome, superfemale syndrome (XXX) and XYY.

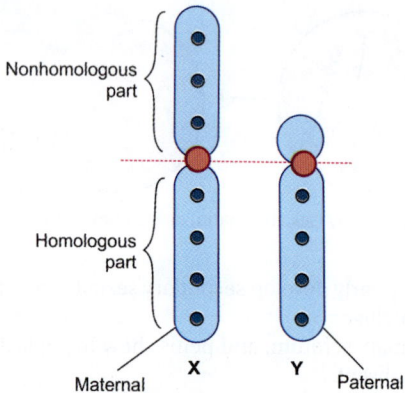

Fig. 8.8: Sex chromosome

ALLELIC GENE (FIG. 8.9)

Genes are units of heredity. The position of gene in a chromosome is called locus. Usually genes do not change their loci. But in recombination during crossing over or in alteration of chromosomal morphology, loci are changed. The gene occupying in a pair of homologous chromosomes is called allelic gene or allelomorph. These

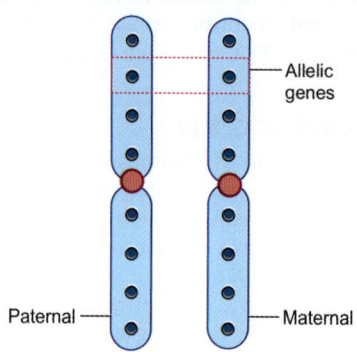

Fig. 8.9: Allelic gene

allelic genes regulate different physical and biochemical characters of an individual when allelic genes work in same direction (e.g. height) they are called homozygous; when working in the opposite direction (one tall and other short), the allelic genes are heterozygous. Sometimes, a pair of allelic genes may influence more than one character; this is known as pleiotropy.

TRANSLOCATION
- It is a type of disorder of chromosome when there is exchange of segment between two nonhomologus chromosomes.
- This is done by break of a portion of chromosome and then resealing of chromosome after exchanging of segments.
- Mainly occur in D and G group of chromosomes:
  - 22 and 21 chromosomes
  - 21 and 21 chromosomes.
- This type of disorder leads to different clinical conditions.
- Type:
  Pericentric → when translocation involves centromere
  Paracentric → when translocation not involve centromere.

Example of Translocation
1. Robertsonian translocation.
   - Chromosomal segment exchange between Chromosomal-21 and Chromosomal-14

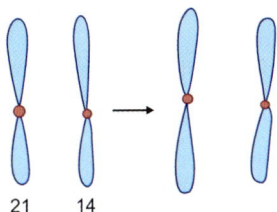

21   14

   - This leads to Down's syndrome due to trisomy 21 though chromosome number remain 46, not 47.
   - This accounts for 5% cases of Down's syndrome
   - If mother has translocated chromosome then there is chance of recurrent birth with Down's syndrome.

2. Philadelphia chromosome.
    - It is seen in chronic myeloid leukemia.
    - Translocation both chromosome 9 and 22
    - Long arms of both chromosomes joins to each other to form translocated chromosome → philadelphia chromosome and the short arms of them are lost.

PHILADELPHIA CHROMOSOME

It is a chromosomal disease affecting autosome. The long arm of chromosome 22 is detached and gets attached to chromosome 9. It is an example of translocation.

Clinical Manifestations
- It is associated with chronic myeloid leukemia (blood cancer in 95% of the cases).
- They are sensitive to chemotherapy.

ALBINISM

In this condition, there is partial or complete absence of pigments in the skin, hair and eyes. In normal human being, tyrosine is converted to melanin (a pigment) by an enzyme tyrosinase. But if tyrosinase is absent, melanin is not produced and results in albinism. Albinism is an autosomal recessive disorder.

Clinical Features
- Absence of pigment from hair, eyes, and skin (known as oculocutaneous albinism).
- There is photophobic (intolerance to light).
- Nystagmus (jerky rapid eye movement).
- Squint.
- Decreased equity.
  Life expectancy is not affected in this disorder.

Treatment

The patients are advised:
- To avoid sun.
- To use sunglasses to reduce photophobia.
- To completely cover the body with clothing when exposed to sun.

ABNORMALITIES DUE TO ALTERATION OF CHROMOSOMAL MORPHOLOGY

Each chromosome contains numerous genes which are arranged in linear series. Centromere is devoid of genes. The position of genes in a chromosome is known as locus which is mentioned in reference to centromere. Genes do not change their position except in alteration of morphology. The different types of morphology are:

- ***Deletion (Fig. 8.10A):*** It means loss of a part of a chromosome with genes. Altered position of genes may have bad effect on the organism. Short arm is indicated by p and long arm by q. Deletion of short arm is symbolized by p- and that of long arm is q-.
    - ***Cri-du-chat syndrome***: Characterized by moon face in appearance, child's cry similar to cat's cry and they are physically and mentally handicapped, die in early childhood.
    - ***Philadelphia chromosome (Ph)***: The karyotype shows deletion from q arm of chromosome 21 or 22. The abnormal chromosome was first discussed in Philadelphia and hence the name.
- ***Translocation***: When the broken segment of one chromosome unites with a part of nonhomologous chromosome, it is known as translocation. Many examples of translocation are seen in human like Down's syndrome (mongolism). Here a segment of chromosome 21 is transferred to shorter arm of any member of group D (13–15).
- ***Isochromosome (Fig. 8.10B)***: During anaphase of normal division, the centromere splits longitudinally. In isochromosome, it splits transversely instead of longitudinal splitting resulting in two unequal chromosomes with duplication of genes.
- ***Ring chromosome (Fig. 8.10C)***: A ring-like chromosome is observed when a chromosome is deleted at both ends and the sticky ends adhere to each other to form a ring. Manifestation depends on deletion of specific genes.

The patient suffers from chronic myeloid leukemia:

- ***Duplication:*** It is the process of addition of a portion of chromosome from another homologous chromosome with duplication of genes. It is rare in human.
- ***Inversion***: A part of chromosome is detached which later reunites in inverted position. Genes are not lost but placed in altered position.

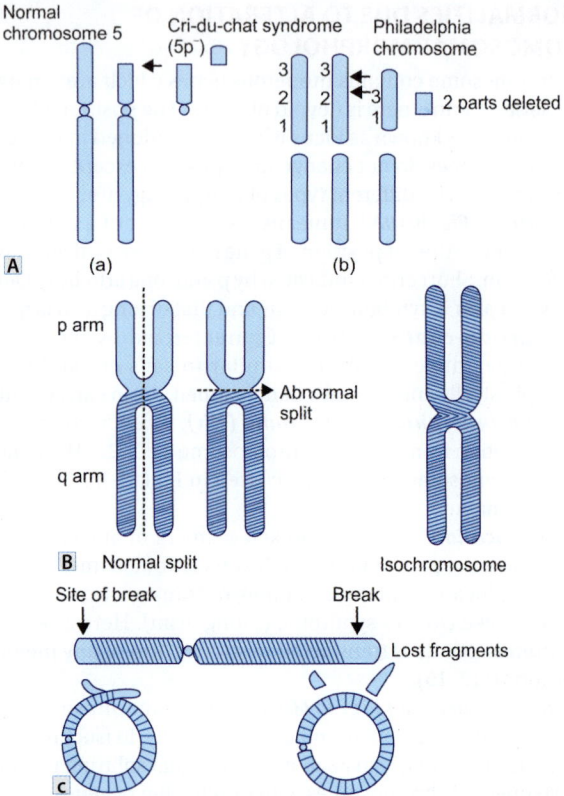

Figs 8.10A to C: (A) Cri-du-chat syndrome and Philadelphia chromosome; (B) Isochromosome; and (C) Ring chromosome

EXPLANATORY NOTE

Q1. An elderly female (38-year-old) gave birth to a baby who is examined to have a rounded face, epicanthic folds and a characteristic single palmar crease. Explain the genetic cause of the event.

Ans.
- The genetic disorder that leads to the given symptoms is Down's syndrome.

- Genetic cause.
- Majority of the bodies with Down's syndrome have 47 chromosomes with trisomy 21, but about 3% have normal 46 chromosomes with translocations.
- Trisomy 21 baby is usually born to an aged mother (35-year-old or above); increased maternal aged predisposes to nondisjunction carrying two 21 chromosomes instead of one in gametogenesis. The banding patterns of chromosome have revealed that about one-third of cases are of paternal origin, suggesting also significant paternal age effect.

Q2. Marriage between the first cousin is not advisable. Explain.

Ans. Consanguineous marriage or marriage between the cousins may result in genetic disorders in the family has a history of presence of dominant or recessive genetic disorder.

So better to avoid consanguineous marriage.

Example:
- Color blindness
- Thalassemia.

Q3. Define double barr body in klinefelter's syndrome.

Ans. According to Lyon's hypothesis the number of Barr body = n – 1, n = Total number of X chromosome.

In Klinefelter's syndrome, the genetic set-up is 47XXY and sometimes, 48XXXY. So, the number of Barr body is 2 – 1 = 1 (in 47XXY) or 3 – 1 = 2 (in 48XXXY). So, double Barr body may be seen in Klinefelter's syndrome.

TERMS USED IN GENETICS (GLOSSARY)

- *Adenine*: It is a purine base in DNA and RNA.
- *Allograft*: A graft, where both donors belong to same species, but not genetically identical.
- *Amniocentesis*: A procedure by which amniotic fluid is obtained for prenatal diagnosis. It is performed between 14 weeks and 16 weeks because sufficient amount of amniotic fluid is available for tapping, without harming the conceptus.
- *Chimera*: An individual with two genetically different cell populations derived from different zygotes.
- *Control gene*: A gene that can turn other genes on or off.

- ***Consanguinity***: A relationship by descent through a common ancestor.
- ***Dominant gene***: An allele that is always expressed both in homozygous or heterozygous combination.
- ***Euchromatin***: Active, lightly stained form.
- ***Genome***: Complete set of gene, characteristic of species.
- ***Gene***: It is a segment of DNA molecule possessing codes for amino acid sequence of a polypeptide chain.
- ***Heterochromatin***: Inactive highly condensed, densely staining form.
- ***Human leukocyte antigen (HLA)***: It is present on the surface of cells including lymphocytes.
- ***Human leukocyte antigen complex***: Genes on chromosome 6, responsible for determining the cell surface antigens. They are important in organ transplantation.
- ***In vitro***: In the laboratory.
- ***In vivo***: In the cell, actually means in the living organism.
- ***Mosaicism***: Two or more different karyotypes in an individual derived from single zygote are called mosaicism.
- ***Mutation***: A change in sequence of genomic DNA.
- ***Recessive gene***: An allele that is expressed only when it is homozygous.
- ***Satellite***: A distal part of chromosome separate from the rest of the chromosome by narrow stalk.

Points to Remember

- Cytoskeleton maintains the shape of the cell (as in muscle contraction)
- Lysosome autophagocytose old, worn out organelles
- Cilia beat and cause movement of the surrounding media
- Function of flagella is to beat and cause movement of cell itself
- Besides being within the nucleus, chromosomes are also present in mitochondria. It is a circular chromosome inherited by an individual from maternal ovum
- Chromosomes are best seen when they are maximally coiled. This takes place during metaphase of mitosis and meiosis
- Gene is made up of varying length of DNA
- In autosomal dominant inheritance trait expressed in both homozygous and heterozygous state.

Contd...

Contd...

- In autosomal recessive inheritance trait expressed only in homozygous state
- In X-linked dominant inheritance when an affected male marries a normal female, he will transmit the trait to all his daughters but not to none of his sons, e.g. Vitamin D-resistant rickets
- Mutation is any sudden, heritable, and structural change in DNA
- Immunogenetics deals with the genetic aspect of antigen, antibodies and their interaction
  Example:
    - Blood group and related problem in compatibility
    - Organ transplant
    - Immune deficiency diseases
    - Autoimmune diseases
- Genes involved in embryogenesis as a result of "genetic switches" like:
    - Fibroblast growth factor family (FGF3)
    - Hedgehog family
    - Wingless family (Wnt), etc.
- ***Inborn error of metabolism:*** It is genetically determined biochemical disorders in which a specific enzyme produces a metabolic block resulting in abnormal metabolism, e.g. phenylketonuria.

Embryology

CHAPTER OUTLINE

- Spermatogenesis
- Oogenesis
- Capacitation
- Morula
- Blastocyst
- Zona Pellucida
- Notochord
- Chorion
- Allantois or Allantoenteric Diverticulum
- Gastrulation
- Different Types of Placenta
- Placenta Previa
- Placental Barrier
- Umbilical Cord
- Amnion
- Meckel's Diverticulum
- Ectopic Pregnancy
- Somite
- Septum Transversum
- Physiological Umbilical Hernia
- Nonfusion of Müllerian Duct
- Abnormal form or Teratology
- Development of Certain Important Organs (Special Embryology)
- Nerves

SHORT NOTES

SPERMATOGENESIS (FIGS 9.1A AND B)

It is a series of process by which spermatogonia are changed to spermatozoa (sperms) (Figs 9.1A and B). The spermatogenesis is divided into three phases—(1) spermatocytosis, (2) meiosis, and (3) spermiogenesis. Primordial germ cells divided by mitosis repeatedly to provide a continuous reserve of sperm cells. Some of the spermatogonia are specialized and form type B spermatogonia, from where primary spermatocyte (contains diploid chromosome) is derived by mitosis division (spermatocytosis). The large primary spermatocyte undergoes first meiotic division and forms secondary spermatocyte with haploid number of chromosome. After completion of meiosis, one secondary spermatocyte gives rise to four equal sized spermatids; out of which, two bear the X chromosome and two bear the Y chromosome. The changeover of spermatids to mature spermatozoa is known as spermiogenesis. These changes include: (1) shedding of excess cytoplasm (which is engulfed by Sertoli cells, (2) condensation of nucleus, (3) formation of acrosomes at the head, which contains a number of important enzymes, and (4) formation of neck, middle piece and tail. In human the time required for a spermatogonium to develop into a mature spermatozoon is approximately 64 days. This spermatozoa is ejaculated during sexual act. The emitted material is known as semen. The amount varies from 2cc to 5cc. It comprises of sperm, secretion of seminal vesicles (60% of volume), secretion of prostate gland (30% of seminal fluid volume) and secretion of bulbourethral gland. In males, *differentiation of primordial germ cells begins at puberty* within seminiferous tubule. P.G.E.

OOGENESIS

In female, the maturation of primitive germ cells to mature gamete is known as oogenesis (Fig. 9.2). Oogenesis starts in prenatal life. It includes three processes:

1. *Repeated mitosis*: It produces a number of oogonia.
2. Specialization of some oogonia into primary oocyte (with diploid number of chromosome).
3. Meiotic division starts before birth of baby and completed (formation of secondary oocyte), if there is fertilization.

The oocyte with follicular cells surrounding them is known as primordial follicle. The primary oocyte does not complete their first

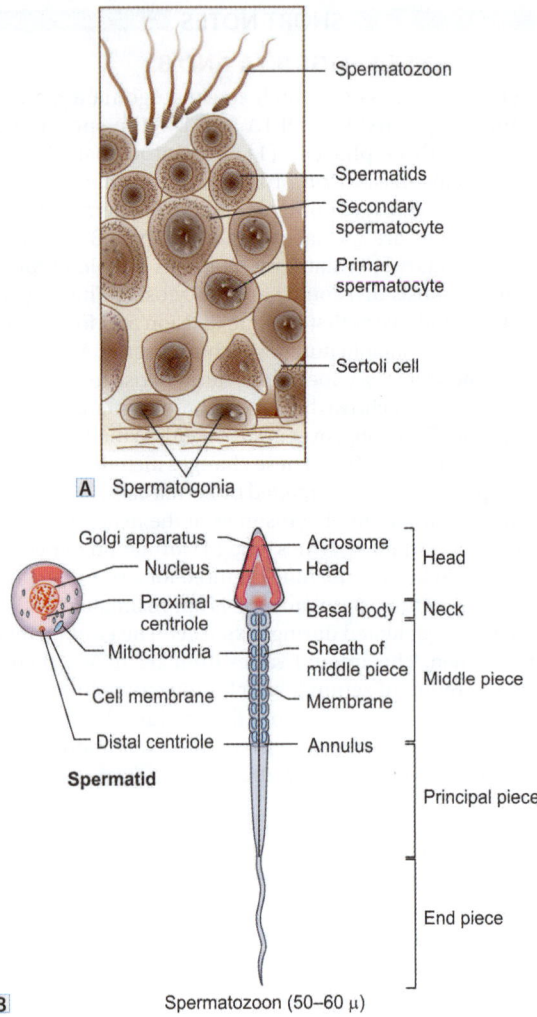

Figs 9.1A and B: Spermatogenesis

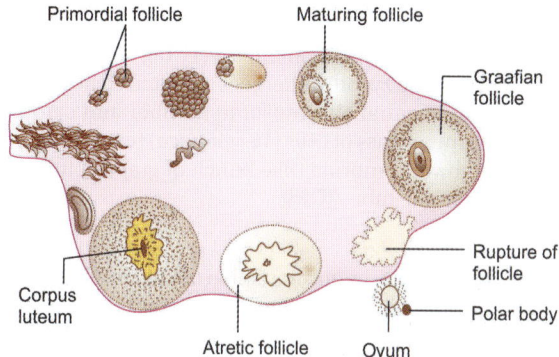

Fig. 9.2: Oogenesis

meiotic division and remains in diplotene stage until puberty. With the onset of puberty, a number of follicles begin to mature, with each ovarian cycle, but only one of them reaches to full maturity. During the process, one primary oocyte gives rise to one ovum (instead of four) and three polar bodies. Mature ovum with its follicular cells is known as Graafian follicle, which lies at the surface of the ovary and can be examined by laparoscope.

CAPACITATION

It is the final step of maturation of spermatozoa in the female genital tract in the process of fertilization. It requires 7 hours of time.

- *Mechanism*: After approximation of gametes (sperm and ovum) in the female genital tract the direct contact between them is necessary to break the three barriers of ovum (corona radiata, zona pellucida, and vitelline membrane). In this process, prior to penetration sperm has to undergo capacitation.
- Exact mechanism is unknown.
- The antigenic coating on the surface of the sperm may be involved to produce an immunological reaction between fertilizin derived from the oocyte and antifertilizin derived from spermatozoa.
- *Effects*: After capacitation sperm can undergo acrosomal reaction which is the next step to disintegrate the female gamete. In vitro fertilization capacitation is done by adding albumin (protein) in culture media.

MORULA (FIG. 9.3)

The zygote formed after fertilization, is very big cell. To restore the normal size of cell, the zygote undergoes repeated cleavage division. Each cell contains equal chromosome number and cytoplasmic volume. This forms a mass of cells (16 cell stage) resembling a bunch of mulberry, known as morula (like bunch of grapes). It lies within the isthmus of uterine tube. P.G.E.

BLASTOCYST (FIG. 9.4)

It is derived from morula by accumulation of fluid inside it. It has two parts—one is trophoblast and other embryoblast. Implantation on

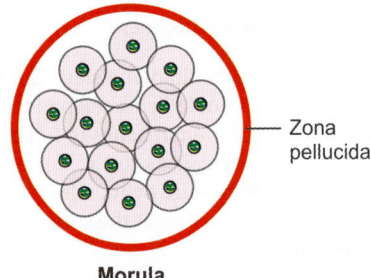

Morula

Fig. 9.3: Segmentation of the fertilized ovum

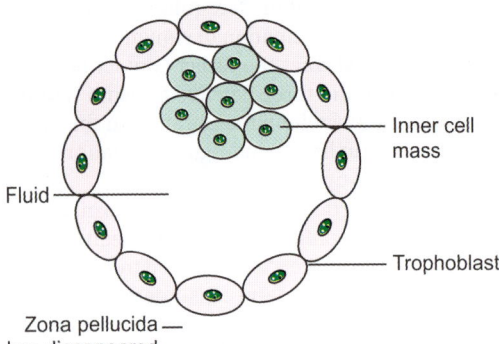

Fig. 9.4: Formation of blastocyst (early stage)

blastocyst in uterine body takes place on sixth or seventh day after fertilization. Implantation anywhere in the upper part of uterine cavity is considered as normal. Sometimes blastocyst is embedded in abnormal situation which may be extrauterine and intrauterine. If blastocyst is implanted in lower uterine segment, it gives rise to placenta previa and if occurs in uterine tube, it is known as tubal pregnancy.

ZONA PELLUCIDA (FIG. 9.4)

It is a covering, surrounding the secondary oocyte.
- *Nature*: Chiefly polysaccharide.
- *Appearance*: After adolescence when the secondary oocytes formed in the ovary zona pellucida appears.
- *Disappearance*: Normally it disappears on 5th day after fertilization and then the blastocyst undergoes implantation.

NOTOCHORD (FIG. 9.5)

It is a flexible rod that defines in the midline of embryo. It is the forerunner of vertebral column and extends from prochordal plate up to primitive tail end of embryo. It is formed by differentiation of head process. The notochordal process undergoes different changes that convert it first into a canal and finally back into rod-like solid structure which gives some amount of rigidity. Most of the notochord disappears in future. In adults remnants of notochord persist as apical ligament of odontoid process and nucleus pulposus of intervertebral disc.

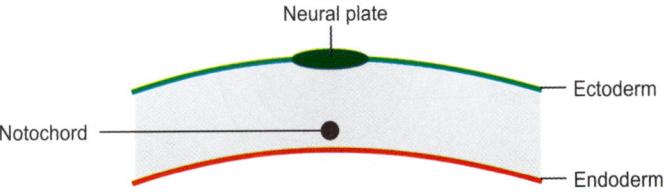

Fig. 9.5: Development of neural tube anterior and posterior neuropores. Note the circulation of the amniotic fluid into the cavity of the neural tube when the neuropores get closed. The amniotic fluid gets trapped within embryonic body

CHORION

Literally chorion means skin (outer covering) (Figs 9.6A and B). It is an important membrane, which surrounds embryo. It is formed by parietal layer of extraembryonic mesoderm and the trophoblast. The chorion plays an important role in childbirth. It appears in 24 days of development. It consists of chorion frondosum and chorion

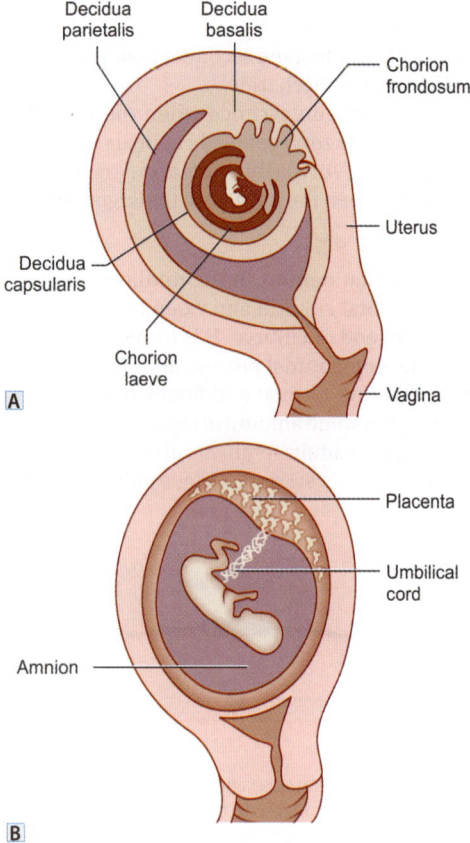

Figs 9.6A and B: Chorion

laeve. Chorionic frondosum forms placenta and gives nutrition to developing embryo. Abnormal growth of chorion is known as hydatidiform mole with nondevelopment of embryo. Most moles are benign but 15% invades and destroy myometrium.

ALLANTOIS OR ALLANTOENTERIC DIVERTICULUM (FIG. 9.7)

It lies first within the body stalk and later within umbilical cord. It is diverticulum from dorsocaudal part of yolk sac. It appears on 15th day of development. Vascularization of embryo starts first in this region. Allantois is vestigial organ in human. Its remnant is known as urachus. Its abnormalities are, patent urachus, urachal cyst, and urachal fistula (Fig. 9.7).

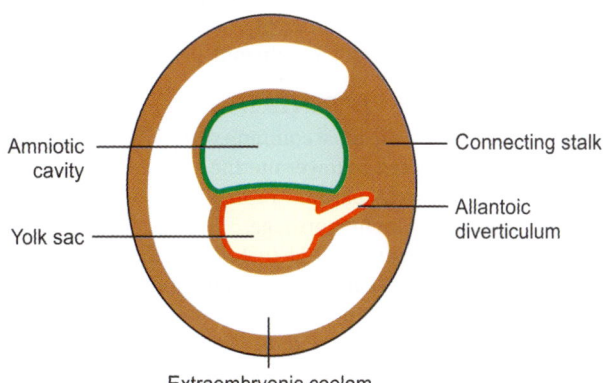

Fig. 9.7: (A) Allantoenteric diverticulum arising from yolk sac; (B) Allantoenteric diverticulum projecting from hindgut into the connecting stalk

GASTRULATION

The appearance of three germ layers are known as gastrulation (i.e. ectoderm, mesoderm and endoderm).

Embryoblast (Inner Cell Mass) Derivatives P.G.E.

- Ectoderm gives rise to:
  - Central nervous system

- Peripheral nervous system
- Sensory epithelium of eye, ear and nose
- Skin (includes hair and nails)
- Pituitary, mammary and sweat glands
- Enamel of teeth
- Mesoderm gives rise to:
  - Dermis of skin and subcutaneous tissue
  - Cartilage and bones
  - All supporting tissue of body
  - Vascular system (arteries, veins, lymphatic channel)
  - Urogenital system (except urinary bladder)
  - Spleen, cortex of suprarenal glands
- Endoderm gives rise to:
  - Epithelial lining of gastrointestinal tract, respiratory tract and urinary bladder, tympanic cavity, auditory tube
  - Parenchyma of thyroid, parathyroid, liver and pancreas.

DIFFERENT TYPES OF PLACENTA (FIG. 9.8)

1. *Placenta previa*: It is the most common variety. They are (1 in 250 births). It is implanted in lower uterine segment that gives rise to placenta which may partially or totally block the internal os producing antepartum hemorrhage.
2. *Placenta succenturiata rare (1 in 1,000 births)*: One or more small lobes (accessory) lies away from main mass connected by membrane containing umbilical blood vessels.
3. *Large placenta (weight more than 500 g)*: It is seen in case of maternal diabetes, Rh incompatibility and syphilis.
4. *Circumvallate placenta*: The fetal membrane instead of being attached to extreme periphery of the placenta there is whitish strong band lies in the periphery. The central part of fetal surface is normal.
5. *Battledore placenta (1 in 1,000 births)*: The umbilical cord is attached in eccentric position instead of middle.
6. *Velamentous insertions of cords (1 in 5,000 births)*: When umbilical cord is attached to fetal membrane.
7. *Bipartite or tripartite*: It shows two or three almost equal lobes lying each other with connecting vessels.

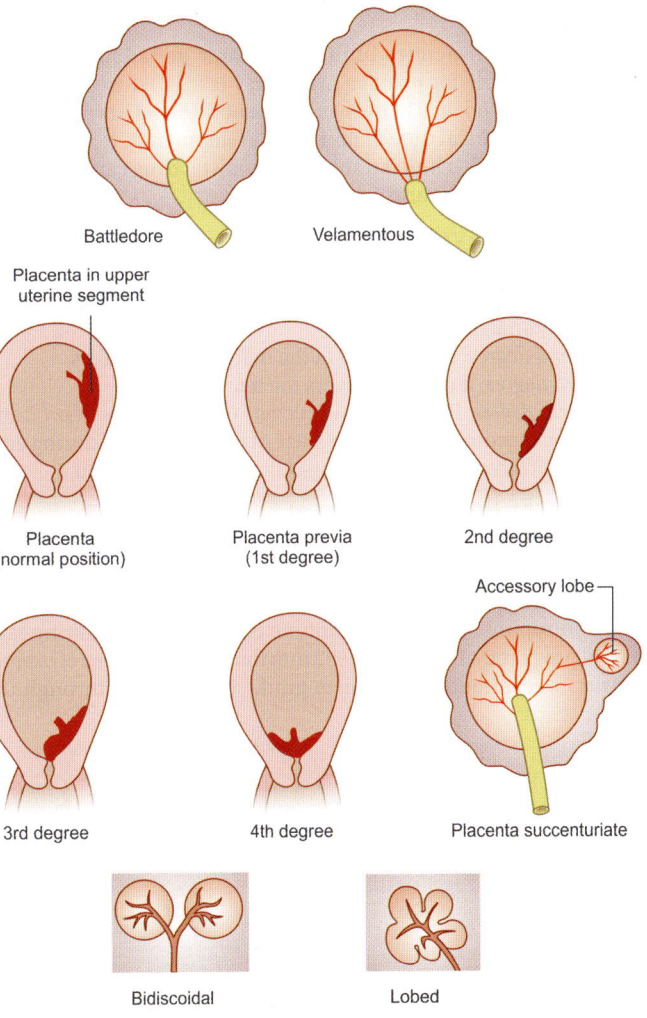

Fig. 9.8: Different types of placenta

Clinical Anatomy

1. Trophoblast secretes human chorionic gonadotropin which is responsible for positive pregnancy test in 1st week, after the missed period. It is known as pregnancy test or Gravindex test.
2. The most critical time of prenatal development is from 4th week to 8th week. So clinician should administer drug carefully in this period to prevent organ anomaly.

PLACENTA PREVIA (FIG. 9.8)

There are four types of placenta previa:
1. *First degree*: It occupies the lower uterine segment but fails to reach the internal os.
2. *Second degree*: It is situated at the margin of internal os.
3. *Third degree*: It partially covers the internal os.
4. *Fourth degree*: Placenta totally covers the internal os. It produces severe bleeding during early stage of pregnancy and during early stage of labor. Fourth degree requires cesarean section.

PLACENTAL BARRIER (FIG. 9.9)

Placental barrier is the membrane that separates fetal blood from maternal blood (Fig. 9.9). It is made up of endothelium of fetal blood vessels, surrounding mesoderm, cytotrophoblast and syncytiotrophoblast. This membrane is very thin and during later part of pregnancy, it is about 0.002 mm thick. Interchanges of oxygen, nutrition, respiration, and waste product takes place through this

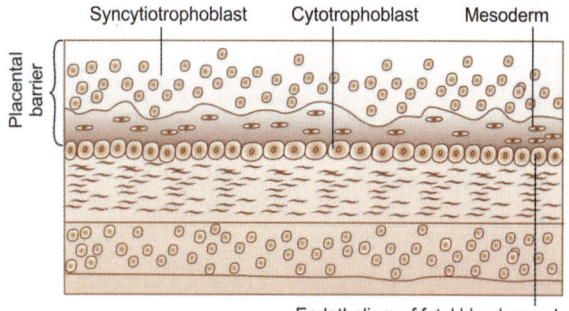

Fig. 9.9: Placental barrier

membrane. Maternal antibody passes to fetus which protects the fetus from bacterial infections. But viruses like rubella and herpes simplex can diffuse across placenta from mother and form malformation of fetus. Certain drugs like thalidomide, tetracycline, etc. can pass through the barrier and can damage the fetal tissue. So one should take precaution about drug administration during pregnancy.

UMBILICAL CORD (FIG. 9.10)

It connects abdominal wall of fetus with the fetal side of placenta (Fig. 9.10). At full term, it measures about 50 cm in length and 2 cm in breadth. The cord is twisted and presents false knots. Umbilical cord is formed from body stalk (Fig. 9.10). It appears as 5th week of intrauterine life and a vascular pathway between fetus with placenta. It consists of two umbilical arteries and a vein surrounded by Wharton's jelly. It is cut off after birth. Too short cord or too long cord may produce difficulty during birth of baby. Too long cord may encircle the fetal neck and produce fetal distress. The blood in the umbilical cord is rich in stem cells (blood forming cells). It has got great clinical importance. It will replace the bone marrow transplant and is more easy method.

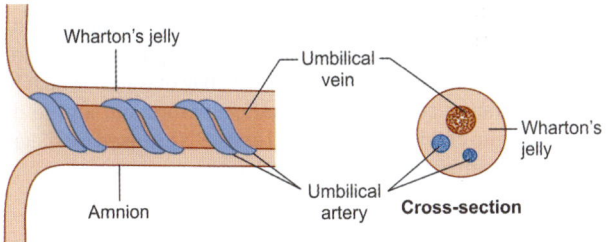

Fig. 9.10: Umbilical cord

AMNION (FIG. 9.11)

A thin membrane which encloses embryo and umbilical cord. Amniotic sac is membranous sac, filled with amniotic fluid and present on fetal surface. It appears at the beginning of 2nd week. The membrane is known as amnion, the cavity it encloses is called amniotic cavity. The

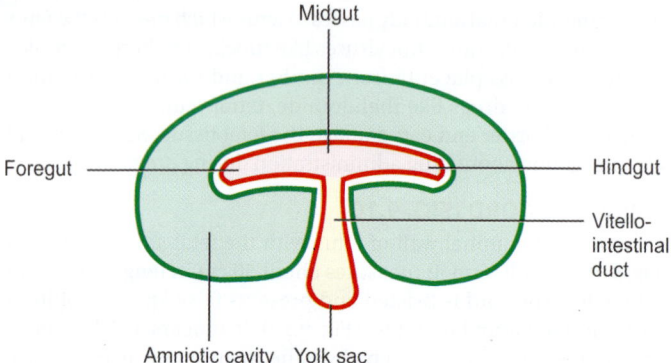

Fig. 9.11: With formation of head and tail folds, foregut, midgut and the hindgut are formed. Note that the amniotic cavity covers the embryonic disc on all sides except at the umbilical opening

fluid inside it is amniotic fluid. With the folding of embryo, amniotic cavity enlarges and encroaches on all aspects of embryo. The amniotic fluid is secreted first by amniogenic cells, the fetal urine and slight secretion from fetal tracheobronchial tree are added in its volume. At the full term, the amniotic fluid measures about 1,500–2,000 cc. The amniotic fluid more than 2,000 cc is known as hydramnios and less than 1,000 cc is known as oligohydramnios (oligo means "scanty"). Obstetrician terminology of amnion is "the bag of water" which helps fetus to maintain a constant hydrostatic environment and to dilate cervix during the childbirth. Both fluid and cells are used for diagnosis of genetic abnormalities of embryo and fetus.

MECKEL'S DIVERTICULUM (FIG. 9.12)

The extraembryonic part of yolk sac is connected with the midgut by vitellointestinal duct. This part normally disappears. But when it is present, the persistent proximal part is known as Meckel's diverticulum. It is present in 2% of cases, 2 inch in length, attached 2 feet away from ileocecal junction at antimesenteric border.

Clinical Importance

It is the site of development of peptic ulcer when gastric tissue are present in it. It may cause intestinal obstruction and its acute

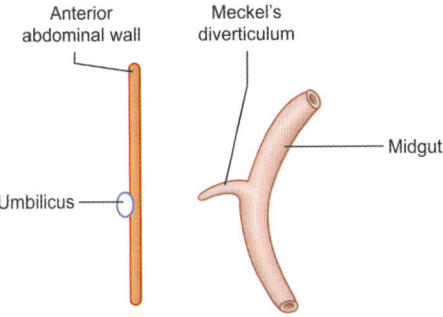

Fig. 9.12: Meckel's diverticulum

infection may resemble appendicitis. When there is patent Meckel's diverticulum small intestinal contents may be discharged at the umbilicus.

ECTOPIC PREGNANCY (FIG. 9.13)

It means pregnancy in abnormal position. It may be intrauterine or extrauterine. 90% of ectopic pregnancy is tubal pregnancy. Other

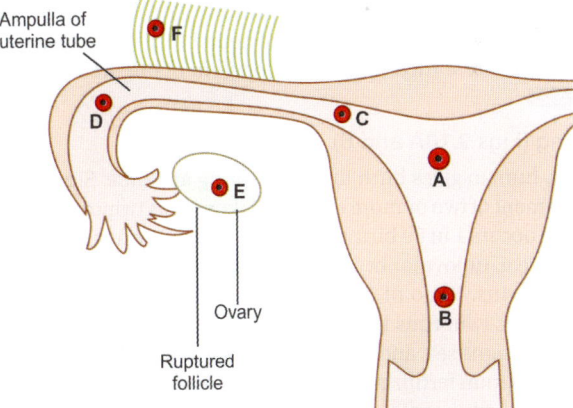

Fig. 9.13: Sites of abnormal implantation of the fertilized ovum, A- Normal, B- Placenta previa, C - Interstitial type, D- Tubal, E- Ovarian, F- Peritoneal

varieties are pregnancy at internal os, mesentery or omentum and ovary. In tubal pregnancy embryo does not survive beyond 2 months of gestation. After 2 months there is rupture of tubal pregnancy which causes severe pain in abdomen and alarming hemorrhage leading to the state of shock. Emergency operation of removal of uterine tube at affected site may save the patient.

SOMITE (SEE FIG. 9.15)

Concomitant to ectodermal development, intraembryonic mesoderm shows three subdivisions by the appearance of a groove on the medial aspect. The part medial to the groove, mesoderm is cubical, known as *paraxial mesoderm which later forms somite*. It extends from cranial end of notochord to coccygeal end. Total number of somite may be 42–44. Out of which 4 are occipital, 8 cervical, 12 thoracic, 5 lumbar, 5 sacral, and 8–10 coccygeal. Age of the embryo can be determined as presomite stage, somite stage and postsomite stage. The somite divides into:

1. *Sclerotome*: Ventromedially forms vertebrae and ribs.
2. The *dermomyotome* or the muscle plate dorsolaterally. It produces the muscles of body wall and the dermis of skin.

Clinical Anatomy
- *Spina bifida*: When two-halves of neural arch fail to fuse.
- *Hemivertebra*: Incomplete development of one-half of vertebra.
  P.G.E.

Twining (Figs 9.14A and B)

Usually, human gives birth to one offspring at a time. Simultaneous development of two or more embryos is known as twining or multiple births. It occurs 1 in 80 births (approximately). Twins are of different varieties, e.g. uniovular or monozygotic, binovular or dizygotic and conjoint twins. Ratio of dizygotic and monozygotic twin is 70:30. Monozygotic twin runs in family (hereditary character) and the two twins are of same sex, and appearance, of same blood group. Dizygotic twin results from fertilization of two ova by two separate sperms. The twins are usually not of same sex and their appearance and character is different. Conjoint twins are those monozygotic twins which are joined with each other to a small or large extent due to incomplete

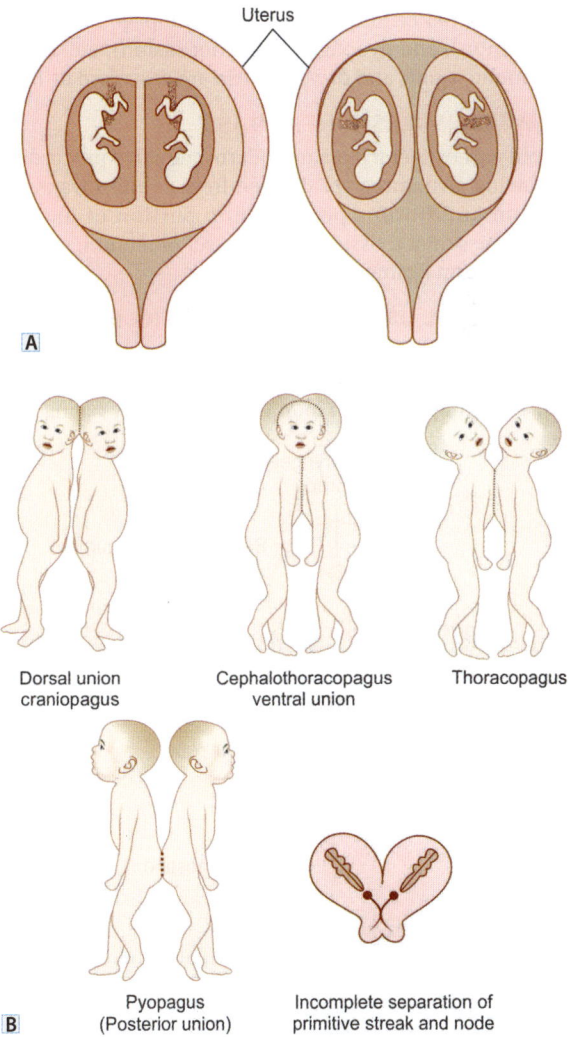

Figs 9.14A and B: Twining

separation of inner cell mass. They are craniopagus, thoracopagus (most common), and pyopagus (posterior fusion), etc. Difference between monozygotic and dizygotic twin are described in Table 9.1.

SEPTUM TRANSVERSUM (FIG. 9.15)

It is unsplit part of lateral plate mesoderm cranial to procordal plate. The following structures are derived from septum transversum: epicardium and fibrous pericardium; portion of diaphragm; esophageal mesentery; tissues within lesser omentum; sinusoids of liver and falciform ligament.

PHYSIOLOGICAL UMBILICAL HERNIA (FIG. 9.16)

There is a stage of embryonic life when a portion of coelomic cavity exists outside the body in the umbilical cord, known as extraembryonic coelom. The midgut forms a loop with a convexity facing forward.

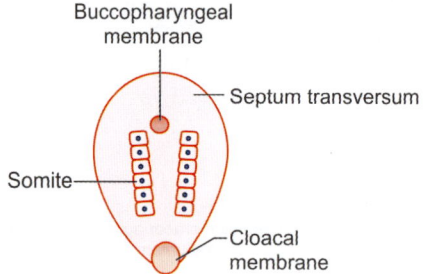

Fig. 9.15: Mesodermal plate

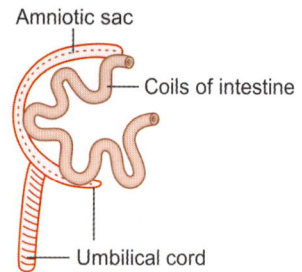

Fig. 9.16: Physiological umbilical hernia

Table 9.1: Differences between monozygotic and dizygotic twin

Monozygotic twin	Dizygotic twin
1. Single ovum and single sperm fertilize	1. Different ovum are fertilized by two different sperm
2. Shares the same placenta	2. Two embryology form their separate placenta
3. Have the same chromosomal karyotype	3. Have different chromosomal karyotype
4. Are always of the same sex	4. They may be of the same sex or different sex

It grows so rapidly and the developing liver is too large that the intraembryonic coelom is small to accommodate them. So, a part of the loop comes out into the extraembryonic coelom in the umbilical cord forming a temporary physiological umbilical hernia.

When physiological umbilical hernia persists abnormally, the child is born with loops of intestine hanging out of the umbilicus. This condition is called "exomphalos or omphalocele".

In this congenital hernia, the muscle layer and skin are absent in the region of umbilicus. The contents of the intestine are covered by peritoneum and amnion only.

NONFUSION OF MÜLLERIAN DUCT

Both sided Müllerian duct fusses to form uterus and part of vagina in female. If there is defect in fusion of Müllerian duct of both side along the normal fusion line, thus may leads to formation of defective uterus and vagina depending up to the degree of nonfusion as follows (Fig. 9.17):

- Double uterus: It occurs when there is complete nonfusion of the Müllerian ducts. It may be associated with or without double vagina.
- *Septate uterus*: Sometimes uterus looks normal externally but is separated internally by a thin septum due to defective fusion.
- *Bicornuate uterus*: Nonfusion involves only the upper part and duplicate occur only in upper part of the body of the uterus.
- *Bicornuate uterus with rudimentary horn*: When growth of one paramesonephric duct is retarded and does not fuse with other one this happens. The rudimentary horn may not communicate with uterine cavity.

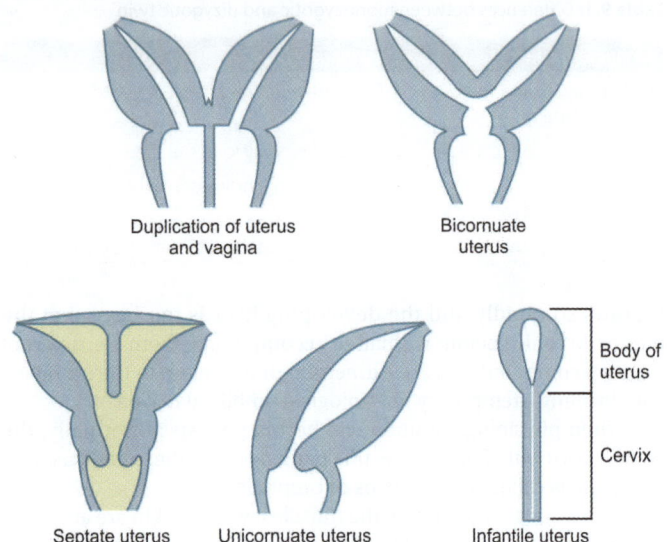

Fig. 9.17: Anomalies of the uterus

ABNORMAL FORM OR TERATOLOGY

Introduction

Teratology is a branch of science that deals with abnormal prenatal development. Factors that cause anomalies are known as teratogens.

- The normal development is an integrated process of cellular differentiation, increase in number of cells, and growth. The overall processes and induction of particular organizer is performed by genes of zygote (form blue print of life) and guided by environment both internal and external.
- The susceptibility to a teratogen and the degree of damage depends upon the stage of embryonic development.
- Teratogenic agents act by influencing metabolic processes.
- The first two weeks, i.e. germinal period is more or less resistant to teratogens.
- From 3rd to 8th weeks, i.e. the period of organogenesis, this period is highly susceptible to teratogen. Organ deformity limbs anomalies like amelia and meromelia may develop.

Embryology

- The agents that act as teratogens are as follows:
  - *Viruses*:
    - HIV
    - Rubella
    - Cytomegalovirus
    - Influenza virus.
  - *Bacteria*: Syphilis producing bacteria
  - *Radiation*
  - *Drugs:*
    - Vitamin A and analogs
    - Thalidomide (antiemetic)
    - Anticonvulsants
    - Antipsychotics
    - Social drugs like cigarette, alcohol and Phencyclidine (PCP)
    - Anticoagulant like warfarin.
  - *Maternal hormones*:
    - Androgenic agent
    - Maternal diabetes.

DEVELOPMENT OF CERTAIN IMPORTANT ORGANS (SPECIAL EMBRYOLOGY)

Development of Heart (Fig. 9.18)

Heart is a hollow muscular organ, which pumps blood continuously throughout the body, till death. The development of heart takes place in cardiogenic area below the stomodeum. Primitive angioblastic tissues fuse together to form two paramedian heart tubes (Fig. 9.10).

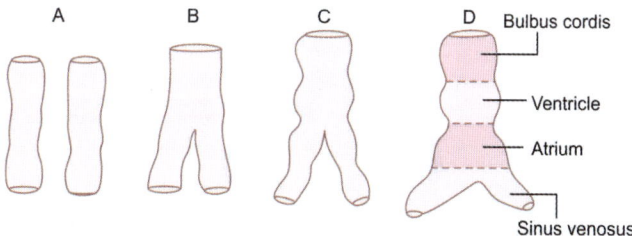

Figs 9.18A to D: (A) Right and left heart tubes. (B to D) Progressive fusion of tubes from cranial to caudal end. Fusion of sinus venosus is partial

Two tubes fuse to form a single heart tube. Single heart tube undergoes enormous expansion and five chambered heart is formed. From caudal to cranial aspect, they are sinus venosus, primitive atrium, primitive ventricle, bulbus cordis and truncus arteriosus. Further growth within this limited area (pericardial cavity) produces bending of heart tube. As a result of bending, the venous end is carried dorsally and in cephalic position. The bulbus cordis tends to lose its identity and to merge with ventricle on one hand and truncus arteriosus on other hand. The common atrium is partitioned into primitive right and left atria by means of development of interatrial septum and primitive ventricle is divided by development of interventricular septum (Figs 9.18 and 9.19). Cardiac development is controlled by a group of regulatory genes and transcription factor.

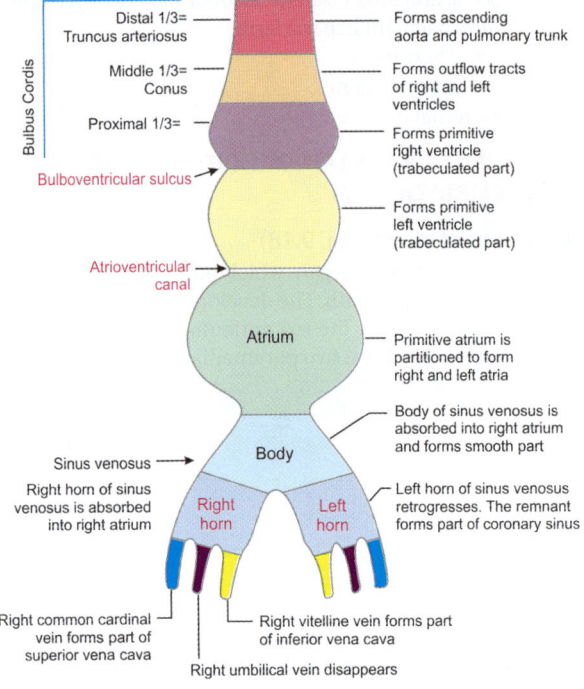

Fig. 9.19: Main subdivisions of heart tube and their fate

Development of Interatrial Septum (Figs 9.20 and 9.21)

It is developed from three sources: (1) septum primum, (2) septum intermedium, and (3) septum secundum. Atrium communicates with primitive ventricle through atrioventricular opening. There is development of two swelling from the dorsal and ventral aspect of atrioventricular orifice known as ventral and dorsal endocardial cushion. The cushion fuses to form a broad anteroposterior partition—the septum intermedium. During the same time (6th week) from the roof and dorsal wall of primitive atrium septum primum (an endocardial fold) develops and it grows caudally. Its lower margin is free and concave. The two ends of the septum fuses to the anterior and posterior ends of septum intermedium and a foramen exists in the middle—named ostium primum. Gradually, there is closure of ostium primum in 7th week. The foramen secundum permits a transseptal blood flow in both directions, but it is necessary to convey most of the blood to left atrium in order to develop left half of heart. The function of fetal lung is nil. There is disintegration by apoptosis of upper and posterior part of septum primum and formation of ostium secundum. So in the later part of fetal life, ostium secundum is guarded by a flap

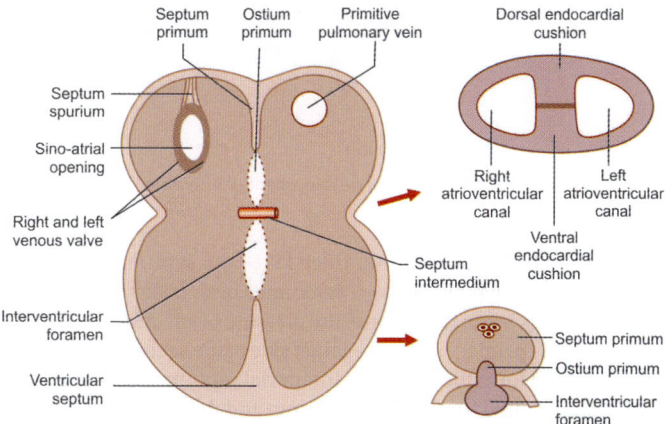

Fig. 9.20: Development interatrial and interventricular septum in various stages

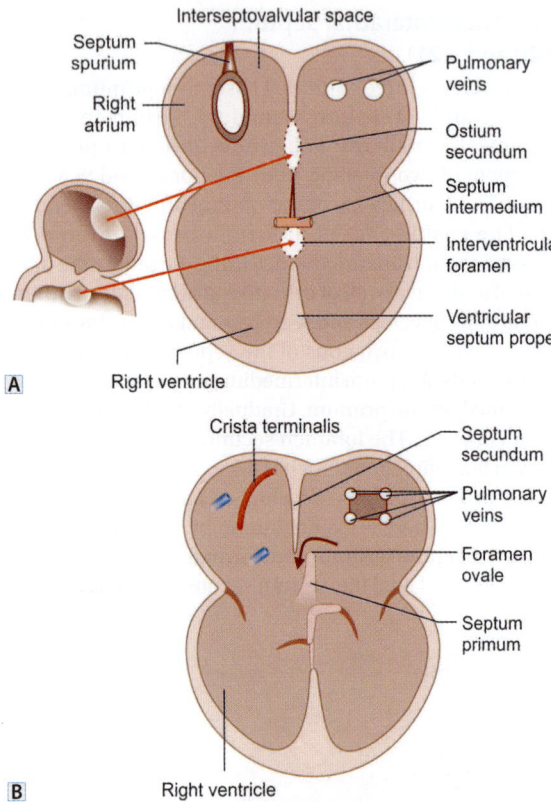

Figs 9.21A and B: Stages of development of interatrial septum

valve due to growth of another thick fold—the septum secundum. Ostium secundum then is known as foramen ovale. After birth of baby, when the lungs begin to function, the pressure of left atrium increases and forces the primary septum against side of the secondary septum. They fuse and form the complete interatrial septum. P.G.E. The fossa ovalis is developed from septum primum and the limbus fossa ovalis developed from lower free margin of the septum secundum.

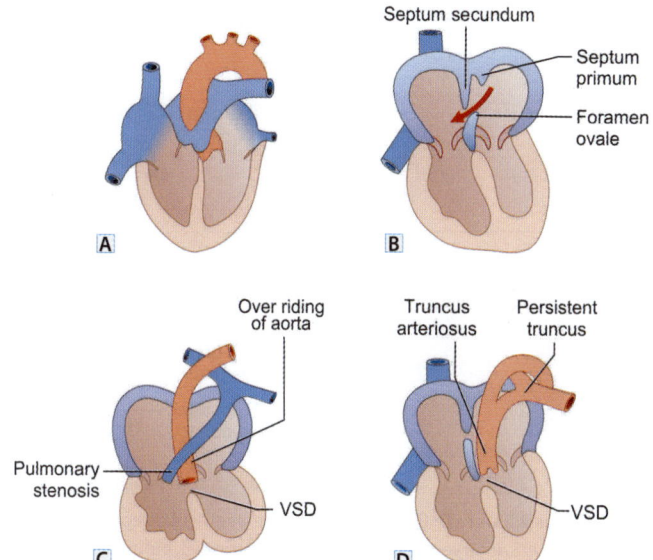

Figs 9.22A to D: Various anomalies of heart (A) Normal heart; (B) Atrial septal defect; (C) Fallot's tetralogy; (D) Persistent truncus arteriosus
Abbreviation: VSD, Ventiricular septal defect

Clinical Anatomy

- Common type of malformation is atrial septal defect (ASD) (Fig. 9.22). In 25% of individuals small opening exists, known as probe patency of foramen ovale. It is insignificant clinically.
- When the defect is large, the left atrial blood passes to right atrium and 50% cases die. If the right atrial blood passes to the left, there is cyanosis (bluish discoloration). Ratio of preponderance is female : male = 2:1.

Development of Interventricular Septum (Figs 9.23A to D)

It is developed from three sources:

1. *Ventricular septum proper*: Develops from floor and ventral wall of primitive ventricle. It forms muscular part of interventricular septum. It does not grow as far as septum intermedium. A foramen exists in between them.

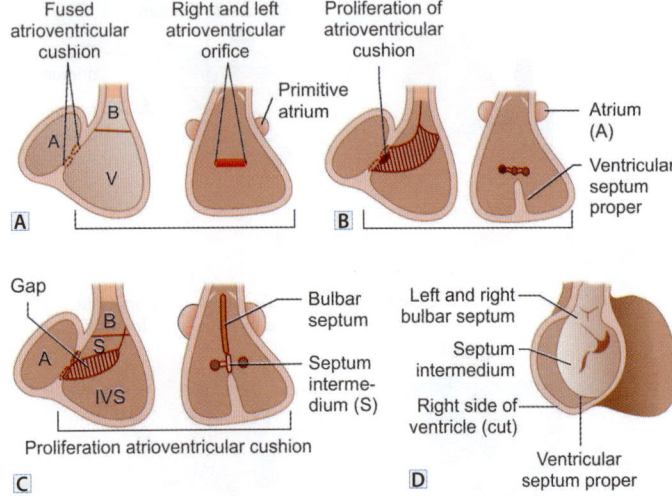

Figs 9.23A to D: Development of interventricular septum
Abbreviations: IVS, interventricular septum, V, ventricle; B, bulbus cordis

2. *Proximal bulbar septum*: This septum partially closes the upper part of ventricular foramen.
3. *Septum intermedium*: The area between ventricular septum proper and proximal bulbar septum is closed by growth of right edge of septum intermedium.

Clinical Anatomy

- *Persistent interventricular foramen*: It is due to the defect in development of membranous part. It may be associated with other cardiac defect. Blood flow from left to right. Small opening is asymptomatic. Large defect can shorten life. It is a congenital malformation (10% of all congenital heart disease).
- *Fallot's tetralogy* P.G.E. *(Fig. 9.22)*: Here four cardiac anomalies are seen—(1) pulmonary stenosis, (2) displacement of aortic orifice, (3) ventricular septal defect (VSD), (4) hypertrophy of right ventricle. It is associated with dextrocardia and right-sided aortic arch. It is due to unequal division of conus cordis.

Aortic Arches and Its Derivatives (Figs 9.24A to D)

The entire cardiovascular system is developed from mesoderm. Pharyngeal arches develop during 4th week. Primitive aorta

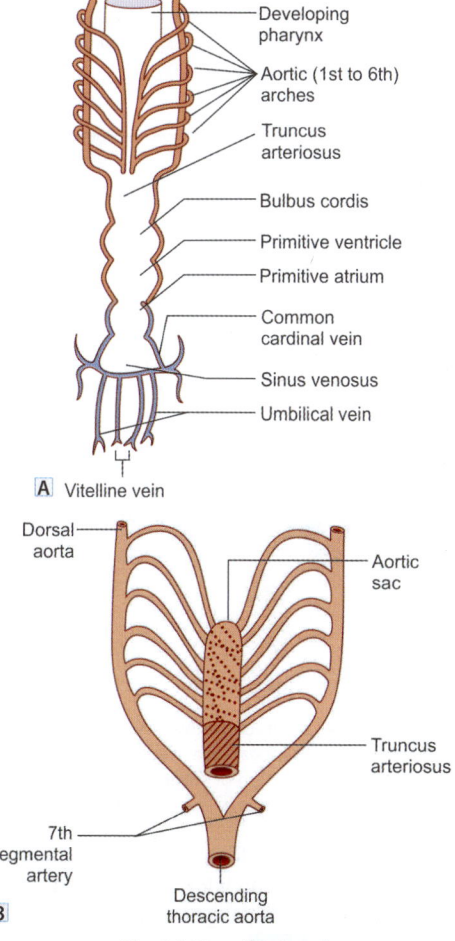

Figs 9.24A and B: Contd...

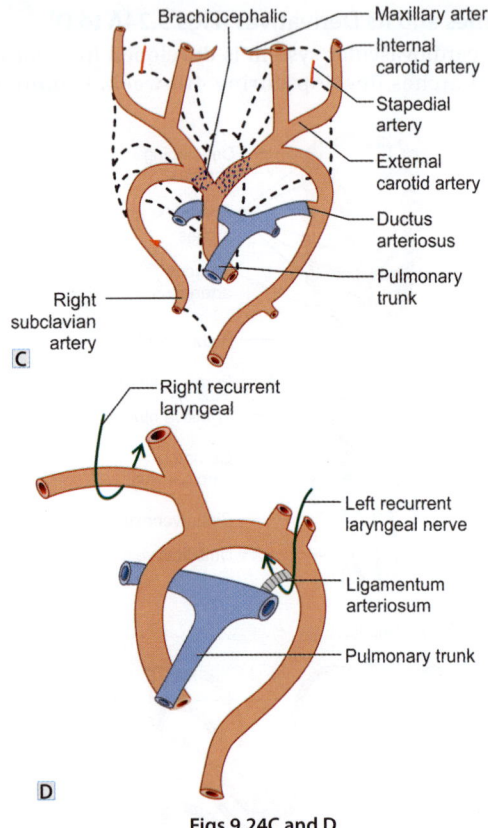

Figs 9.24C and D

Figs 9.24A to D: Aortic arches and its derivatives. (A) The formation of aortic arch arteries; (B) Aortic arches; (C) Disappearance of aortic arches are represented by dotted line; and (D) Changing pattern of aortic arches and relations of nerves with them

develops on either side of developing vertebral column encircling the developing pharynx. They arch forward and connected with the developing heart. There are six pairs of aortic arches but they do not develop at the same time. P.G.E.

Embryology

- 1st aortic arch disappears and in adult it persists as part of maxillary artery. P.G.E.
- The 2nd arch also disappears. It persists as stapedial artery.
- The 3rd arch forms common carotid artery and proximal part of internal carotid artery on both sides.
- The 4th arch on the left side forms a part of arch of aorta. On the right side forms a part of right subclavian artery. P.G.E.
- The 5th aortic arch disappears completely.
- The 6th arch is also known as pulmonary arch. On the left side it forms: (1) proximal part of left pulmonary artery, (2) ductus arteriosus (after birth it is transformed into ligamentum arteriosum).
- As the right side 6th aortic arch forms:
  - Proximal part of right pulmonary artery
  - The regression of dorsal part of the right 6th aortic arch causes the right recurrent laryngeal nerve to hook around the right subclavian artery as in left where arch (6th) due to persistence of dorsal part the left recurrent laryngeal nerve hooks the ligamentum arteriosum.
- During 8th week these are transformed into the final fetal arterial arrangement.

It develops at the end of 4th week of intrauterine life from mesoderm ventral to the foregut sources. It is developed from three sources (from before backward):

1. *Left horn of aortic sac*: It forms the part of the arch between brachiocephalic trunk and left common carotid artery.
2. *Left 4th aortic arch*: It forms the part of arch of aorta between left common carotid artery and ductus arteriosus.
3. *Left dorsal aorta*: It forms the rest of the arch up to ascending aorta.

Clinical Anatomy

4. Coarctation (narrowing) of aorta. It may be preductal or postductal.
5. *Aortic knuckle*: A convex margin is found in plain chest X-ray known as aortic knuckle. It is formed by the distal part of the arch of aorta.

Development of Alimentary System (Figs 9.25A and B)

Most of the alimentary system is developed from endoderm of definitive yolk sac during folding of embryo at 4th week of intrauterine life. The part within the head fold of embryo forms foregut, within the tail fold is the hindgut, in between two lateral folds forms midgut (Figs 9.25A and B). Foregut is initially separated from stomodeum by

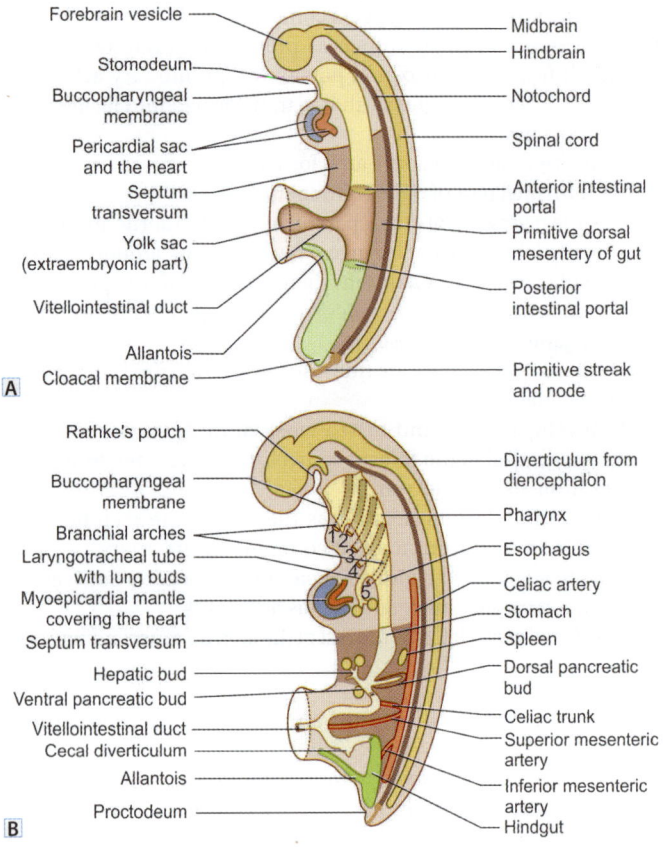

Figs 9.25A and B: Alimentary system

buccopharyngeal membrane. It ruptures by the end of 4th week. P.G.E. The mucous membrane of gut is formed from endoderm, muscle coat and outer coat is formed by invading splanchnopleuric layer of lateral plate of mesoderm. The glandular accessory organs (liver, pancreas, salivary glands, and gallbladder) are formed from outpocketing of foregut endoderm. Development of individual organs are discussed on page 337.

Development of Face (Fig. 9.26)

Face is developed as a result of changes around the stomodeum (oral) aperture. In the 5th week of intrauterine life, the stomodeum is deepened by the appearance of five processes around it. The process of elevations are the frontonasal process above, the right and left maxillary process (arising from first arch) from sides, and right and left mandibular process below. Within the frontonasal process, two swellings (olfactory) appear which divide the process into one median nasal and two lateral nasal processes. Median nasal process gives rise to philtrum of upper lip, premaxilla with four incisor teeth and nasal septum. The right and left mandibular processes meet in the midline and form lower lip and lower jaw. Fusion of frontonasal process with right and left maxillary process forms upper lip. The cheeks are formed by fusion of the posterior part of maxillary and mandibular process.

Clinical Anatomy
Failure of fusion completely of partly leads to various forms of harelip.

Development of Palate (Figs 9.27 and 9.28) P.G.E.

Palate is developed by fusion of right and left shelf-like palatine process which arises from maxillary processes (secondary palate) with premaxilla (developed from frontonasal process (primary palate). The two palatal processes unite with each other and with nasal septum from before backward. Deficiency in fusion leads to various forms of cleft palate. It may be partial or complete. Arrest in union varies from uvula to gum. In the latter case, the cleft runs between lateral incisor and canine teeth. Complete cleft palate produces nasal regurgitation of milk and needs early repair. The cleft palate is due to administration of teratogen during 7th–8th week of intrauterine life. The cleft lip and palate are the most common congenital anomalies of head and neck. It occurs in 1 per 750 live births.

330 Surgical Anatomy

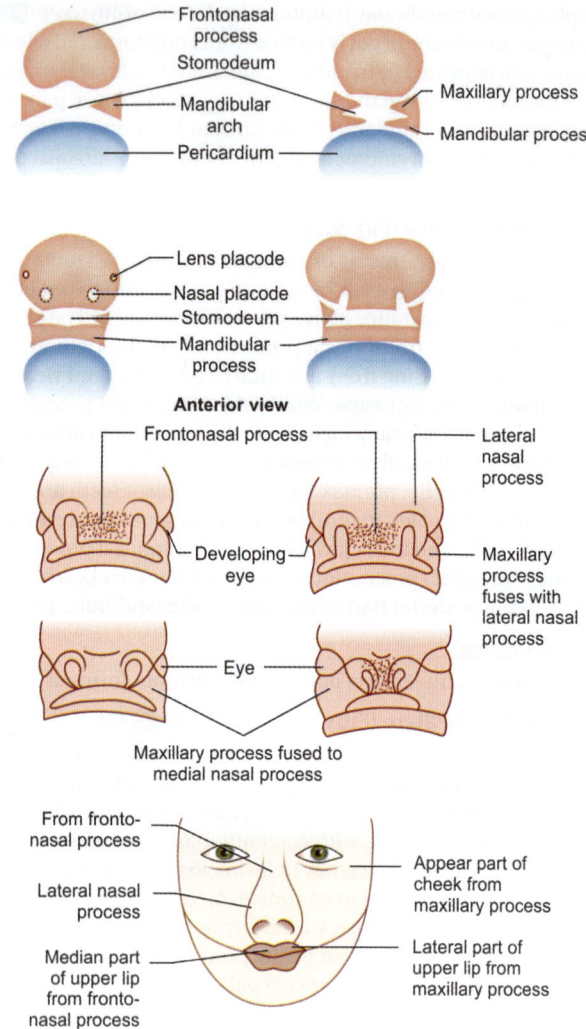

Fig. 9.26: Development of face

Embryology

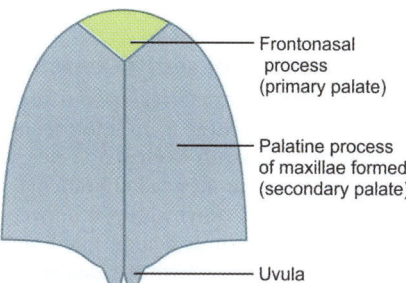

Fig. 9.27: Development of palate

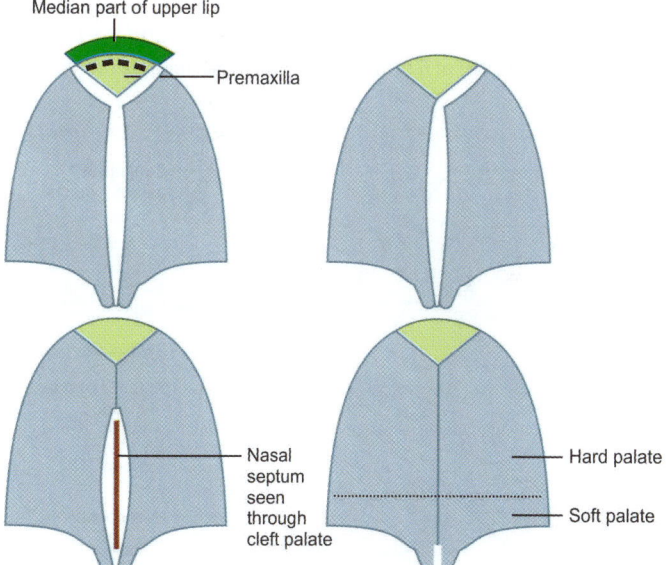

Fig. 9.28: Types of cleft palate

NERVES

Branchial (Pharyngeal) Arches and Its Derivatives (Fig. 9.28)

The secondary mesoderm of the neck region consists of only paraxial and lateral plate mesoderm. There is no intermediate mesoderm. Lateral plate mesoderm has no cavity. A series of condensed mesoderm forms six pairs of arches called branchial arches which pushes the pericardial cavity downward. In between the arches, there are gaps which have got only ectodermal lining outside and endodermal lining within. Due to growth of mesodermal arches, 5 cleft develop externally known as branchial cleft (one on each side), while endodermal furrows on the inner aspect forms 5 pairs of pharyngeal pouches. Each branchial arch gives rise to skeletal element, myotome, nerve of the arch, and artery of the arch.

Derivatives (Fate) of 6 Branchial Arches (Figs 9.29 and 9.30)

The derivatives (fate) of 6 branchial arches described in Table 9.2.

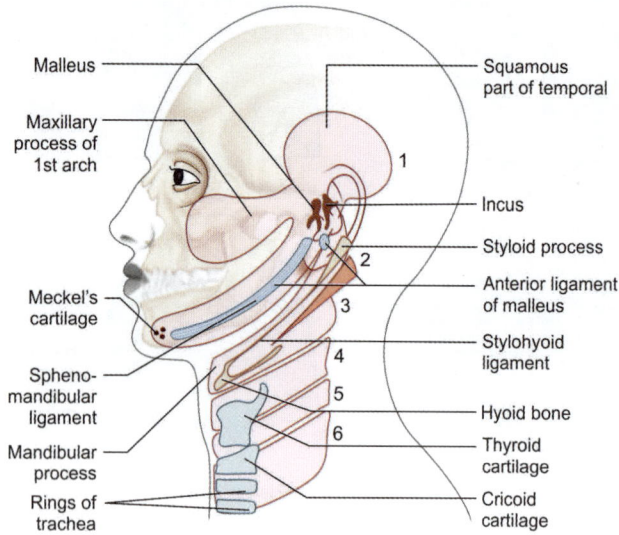

Fig. 9.29: Derivatives of branchial arch

Table 9.2: Derivatives (fate) of 6 branchial arches

Nerves	Skeletal derivative	Muscular derivative	Nerve	Artery
First arch	Meckel's cartilage—from which *incus and malleus is developed*. Anterior ligament of malleus, sphenomandibular ligament, *body of mandible and maxilla also developed*. P.G.E.	Muscles of mastication, mylohyoid, anterior belly of digastric, tensor veli palati, tensor tympani	1. Mandibular 2. Chorda tympani	Maxillary
Clinical anatomy	Treacher Collins syndrome: Unilateral agenesis of mandible shows weakness of muscle of mastication and there is facial asymmetry			
Second arch	Reichert's cartilage from which stapes, styloid process, stylohyoid ligament lesser cornu and superior part of hyoid bone is developed	Muscles of facial expression, stapedius, stylohyoid, and posterior belly of digastric	Facial	Stapedial artery
Third arch	Greater cornu and inferior parts of body of hyoid bone P.G.E.	Stylopharyngeus muscle	Glossopharyngeal	Common carotid and proximal part of internal carotid
Fourth arch	Thyroid cartilage and cuneiform cartilage	Cricothyroid muscle	Superior laryngeal	Left fourth arch forms part of arch of aorta and right fourth arch form part of right subclavian artery
Fifth arch	Disappear	No important remnant		
Sixth arch	Cricoid, epiglottis, and arytenoids cartilage	All intrinsic muscles of larynx except cricothyroid	Recurrent laryngeal	Ventral part both sides of right and left form pulmonary artery. Dorsal part form ligamentum arteriosum. Dorsal part of right disappears

Embryology

Development of Tongue (Fig. 9.30)

Tongue has composite origin. It is formed by different elements which do not appear simultaneously. Ventral end of first branchial arch are swollen and form the lingual swelling. Another swelling called

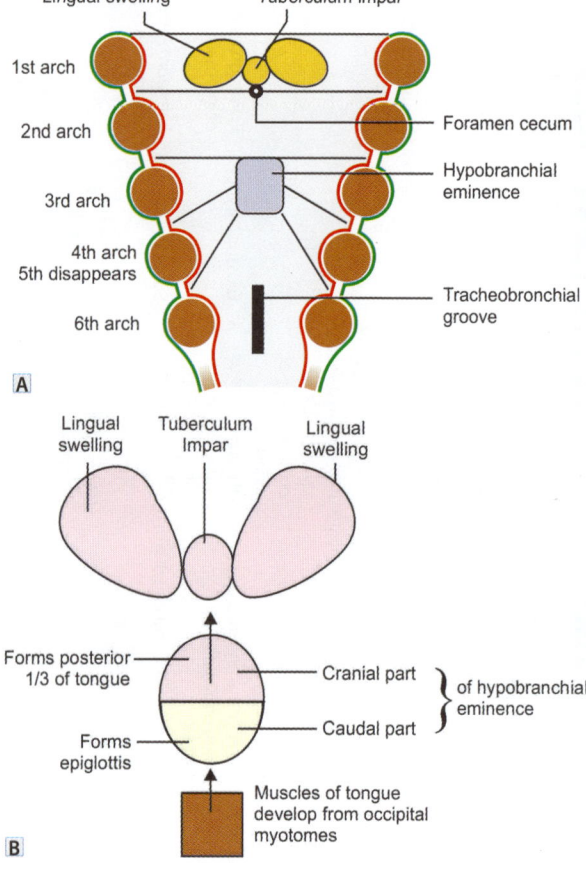

Figs 9.30A and B: (A) Development of tongue; (B) Diagrammatic

Table 9.3: Fate of pharyngeal pouches

Name of pouch	Derivatives
First: Ventral	Atrophy
Dorsal	Tubotympanic recess forming auditory tube, middle ear, mucous lining of tympanic membrane
Second: Ventral	Atrophy
Dorsal	Palatine tonsil and along with first pouch form part of tubotympanic recess
Third: Ventral	Thymus
Dorsal	Parathyroid (lower)
Fourth: Ventral	Lateral lobe of thyroid
Dorsal	Parathyroid (upper)
Fifth: Ventral P.G.E.	Ultimobranchial body: It forms parafollicular 'C' cells of thyroid

tuberculum impar appears in the floor of first pharyngeal pouch. These lingual swelling and tuberculum impar fuse to form anterior two-thirds of tongue. The posterior one-third of tongue develops from a cranial part median swelling called hypobranchial eminence (which is formed by fusion of mesoderm of ventral ends of second, third, and part of fourth branchial arches). At first, the regions of tongue, teeth, and lip are not demarcated from each other. Soon tongue forms a big mass, which is separated from rest of the mandibular process by formation of linguogingival sulcus. Gradually, this sulcus deepens and makes the inferior surface free from floor of mouth in anterior part. Muscles are developed from migrated occipital myotome, but some embryologist say muscles are developed from regional mesoderm. Taste buds are developed from nerve endings (Table 9.3).

Clinical Anatomy

- *Ankyloglossia or tongue tie*: It is due to deficiency in formation of alveolingual groove. Here frenulum is short. There may be certain difficulty in speech according to the degree of tie.
- *Bifid tongue*: A split in the anterior two-thirds due to failure of fusion of two lingual swellings.
- *Macroglossia*: Large tongue, due to enlarged plexuses and tissue spaces. In all these cases, there is difficulty in speech.

Development of Individual Organ in Short (Special Embryology) (Table 9.4)

Table 9.4: Development of individual organ

Names	Anatomical positions
Esophagus	It is developed from the part of foregut between pharynx and stomach. It is elongated during the formation of neck and caudal migration of septum transversum. Upper one-third musculature is developed from musculature of branchial apparatus. That's why upper one-third musculature is for voluntary type; rest is involuntary
Clinical anatomy	• *Tracheoesophageal fistula:* It communicates with trachea due to failure of caudal growth of tracheoesophageal septum • *Cardiospasm (achalasia):* It is due to neuromuscular in coordination at cardioesophageal junction. As a result proximal part dilates and distal part narrows down
Stomach	It is developed from fusiform dilatation from lower part of foregut during 4th or 5th week. It lies initially in the median plane. There is rapid growth of dorsal border which forms the greater curvature. Due to differential growth, there is alteration in size and shape of stomach. The original ventral border face upward and to the left and right surface becomes the anterosuperior surface and left surface becomes the posteroinferior surface, due to rotation of stomach about 90° around vertical axis
Clinical anatomy	Congenital hypertrophic pyloric stenosis. It is more common in male. Here the circular muscular coat undergoes hypertrophy and there is also neuromuscular in coordination. The child suffers from progressive vomiting. A mass is felt in the transpyloric plane 1 cm right to midline
Duodenum	The part of duodenum above the orifice of common bile duct is developed from foregut. The part below it is developed from proximal part of midgut
Jejunum and ileum	Midgut loop has got two segments. Above the superior mesenteric artery is known as prearterial segment and below the artery is known as postarterial segment. The whole of jejunum and most of the ileum have developed from prearterial segment. The terminal part is developed from postarterial segment near the cecal bud

Contd...

Embryology

Contd...

Names	Anatomical positions
Cecum and appendix (Fig. 9.31)	Developed from cecal bud which is developed from postarterial segment of midgut within 5th–10th week. In order to reach the right iliac fossa cecum and appendix undergoes 210° rotation. Within the abdomen cecum and appendix pass successively through the left iliac fossa, umbilical, subhepatic, right lumbar and finally reach the right iliac fossa
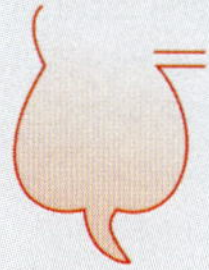 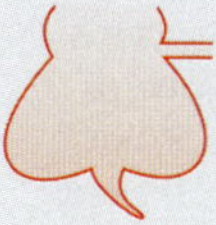 Clinical anatomy 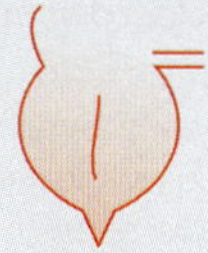	• According to shape adult cecum are of four types: (1) Fetal type (2%)—cecum is conical and appendix comes out from tip. (2) Infantile type (3%)—the two saccules of cecum are of equal in sizes, develops from each side of base of appendix. (3) Adult or normal type—in this case, the right saccules enlarges more than left one and appendix is located 2 cm below the ileocecal junction. (4) Exaggerated type—in this case, the right saccules enlarges and the left saccules atrophies. The appendix lies close to ileocecal junction • According to position (due to defect in the rotation of gut): The cecum with appendix may be in the following position—(1) in the left hypochondrium, and (2) below the right lobe of liver and left iliac fossa due to reverse rotation of the gut 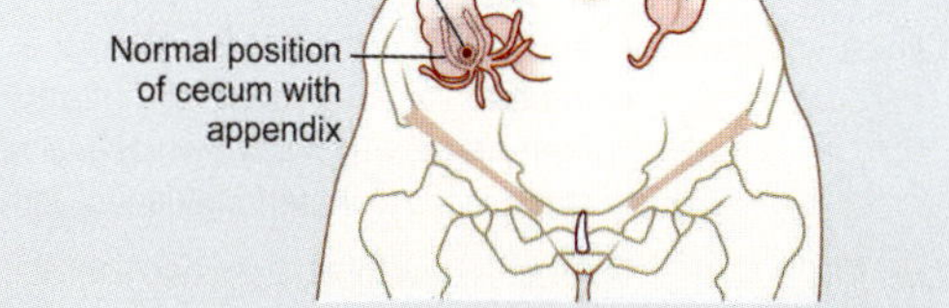

Fetal type

Normal type

Infantile type

Fig. 9.31: Normal and abnormal position of cecum with appendix

Contd...

Contd...

Names	Anatomical positions
Transverse colon: Right two-thirds of transverse colon	It is developed from two sources. Right two-third from caudal part of midgut loop and left one-third from proximal part of hindgut loop Endothelium of mucous membrane including the glands is developed from endoderm of the midgut. Rest of the layers including the musculature is developed from splanchnic mesoderm
Left one-third of transverse colon up to pelvic colon	Endothelium is developed from endoderm of hindgut. Rest of the layers including the musculature is developed from splanchnic mesoderm
Rectum	The caudal part of the gut is dilated to form the endodermal cloaca. The mesoderm between gut and allantois invaginated the wall of endodermal cloaca and divides into two parts: (1) dorsal part forming rectum and anal canal, and (2) ventral part with allantois for urinary bladder. The preallantoic part gives rise to rectum above the third Houston valve. Rest part of rectum including the musculature is developed from the postallantoic part
Anal canal: Above pectinate line	• Mucosa of part of the anal canal above pectinate line is developed from caudal part of dorsal portion of the endodermal cloaca. Rest of the layer develops from splanchnic mesoderm. So internal anal sphincter is involuntary and supplied by the autonomic nerve
Below pectinate line	• It is developed from ectodermal cloaca. So lining membrane is skin (i.e. stratified squamous). The rest of the layer including musculature is developed from somatic mesoderm. So sphincter ani externus is innervated from the somatic nerve
Clinical anatomy	• Agenesis of rectum and anal canal • Imperforate anus: Failure of rupture of cloacal membrane, which is known as anal septum in the fetal stage, leads to imperforate anus. Corrected by surgery
Liver (Fig. 9.32)	The liver is developed from two sources: 1. An endodermal diverticulum grows within the mesoderm of ventral mesogastrium, at the junction of foregut and midgut. This form the parenchyma of liver 2. The fibrous architecture of liver is developed from the mesenchyme of the septum transversum

Contd...

Contd...

Names	Anatomical positions

Pancreas (Fig. 9.32) P.G.E.	It develops in two parts:
	1. Ventral pancreatic diverticulum: It develops from bile duct diverticulum. It forms the lower part of head of pancreas and uncinate process
	2. Dorsal pancreatic diverticulum: It extends within dorsal mesentery of the gut from bile duct diverticulum. This diverticulum form upper part of the head, whole of the neck, body and tail of the pancreas.
	   – (a) The main pancreatic duct develops from a distal part of duct of dorsal bud, (b) duct of ventral bud, and (c) cross communication between the two ducts
	   – The accessory pancreatic duct develops from proximal part of dorsal pancreatic bud

Contd...

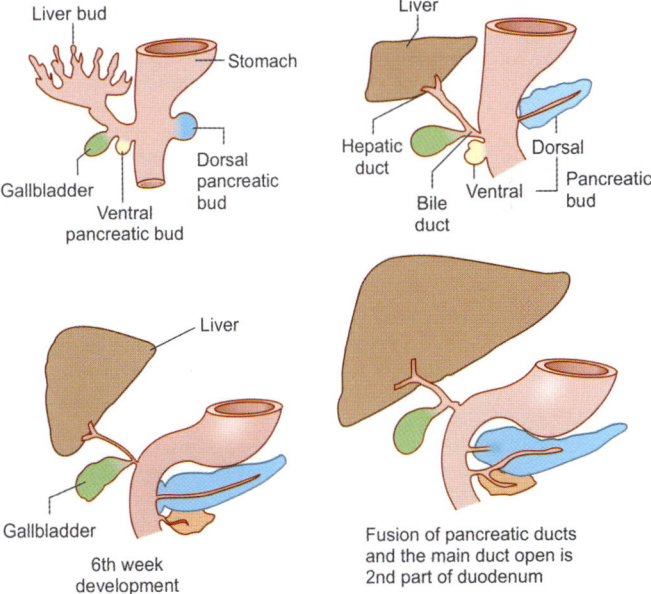

Fig. 9.32: Stages of development of liver pancreas

Contd...

Names	Anatomical positions
Clinical anatomy	• *Annular pancreas:* The original structure of ventral pancreatic bud sometimes failed to fuse with dorsal pancreatic bud to form single mass. In this condition two lobes develop in opposite directions • *Accessory pancreatic tissue:* Heterotrophic nodules of pancreatic tissue may be found in the duodenum, gallbladder and in Meckel's diverticulum
Spleen	It develops from mesoderm within dorsal mesogastrium as lobular pattern. Gradually the lobules are fused and form a single mass but the lobulated origin is represented by notches at superior border of spleen
Kidney (Fig. 9.33A) P.G.E.	Three different sets of kidneys develop from intermediate cell mass. During the 4th week of development pronephros appears (first tubular system). It degenerates gradually after the development of second set. It is never functional and disappear completely by the 6th week. The pronephric duct persists. It is utilized by second duct system that is mesonephros. It utilizes the pronephric duct and now, known as mesonephric duct. The mesonephric kidney disappears once again and finally third set metanephros develops. It persists as adult kidney along with ureteric bud. The ureteric buds push superiorly from the mesonephric duct. The distal end of the bud produce renal pelvis collecting tubules; their unexpanded proximal part become the ureter. As the kidneys develop in the pelvis it has to ascends to reach their final position in abdomen. This metanephric kidney excretes urine by the 3rd month of development
Clinical anatomy (Fig. 9.33B)	• *Horseshoe-shaped kidney:* When kidney ascends from pelvis, if the kidneys are very close together, the lower pole fuse together in the midline forming a single horseshoe-shaped kidney. This condition is usually asymptomatic
(Fig. 9.33C and D)	• *Polycystic kidney:* It is inherited disease (autosomal dominant gene) where the kidneys have many urine filled cyst. It results from failure of communication of collecting tubule with proximal part of renal tubule • *Pelvic kidney:* When the kidney fail to ascend. It remains in pelvis with normal functions

Contd...

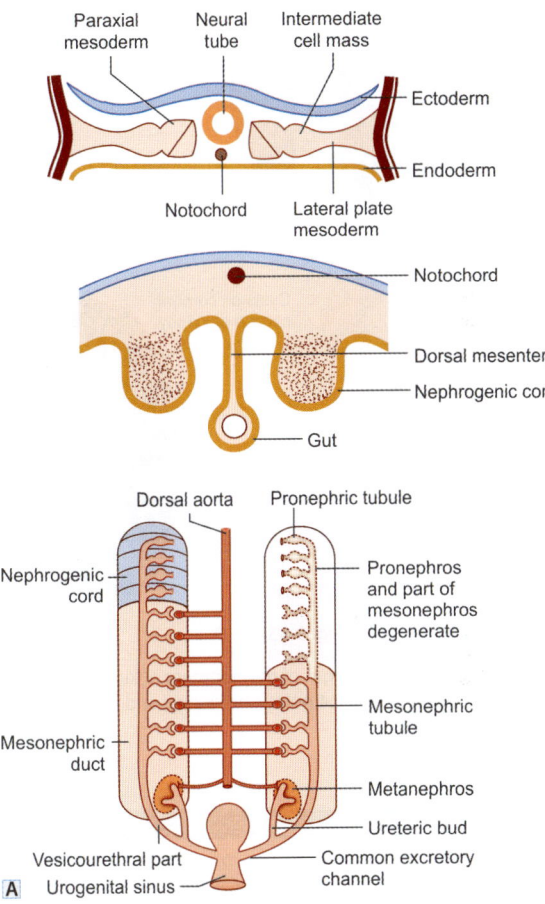

Fig. 9.33A: Contd...

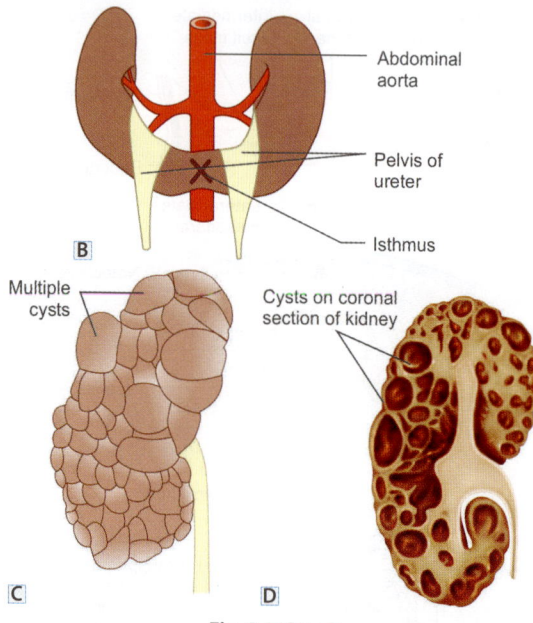

Fig. 9.33B to D

Figs 9.33A to D: (A) Different stages of development of kidney; (B) Horseshoe-shaped; (C) Surface appearance of polycystic kidney; and (D) Coronal sections of polycystic kidney

Contd...

Names	Anatomical positions
Urinary bladder (Fig. 9.34A) **P.G.E.**	The urinary bladder develops from part of endodermal cloaca. The cloaca is divided by urorectal septum (it is mesoderm and its tip touches the cloacal membrane and forms perineal body) into two parts. The ventral part forms the primitive urogenital sinus and the dorsal part forms the anorectal canal. The mesonephric duct opens into primitive urogenital sinus and it divides the urogenital sinus into two parts. The part above the opening is known

Contd...

Contd...

Names	Anatomical positions
	as vesicourethral canal. The epithelium of urinary bladder is derived from endoderm of vesicourethral canal while the other layers of the wall are derived from splanchnopleuric intraembryonic mesoderm. Later the lumen of allantois is obliterated and urachus is formed which extends from apex of urinary bladder to the umbilicus. It is transformed into a ligament—the median umbilical ligament
Clinical anatomy (Fig. 9.34B to D)	• *Urachal fistula:* When lumen persists in whole urachus, a fistula is formed. In this anomaly, urine dribbles through umbilicus. P.G.E. • *Ectopia vesicae:* In this condition, the infraumbilical part of anterior abdominal wall and the ventral wall of urinary bladder does not develop. The posterior wall with trigone of bladder is exposed to the surface. Urine can be seen dribbling from ureteric orifice
Diaphragm P.G.E. (Fig. 9.35)	It is developed from: (1) Septum transversum, (2) pleuroperitoneal folds, (3) dorsal mesentery of esophagus, and (4) body wall

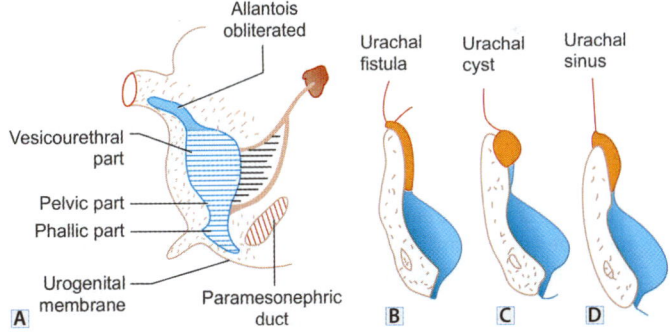

Figs 9.34A to D: Normal development of urinary and congenital anomalies bladder

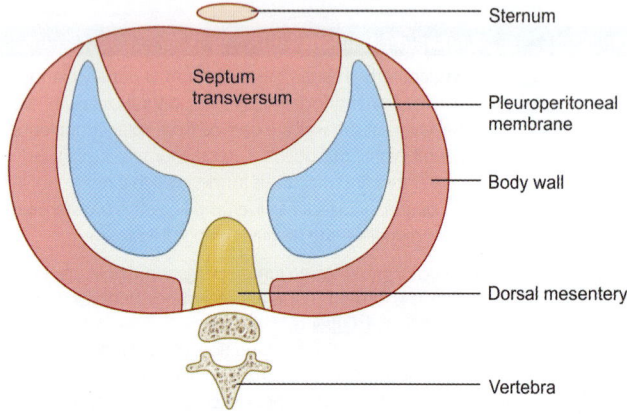

Fig. 9.35: Developmental components of the diaphragm

Branchial Fistula (Fig. 9.36)

Any fistula situated in relation to the sternocleidomastoid muscle in neck is called branchial fistula.

- Branchial fistula may be congenital or acquired.
- *Related embryology*: The external bulging of 1st branchial and 2nd branchial arches are prominent whereas the other arches lies under the bottom of a surface depression below the second arch. The depressions are called cervical sinus.
- This cervical sinus is bounded on cephalic side by the bulging of second arch and dorsally by elevation of premuscle tissue and caudally by epipericardial ridge.
- It is thought that the caudal growth of the second arch eventually meet the epipericardial ridge and closing the cervical sinus.
- *Treatment*: Surgical excision of the fistula tract.

Hypospadias/Orifice at the Base of Glans Penis

These are defects in development of male urethra. The androgen of fetal testis is responsible for the development of genitalia.

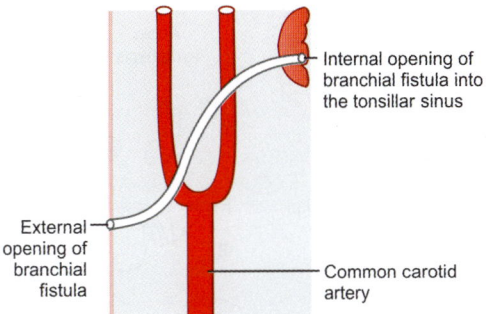

Fig. 9.36: Course of branchial fistula passing through the carotid fork

- In this condition, the external urethral orifice is situated on inferior or ventral aspect of penis instead of at the tip of glans penis.
- It results from failure of fusion of urethral folds.
- Depending upon the location of external urethral orifice the hypospadias are of five types:
  - *Glandular*: When the urethral orifice located at the base of the glans.
  - *Balanic*: When the urethral orifice located at the base of glans penis.
  - *Penile*: The urethral orifice lies anywhere between scrotum and base of glans.

Rectovesical Fistula (Fig. 9.37)

- This congenital, anomaly is due to incomplete development of the urorectal septum leading to the persistence of the cloacal duct.
- Postallantoic part of the hind gut forms a dilated sac—endodermal cloaca bounded caudally and ventrally by bilaminar cloacal membrane. A coronally oriented mesodermal partition arises at the angle between allantois and the hindgut—grows caudally dividing the cloaca into a ventral part (primitive urogenital sinus) and a dorsal part (primitive rectum). At first, urorectal septum does not touch the cloacal membrane. There is a communication

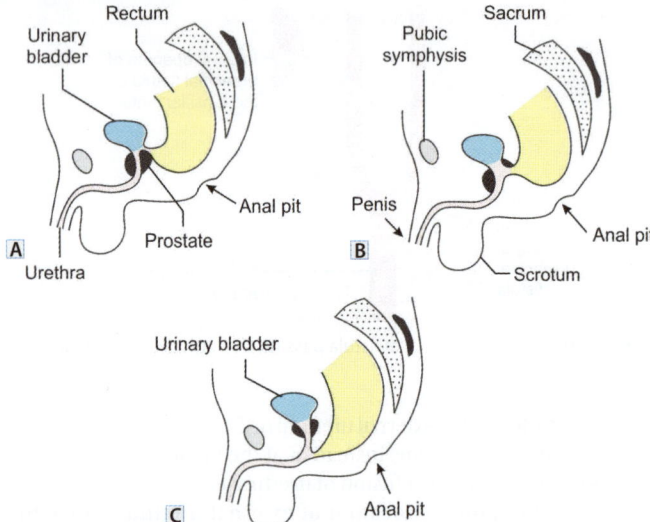

Figs 9.37A to C: Various types of rectal fistulae in the male (A to C). The fistula may be between rectum and urinary bladder (i.e. rectovesical) as in (A), between rectum and urethra (rectourethral) as in (B) and (C)

between the urogenital sinus (forming the bladder) and rectum known as cloacal duct—persistence of which gives rise to congenital "rectovesical fistula". At about the 7th week cloacal duct is closed as the urorectal septum, fuses with the cloacal membrane. The site of fusion is "perineal body".

- Other causes of rectovesical fistula are traumatic, postoperative and rarely nowadays obstructed labor.

Spina Bifida Occulta

The spina bifida occulta is a neural tube defect. It usually occurs in sacrolumbar region. There are various types of this defect. Myeloschisis is more severe anomaly in the back. It is due to unclosure of the particular neuropore. This spina bifida occulta is hidden by a tuft of hair at the surface.

Embryology

EXPLANATORY NOTES

Q1. Ovary experiences incomplete journey of descent. Explain.

Ans.
- *Descent of gonads*: The gonads develop on the posterior abdominal wall bilaterally along the central portion of the mesonephros. Then both gonads descent, the testis lie outside the abdominal cavity and ovary to the pelvis.
- *Testis descent*: The mechanism of testicular descent involves two phases:
  1. *Transabdominal phase*: Each testis lies on the dorsal abdominal wall initially. Testis is attached to the mesonephric fold by mesorchium (a peritoneal fold contains testicular vessels and nerve and a quantity of undifferentiated mesenchyma). It also acquires a secondary attachment to the ventral wall of the abdomen by an inguinal fold of peritoneum within the inguinal fold another chord is created called gubernaculums at the end of the second month the caudal part of the ventral abdominal wall is horizontal but after return of the intestine to the peritoneal cavity it grows in length and becomes progressively more vertical. As the umbilical artery runs ventrally from the dorsal to ventral wall it drags one peritoneal fold which forms the medial boundary of lateral inguinal fossa in which testis projects at the lower end this fossa projects into the inguinal canal up to 10th week, the gubernaculum of male and female is same, but then under the influence of insulin like factor-3 from the Leydig cell male gubernaculums undergoes more enlargement by comparison female gubernaculums is thin and subsequently develops into round ligament of uterus. Female gubernaculum gets one additional attachment to the lateral margin of the uterus near the entrance of the uterine tube. Its lower part caudal to this attachment becomes round ligament of uterus and cranial part becomes ligament of ovary. This new attachment of ovary causes restricted descend of ovary.

2. *Inguinoscrotal phase* of migration is absent in descend of ovary in absence of androgens so gubernaculums develops in female does not extend up to the labia majora corresponds to sacrum in males. So, ovary undergoes incomplete descent.

Q2. Human placenta is hemochorial type. Explain.

Ans.
- Human placenta is considered as hemochorial organ according to tissues forming placental barrier.
- Placental barrier in case of human consists of tissues intervening between fetal blood in chorionic villi and maternal blood in intervillous space.
- Therefore, maternal blood comes in direct contact with fetal chronic villi as endothelium of mouth of uterine vessels (maternal) disappears in decidual plate.

Q3. Why a horseshoe-shaped kidney cannot ascend up to its normal position.

Ans. During development the lower pole of the kidney comes nearby and may fuse with each other. Their ureter comes out from front. But when kidney ascends up, the lower part of the horseshoe-shaped kidney is arrested below the origin of inferior mesenteric artery. So the horseshoe-shaped kidney cannot ascend up to its normal position.

Points to Remember

- Teratoma are tumors of unknown origin that often contain a variety of tissues like bone, hair, muscle or gut epithelium, as this tumor arises from pluripotent cells
- Oogenesis begins before birth and spermatogenesis (male) begin at puberty
- The fertilization occur is the ampullary part of the uterine tube and the results of fertilization are:
    - Restoration of diploid number of chromosome
    - Determination of chromosomal sex
    - Initiation of cleavage division (a series of mitotic division)

Contd...

Contd...

- The 2nd week of development is known as the week of two's
  - The trophoblast differentiates into two cytotrophoblast and syncytiotrophoblast
  - The embryoblast form two layers ectoderm and endoderm
  - Two cavities form one is amniotic cavity and other is yolk sac cavity
  - The extraembryonic mesoderm divides into two layers, i.e. (1) somatopleuric and (2) splanchnopleuric layer
- Third week of development is development of notochord and development of body axis and also intraembryonic mesoderm
- The fetal period extends from the 9th week of gestation up to birth. Total length of pregnancy for a full-term fetus is considered to be 280 days or 40 weeks after onset of the last menstruation or, 266 days (38 weeks) after fertilization
- About 3% of all life born infants have birth defect
- The average size of newborn is 2.5–4 kg with a length of 20 inches. The term low weight refers to a weight less than 2.5 kg regardless of gestation age
- Intrauterine growth retardation (IUGR) is a term applied to infants who do not attain their optimal intrauterine growth. Approximately 1 in 10 babies have IUGR
- Ultrasound can accurately determine fetal age, growth parameter and can detect many malformations
- Bone age can be determined by ossification center appearance. Whether the child has reached his/her maturation age
- Thalidomide disaster may produce abnormalities of limbs like meromelia (partial absence of limb), amelia (total absence of limbs) in one or more extremities, phocomelia (sealed limbs) and micromelia (small limbs)
- A different kind of limb defect affecting the digits. The digits are shortened known as brachydactyly
- Abnormalities of cardiac looping produces dextrocardia where heart lies on the right side instead of left
- Neural crest cells also contribute to craniofacial development, it is common to see facial and cardiac abnormalities in the same individual
- Surfactant is important for survival of premature infant. Absence or insufficient surfactant in premature baby cause respiratory distress syndrome because of collapse of primitive alveoli (hyaline membrane disease).

10

Radiology: Imaging Technique

CHAPTER OUTLINE

- Introduction
- Conventional Radiography
- Standard Position Used in Radiological Examination
- Other Methods of Imaging Technique
- Superior Extremity
- Anteroposterior View of Shoulder Joint
- Elbow Joint
  - Anteroposterior View
  - Lateral View
- Posteroanterior View of Wrist Joint and Hand
- X-ray of Chest (PA View)
- Heart and Aorta
- Lungs
- Abdomen
  - Straight X-ray of Abdomen
- Contrast Radiography
  - Barium Meal X-ray of Stomach
  - Barium Enema Barium Enema of Large Intestine
- Pyelogram
  - Descending Pyelogram
  - Ascending Pyelogram
- Hysterosalpingogram
- Head and Neck
- Cervical Spine
- Inferior Extremity
  - Anteroposterior View of Hip Joint
  - X-ray of Knee—Anteroposterior and Lateral View
  - X-ray of Ankle
  - Lateral View of Foot

INTRODUCTION

Radiology is the study of structures of body by means of radiograph.

CONVENTIONAL RADIOGRAPHY (FIG. 10.1A)

The making of X-ray picture on photo film is known as radiography. It is excellent for high contrast structures like bones and lungs. Normally soft tissues with slight thickness are not visible. So, the contrast media is used to identify soft structures. Contrast media are of two different types:
1. *Translucent*: Air and oxygen
2. *Opaque*: For example, barium sulfate and iodine compound.

The rays when readily absorbed by a substance are known as radiolucent (like soft tissue). The tissue like bone is so dense that X-rays do not pass through it, is known as radiopaque substance. One should get white shadow in radiopaque bone and black shadow in case of gas or air (e.g. lung shadow and fundic gas shadow). Thick soft tissue shadow looks gray.

The orientation of radiograph is marked by incorporating a lead letter into the cassette before exposing a film, such as right side with R.

Advantages

- To diagnose bony deformities and fractures.
- To diagnose a congestion of soft tissue, or space-occupying lesion (tumor, etc.).

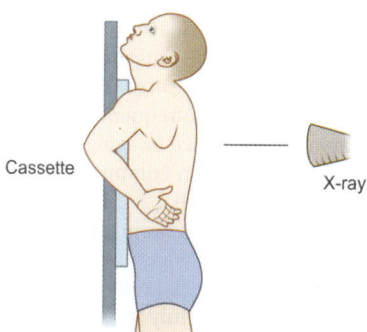

Fig. 10.1A: Technique of X-ray of posteroanterior view

STANDARD POSITION USED IN RADIOLOGICAL EXAMINATION

- ***Anteroposterior view:*** In this view, the source of light is in front of the subject and the film lies behind the subject. Posterior structure is better visualized in this view, e.g. anteroposterior view of hip joint, elbow joint, etc.
- ***Posteroanterior view (Fig. 10.1A):*** Here the source of light is behind the subject and the rays passing posteroanteriorly as the film is in front, e.g. posteroanterior view of the skull and chest.
- ***Lateral view:*** This view is used to assess the depth of structures. The position in this view is at the right angle to anteroposterior and posteroanterior.

OTHER METHODS OF IMAGING TECHNIQUE

- ***Angiographies:*** Visualization of vascular tree by introducing iodinated contrast medium through catheter is known as angiography. It is useful in visualizing tumor vascularity and to assess the position of arteries.
- ***Ultrasound (Fig. 10.1B):*** It is inaudible sound with frequency of more than 20,000 decibels/sec is passed to obtain the image or photograph of an organ and tissue; it is known as ultrasonography, or ultrasound in common language. Ultrasound is difficult in very obese person. It is the most common imaging technique to visualize the condition of fetus and to identify gallbladder disease.
- ***Computed tomography (Fig. 10.1C):*** It permits the study of tissue in slices, by which we can clearly localize the area of lesion and changes produced by it. The procedure is safe and quick.
- ***Magnetic resonance imaging:*** Here magnetic property of H-nucleus is excited by radiofrequency radiation and photograph is taken. Magnetic resonance imaging is safe and structures are more clearly visualized than computed tomography (CT) scan, but it is more expensive than CT. It is the first choice of imaging technique to detect tumor of brain and spinal cord and also disk prolapse.
- ***Mammography:*** It is a special radiographic technique used for imaging of breast tissue, mainly for assessment of palpable lump in the breast or as a screening procedure for suspected malignant disease prior to biopsy.

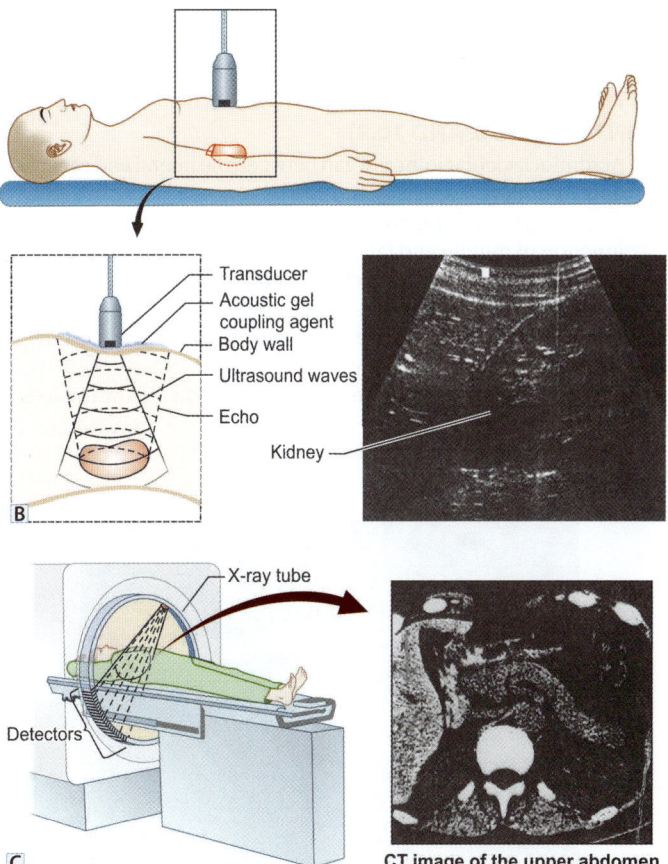

Figs 10.1B and C: (B) Technique for producing an abdominal ultrasound image; (C) Technique of abdominal computed tomography (CT) scan

Tissues sensitive to ionizing radiation: Lymphocytes, leukocytes and reproductive cells.

Here are few conventional X-ray plates which often come in examination.

SUPERIOR EXTREMITY

Refer Figures 10.2 and 10.3.

ANTEROPOSTERIOR VIEW OF SHOULDER JOINT (FIGS 10.2 AND 10.3)

- Acromioclavicular joint as a gap between the lateral end of clavicle and acromion.
- *Anatomical neck of humerus*: Medial portion is on a level with a junction of middle and lateral portion of the glenoid cavity.
- *Clavicle*: Lateral half of the clavicle project a little higher than the upper surface of acromion.
- *Conoid tubercle* shows like a bony prominence on the inferior surface of the clavicle.
- Coracoid process looks like a circular shadow below the lateral third of clavicle.
- Glenoid cavity looks like a narrow ellipse.

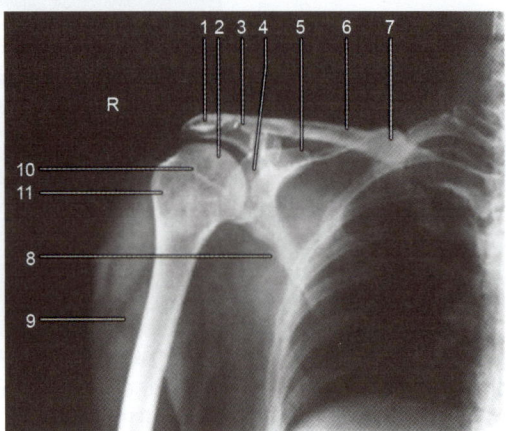

Fig. 10.2: Anteroposterior view of shoulder joint showing: 1. Acromion, 2. Head of humerus, 3. Acromioclavicular joint space, 4. Glenoid cavity, 5. Coracoid process, 6. Clavicle, 7. Superior angle (scapula), 8. Lateral border of scapula, 9. Soft tissue shadow of arm, 10. Anatomical neck of humerus, and 11. Greater tuberosity of humerus. R: Right side

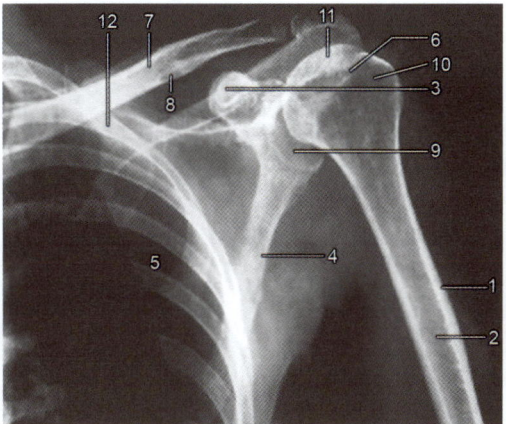

Fig. 10.3: Shoulder joint (anteroposterior view) showing: 1. Cortex, 2. Medullary cavity, 3. Coracoid process (circular shadow), 4. Lateral border, 5. Shadow of lung, 6. Anatomical neck, 7. Clavicle, 8. Conoid tubercle, 9. Glenoid cavity, 10. Greater tuberosity, 11. Head of humerus, 12. Superior angle of scapula

- Greater tuberosity of the humerus as a most lateral bony point of shoulder region.
- Head of the humerus lying against the glenoid cavity.
- Inferior angle of scapula is seen partly superimposed on the lung field at the level of 7th rib.
- Lesser tuberosity and bicipital groove are difficult to identify.
- Superior angle of scapula projects upward in the angle between clavicle and 1st rib.

ELBOW JOINT

Anteroposterior view of shoulder joint showing (Fig. 10.4):
- Elbow joint space as a translucence broad line passing across the ulna between the trochlea and coronoid process. It separates the head of radius from the capitula.
- Head and tuberosity of radius is seen slightly overlapping the ulna.
- Lateral epicondyle of humerus gives a flatter appearance as compared to the medial epicondyle.

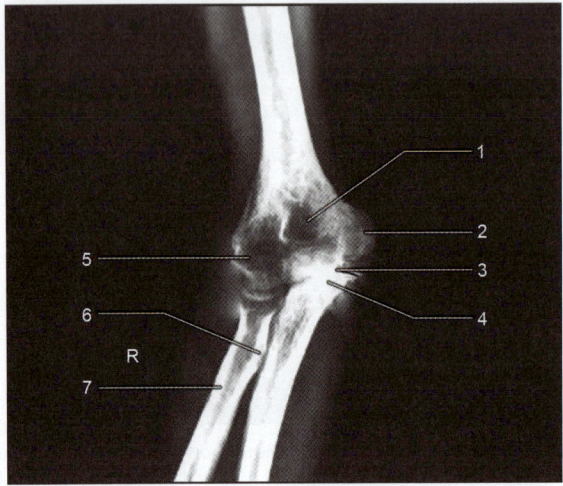

Fig. 10.4: Anteroposterior view of elbow joint showing: 1. Olecranon and coronoid fossae, 2. Medial epicondyle, 3. Olecranon process, 4. Elbow joint space, 5. Lateral epicondyle (flatter appearance), 6. Tuberosity of radius, and 7. Dense cortical shadow of radius. R: Right side

- Medial epicondyle of humerus is seen projecting medially.
- Trochlea is superimposed by ulna.
- Olecranon process is superimposed on the shadow of humerus.

Lateral view of shoulder joint showing (Fig. 10.5):
- Capitulum is seen projecting anteriorly beyond the line of anterior edge of the shaft of humerus.
- Coronoid process partly overlaps the shadow of the head of the radius.
- *Epicondyles*: The shadow of medial and lateral epicondyles is superimposed.
- Head of the radius lies opposite of the capitulum.
- Supracondylar ridges are seen as white lines passing upward from epicondylar shadow.
- Olecranon process is seen projecting backward like a hook.

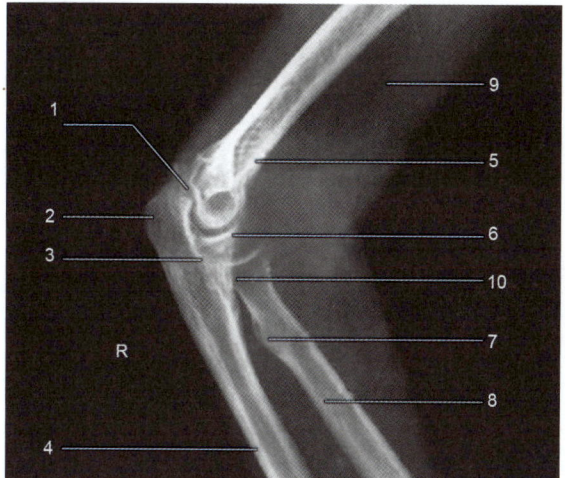

Fig. 10.5: Lateral view of elbow joint showing: 1. Superimposed shadow of two epicondyles of humerus, 2. Olecranon, 3. Elbow joint space, 4. Compact bone, 5. Supracondylar ridge, 6. Coronoid process, 7. Tuberosity of radius, 8. Medullary cavity, 9. Soft tissue shadow, 10. Head of radius, and 11. Supracondylar ridges. R: Right side

POSTEROANTERIOR VIEW OF WRIST JOINT AND HAND (FIGS 10.6 AND 10.7)

Posteroanterior view of hand showing:

Carpals

- Proximal and distal rows of carpal bones which are easily identified by their shape and character.
- Proximal rows from lateral to medial bones are scaphoid, lunate, triquetral and pisiform. Pisiform shadow is superimposed on that of triquetral.
- Distal row from lateral to medial consists of trapezium, trapezoid, capitate and hamate. Hook of the hamate appears as a white denser wing like shadow. Trapezium and trapezoid are slightly overlapped with each other.

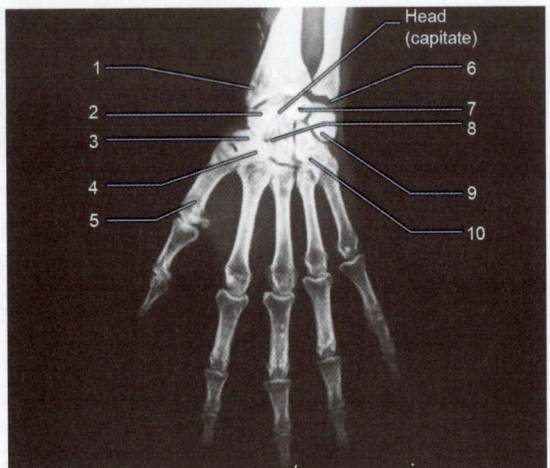

Fig. 10.6: Posteroanterior view of wrist and hand showing: 1. Styloid process of radius, 2. Scaphoid, 3. Trapezium, 4. Trapezoid, 5. 1st metacarpal, 6. Ulnar styloid process, 7. Lunate, 8. Triquetral and pisiform, 9. Capitate, and 10. Hamate with hook

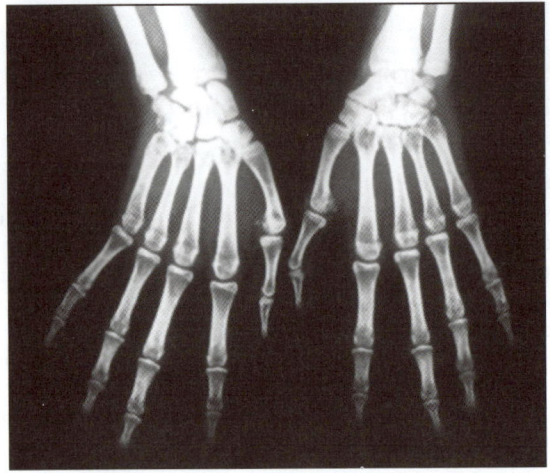

Fig. 10.7: Posteroanterior view of wrist and hand

Metacarpals
- They are miniature long bones. The first metacarpal is placed somewhat lateral.
- The 2nd, 3rd, 4th and 5th outlines are of each is easily define. The bases of the metacarpals tend to overlap.

Phalanges
Phalanges are seen separated by interphalangeal joints. The terminal phalanges give a sped-like appearance.

Styloid Process of Radius and Ulna
- Styloid process of radius extends below the styloid process of ulna.
- Radiocarpal (wrist joint) and intercarpal joint space are clearly seen.
- Sesamoid bone: In the hand the following sesamoid bone are of constant occurrence.
  - The two opposite head of 1st metacarpal in the tendon of flexor pollicis brevis muscle.
  - The 1st or 2nd sesamoid bones are frequently present opposite interphalangeal joint of thumb. They lie of flexor tendon.

X-RAY OF CHEST (FIGS 10.8A AND B) (PA VIEW)
X-ray of chest showing bony thoracic cage and soft tissue shadow. Soft tissue shadows are:
- Lung shadow—looks black
- Mediastinal shadow—formed by heart and mediastinal structure
- Shadow of trachea
- Shadow of diaphragm

Radiopaque bony shadows are:
- Shadow of clavicle—horizontally placed at the root of the neck
- Shadows of rib—outline the first and 2nd rib always come in question. Do not trace the rib up to the sternum as there is gap for costal cartilage.
- Shadow of medial border of scapula.

HEART AND AORTA
The heart lies opposite to 5th, 6th, 7th and 8th thoracic (dorsal) vertebra. About one-third of the heart lies in the right of median plane and two-thirds to the left of median plane. The cardiac apex which is the lowest part of heart lies at the level of space between the 5th rib and 6th rib on left side. Heart size can be expressed as a ratio of maximum

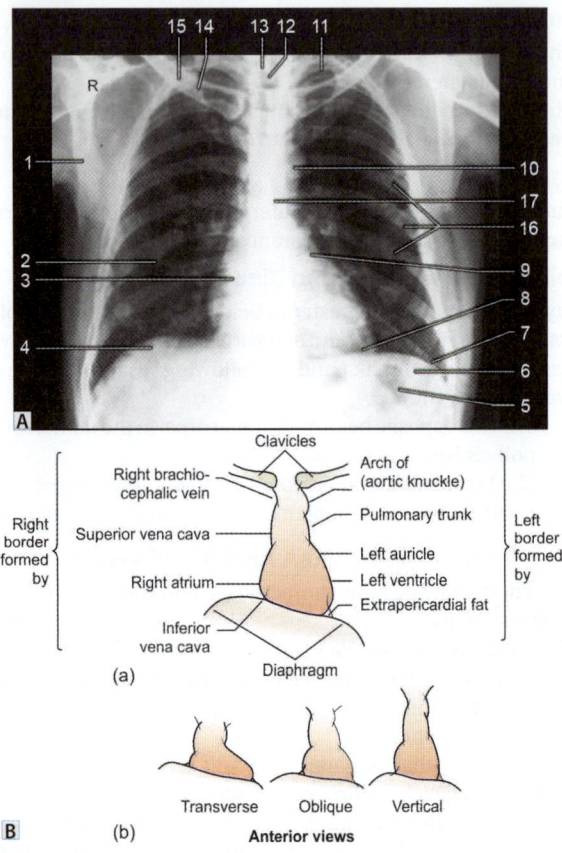

Figs 10.8A and B: (A) Posteroanterior view of chest showing: 1. Lateral border of scapula, 2. Hilar shadow due to lymphoglandular vascular components, 3. Right border of mediastinal shadow, 4. Right dome of diaphragm, 5. Gas in fundus of stomach, 6. Left dome of diaphragm, 7. Costophrenic angle (left), 8. Cardiophrenic angle (left), 9. Left border of mediastinal shadow, 10. Aortic knuckle formed by arch of aorta, 11. Thoracic inlet, 12. Spine of vertebra visualized through shadow of trachea, 13. Shadow of trachea, 14. 1st rib, 15. Clavicle, 16. Ribs, and 17. Pulmonary conus. R: Right side

(B) (a) The composition of the margins of the cardiovascular shadow, (b) Cardiovascular shadows (mediastinal shadows): the common types of normal cardiovascular shadow

transverse diameter of heart to the maximum. Normal ratio is 1 : 2. In small children, this ratio differs.

LUNGS

- The lungs fill and occupy the thoracic cavity.
- The apices of lung extend to a point about 1" (2.5 cm) above the clavicle and lower border or base of the lung reaches almost to the transpyloric plane.
- The roots of the lung are formed by the major bronchi, pulmonary arteries, pulmonary veins and the surrounding lymph nodes. The root lies opposite the bodies of 5th, 6th and 7th thoracic vertebra.

Barium Swallow X-ray of Esophagus (Fig. 10.9)

It delineates the retrocardiac structure. A left anterior oblique view for example will show three shadow oblique show the concave indentation. From above downward they are:

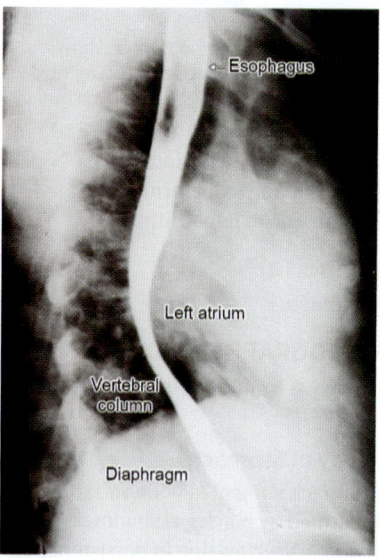

Fig. 10.9: Radiograph taken immediately after the patient had swallowed a suspension of barium sulfate (which is opaque to X-rays). The esophagus is clearly outlined. Any defects in the lumen produced by disease can be made out. An enlarged left atrium (abnormal) produces an indentation on the shadow of the esophagus

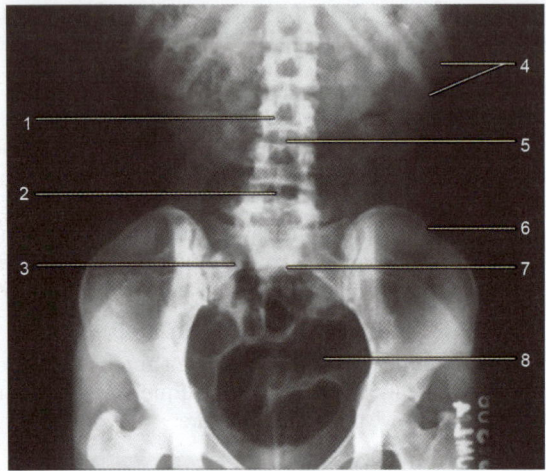

Fig. 10.10: Plain or straight X-ray of abdomen showing: 1. Vertebral body, 2. Intervertebral disk space, 3. Ala of sacrum, 4. Lower ribs, 5. Spine of vertebra, 6. Iliac crest, 7. Sacral promontory, and 8. Gas in large gut

1. First indentation due to aortic arch
2. Second indentation due to left bronchus
3. Third indentation due to left atrium.

ABDOMEN (FIG. 10.10)

Plain X-Ray of abdomen.

CONTRAST RADIOGRAPHY (FIG. 10.11)

Gastrointestinal tract is examined by aid of contrast media barium sulfate.

Barium Meal X-ray of Stomach

- Position of stomach subject to wide variation.
- Fundus is identified by black gas shadow.
- *Greater curvature*: Notches due to persistence wave may be seen in the distal half of greater curvature.
- *Incisura angularis*: Situated at the junction of body with the pyloric antrum.

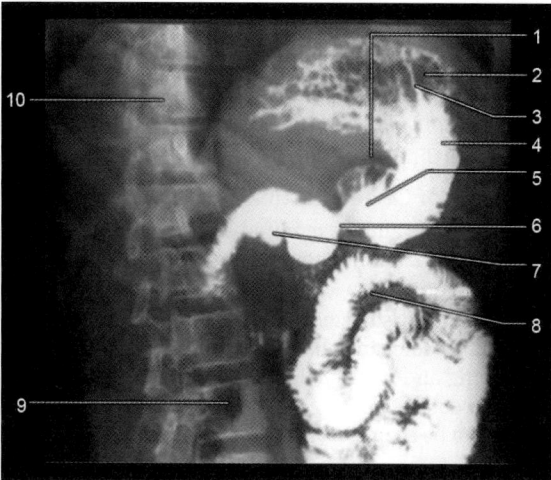

Fig. 10.11: Barium meal X-ray of stomach showing: 1. Lesser curvature of stomach, 2. Fundic gas shadow, 3. Rugae, 4. Greater curvature of stomach, 5. Pyloric antrum, 6. Pyloric canal, 7. Duodenal cap (due to barium in first one inch of first part of duodenum), 8. Feathery intestinal mucosa, 9. Gas shadow in colon, and 10. Shadow of pedicle

- *Lesser curvature*: It runs almost vertically to incisura angularis.
- Pyloric antrum is the wide part of pyloric region, narrows to pyloric canal and the terminal part of which is surrounded by pyloric sphincter.
- *Pyloric canal*: It appears as a column of barium about 2–3 mm wide and 5–8 mm long joining the pyloric antrum.

Duodenum

- *First part*: The first 1 inch of the first part of the duodenum forms a triangular shaped shadow of barium, which is known as duodenal cap.
- *Second part*: It gives a floccular shadow because of folded mucous membrane (Fig. 10.13).
- *Third part*: It is seen running transversely.
- *Fourth part*: It is directed upwards and to the left.
- *Duodenal jejunal flexure*: It is hidden behind the stomach shadow.

- *Jejunum and ilium*: Barium reaches to the jejunum and ilium 1 hour after injection of barium sulfate.
- *Proximal part of small intestine*: The barium shadow remains broken up and shows feather like appearance.
- *Distal part of the ileum*: It forms a more homogeneous shadow, colis are seen line in the pelvis.

Barium Enema of Large Intestine (Fig. 10.12)

The large intestine can be examined either after barium enema or a barium meal but barium enema is chosen, because it gives better shadow of the large gut.

Structure should be visualized:
- Appendix may sometimes be seen arising from the base of the cecum.
- Descending and pelvic colon is narrower than ascending and transverse colon.
- Rectum can be seen closely related to sacrum.

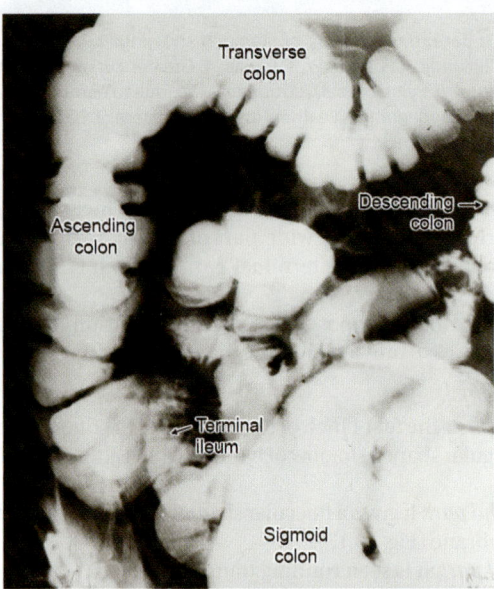

Fig. 10.12: Radiograph of abdomen after a barium enema. The colon is outlined

Barium Meal, X-ray of Stomach and Follow Through Intestine (Fig. 10.13)

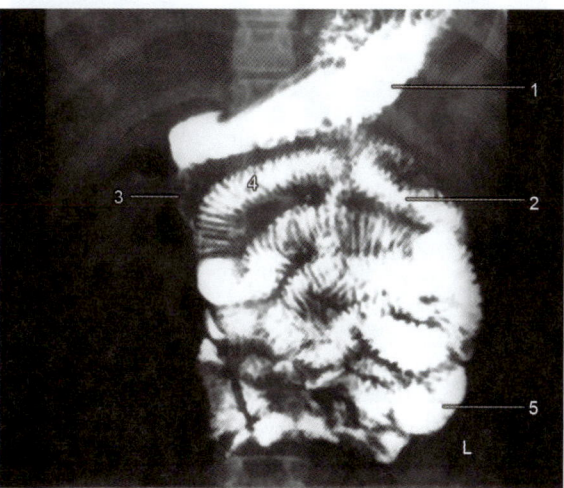

Fig. 10.13: Barium meal X-ray of stomach and follow through intestine showing: 1. Stomach, 2. Feathery appearance of small intestine (due to barium entangle between mucous folds), 3. 2nd part of duodenum, 4. 3rd part of duodenum, 5. distal part of ilium. L: Left side

PYELOGRAM (FIGS 10.14 AND 10.15)

Descending Pyelogram

It is done by injecting 20–40 mL of dye (conray-420) through vein slowly. Descending or excretion pyelogram or intravenous pyelography is done not only the anatomy of kidney but also to assess the functional status of kidney.

Ascending Pyelogram

It delineates the calyces and pelvis of ureters.

Radiographic Appearance

The anatomical details one more clearly visible in ascending pyelogram than excretion pyelogram. The following structures are visualized:

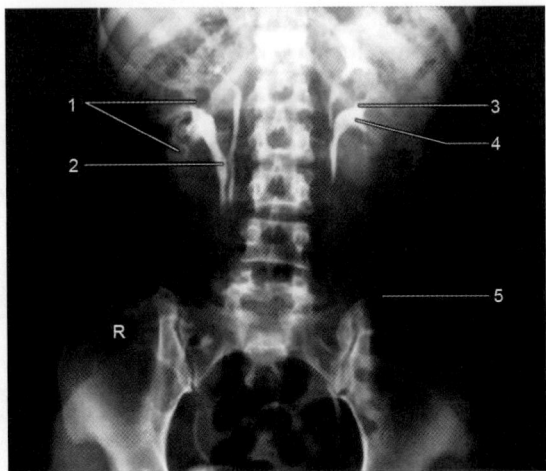

Fig. 10.14: Descending (intravenous) pyelogram showing: 1. Minor calyces, 2. Double ureter on both sides, 3. Major calyces, 4. Pelvis of ureter, and 5. Gas in descending colon. R: Right side

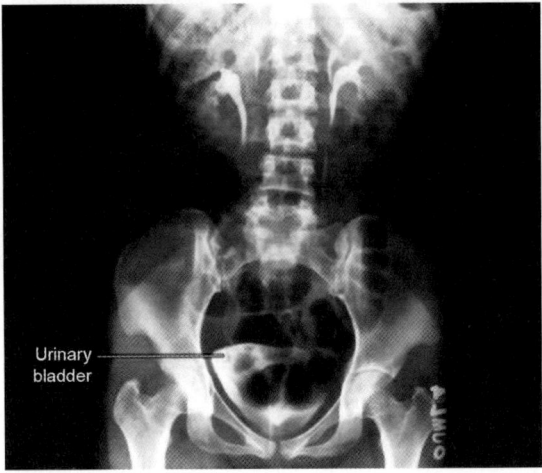

Fig. 10.15: Descending pyelogram showing the dye within concentrated in urinary bladder. R: Right side

- Major calyces
- Minor calyces
- Pelvis of ureter
- Ureter
- Cystoscopy can be seen in urinary bladder.

HYSTEROSALPINGOGRAM

Radiographic appearances are the following (Fig. 10.16):
- *Bladder*: When filled by dye the bladder is clearly shown.
- The calyces major.
- The calyces minor (6–10 cup-shaped area are seen).
- *Pelvis of ureter*: Funnel-shaped.
- The ureters run downward close to the tip of the transverse process of lumber vertebrae.

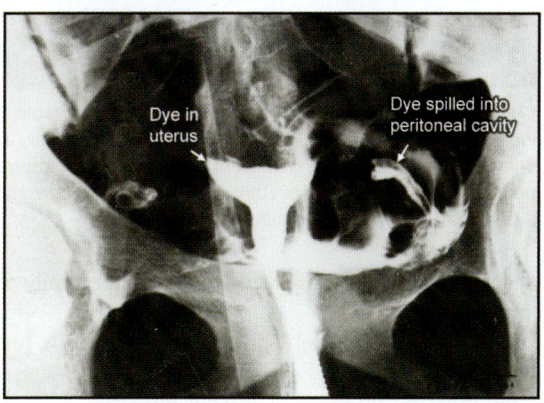

Fig. 10.16: Hysterosalpingography. Contrast medium has been injected into the uterus, and has passed through the uterine tubes to spill into the peritoneal cavity. This indicates that the uterine tubes are patent

HEAD AND NECK

PA view of skull Showing (Fig. 10.17):
- Coronal suture which meets the sagittal suture near the vertex.
- Frontal sinuses appear as translucent areas above and between the orbits. They are unequal in sizes.
- Greater wings of sphenoids and its lateral edges are represented by a white line which descent from lateral part of lesser wings.

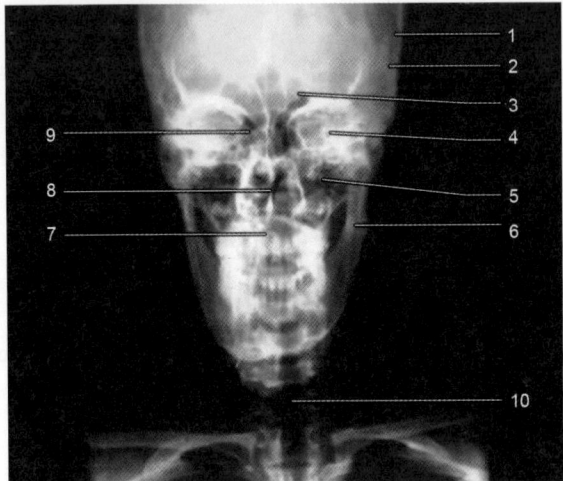

Fig. 10.17: Posteroanterior view (PA) of skull showing: 1. Outer table, 2. Inner table, 3. Frontal air sinus, 4. Petrous part of temporal bone, 5. Maxillary air sinus, 6. Ramus of mandible, 7. Soft tissue shadow of tongue, 8. Nasal septum (upper part formed by perpendicular plate of ethmoid and lower part by vomer), and 9. Ethmoidal air cells, 10. Shadow of trachea

- Lesser wings of sphenoids are seen as a white line extending across the orbital shadow.
- Mandibular condyles can be placed down up to the ramus of mandible.
- Mastoid process and mastoid air cells are visible laterally and inferiorly.
- Maxillary sinuses lies adjacent to the inferior margin of the orbits.
- The petrous temporal shadow is superimposed.
- Orbits are seen clearly below and lateral to the frontal sinuses.
- Petrous temporal forms a dense white shadow running directly medially across the orbits and maxillary air sinuses.
- Nasal fossae are seen on each side of the nasal septum.
- Sphenoidal and ethmoidal sinuses are superimposed. Turbinates are also seen within the nasal aperture.
- Outer table and inner table of the skull is well visualized.

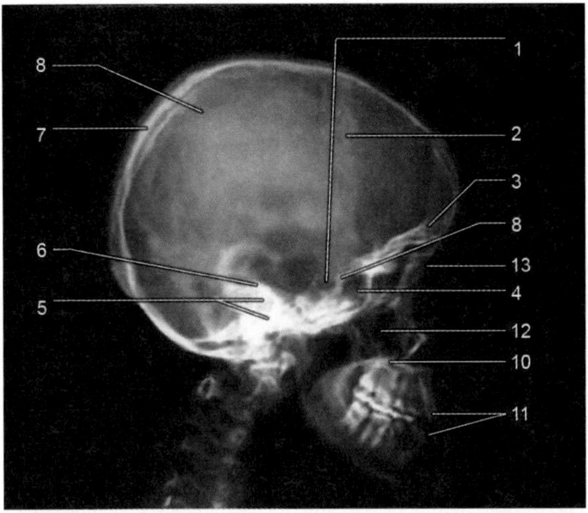

Fig. 10.18: Lateral view of skull showing: 1. Pituitary fossa, 2. Coronal suture, 3. Orbital plate of frontal bone, 4. Sphenoidal air sinus, 5. External auditory meatus, 6. Petrous part of temporal bone, 7. Outer table of parietal, and 8. Inner table of parietal, 9. Anterior clinoid process, 10. Hard plate, 11. Teeth, 12. Maxillary air sinus, 13. Orbit

Lateral view of skull showing (Fig. 10.18):

- Two tables of diploe.
- Anterior clinoid process points posteriorly over the pituitary fossa.
- Anterior cranial fossa is prominent.
- Coronal suture extends as a zigzag line from the vertex.
- External ear soft tissue may cast shadow above the petrous part of the temporal bone.
- External and internal auditory meatus of both side cast a 5 mm ring shadow near the center of petrous temporal.
- Frontal sinuses appear as a triangular black area with the base downward.
- Hard palate and teeth are situated below the maxillary sinus.
- Mastoid air cells appear as honeycomb translucencies line behind the external auditory meatus.
- Maxillary sinuses are seen below the orbits as a black (translucent) area.
- Orbits cast shadow in front of ethmoidal air sinuses.

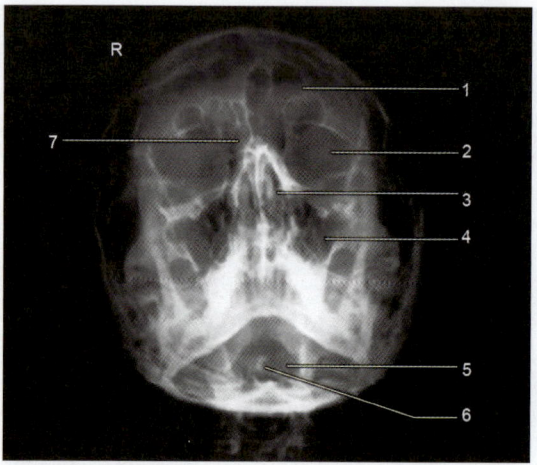

Fig. 10.19: Occipitomental view of sinus for examination of paranasal air sinuses (PNS) showing: 1. Frontal air sinus, 2. Orbital cavity, 3. Nasal cavity, 4. Maxillary air sinus, 5. Foramen magnum, 6. Axis (odontoid process), and 7. Ethmoidal air cells. R: Right side

- Petrous temporal cast a dense triangular shadow.
- Pituitary fossa is seen as a round or oval depression restrict on the sphenoidal air sinuses.
- Posterior clinoid process is seen projecting from each side of the upper margin of dorsum sellae.
- Sphenoidal sinuses are seen as relatively black shadow below and anterior to hypophyseal fossa.

Occipitomental view
Refer Figure 10.19

CERVICAL SPINE

Lateral view of cervical spine is as follows (Figs 10.20 and 10.21):
- Articular facets are imperfectly seen.
- Anterior arch of atlas shadow is seen in front of odontoid process.
- Odontoid process is seen as an upward extension from the body of 2nd cervical vertebra.
- Pedicles from the 3rd cervical vertebra cast a circular or oval shadow on the bodies of the vertebrae.

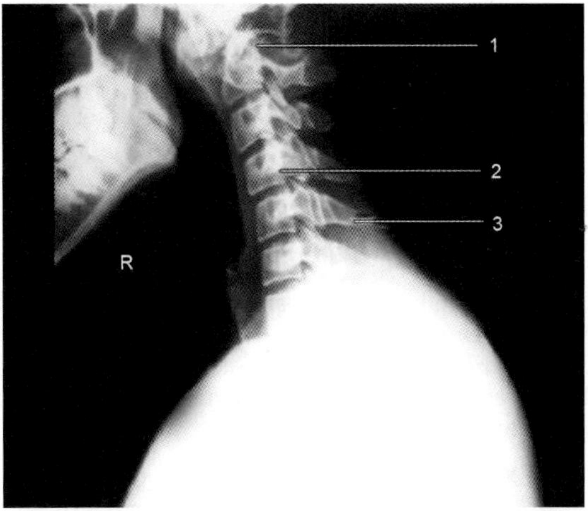

Radiology: Imaging Technique

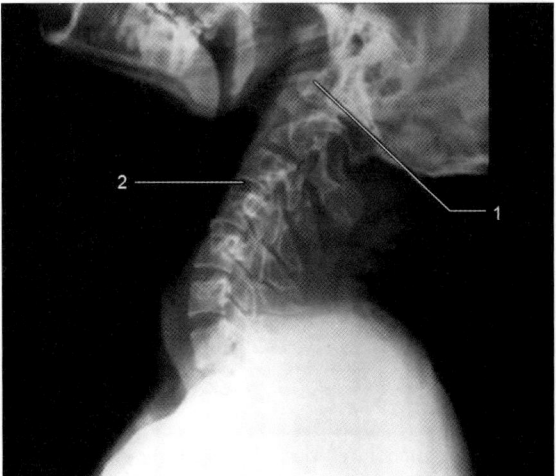

Fig. 10.20: Lateral view of neck (slightly flexed) showing: 1. Dens (odontoid process), 2. Intervertebral foramen, and 3. Spine (cervical). R: Right side

Fig. 10.21: Lateral view of neck (extended) showing: 1. Anterior arch of atlas and 2. Disk space (intervertebral). R: Right side

- Spine of 2nd, 3rd and 4th cervical are sometimes bifid. The spine of 2nd cervical is largest.

Anteroposterior view of cervical spine showing:
- Intervertebral disk are seen as a translucent intervals between the bodies.
- Vertebral bodies appear as rectangular shadows.
- Larynx appears as an abrupt narrowing at the upper end of trachea.
- Mandible shows a superimposed shadow with that of the upper cervical vertebra.
- Thyroid cartilage is seen opposite of the bodies of 4th and 5th cervical vertebrae.
- Transverse process C7 point downwards and laterally in contrast with transverse process of 1st thoracic vertebrae which is projected upwards and laterally.

INFERIOR EXTREMITY

Anteroposterior view of hip joint showing (Fig. 10.22):
- *Acetabulum*: It appears as a curve white line of cortical bone.

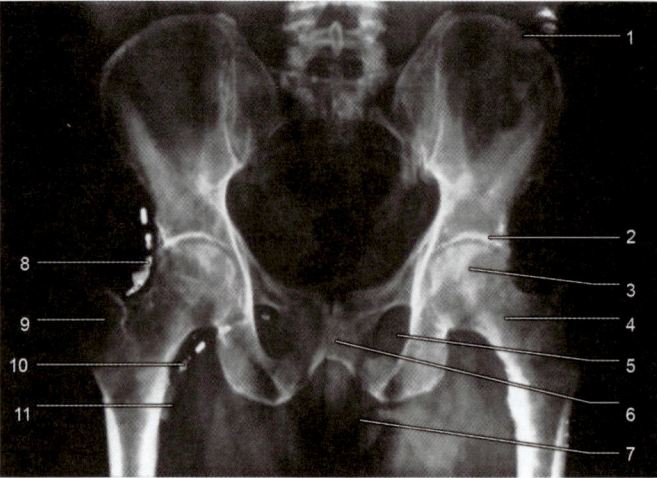

Fig. 10.22: Anteroposterior (AP) view of hip joint showing: 1. Iliac crest, 2. Acetabulum, 3. Head of femur, 4. Neck of femur, 5. Obturator foramen, 6. Symphysis pubis, 7. Soft tissue shadow of external genitalia (by which you can identify sex), 8. Upper curved line, 9. Greater trochanter of femur, 10. Shenton's line, and 11. Lesser trochanter of femur

- *Head of femur*: It cast a white line. Fovea capitis femoris is visible as a small depression on the head.
- *Hip joint space*: Appears as radiolucent interval between the white lines of rim of acetabulum and head of femur.
- *Neck of femur*: The neck of the femur normally makes an angle 25–30° to the coronal plane.
- *Greater trochanter*: The outline of greater trochanter tends to be poorly defined in a usual X-ray of hip region.
- *Lesser trochanter*: It appears as a more prominent projection when the femur is laterally rotated.

The periphery of the normal femoral neck and the pelvic bone produced to regular curvature. They are:
- *Shenton's lines*: The lines of upper margins of obturator foramen follow the same curve as that of undersurface of the neck of the femur.
- *The second line (the unnamed line)*: This line begins from the lateral border of ilium from the anterior superior iliac spine to the superior border of the femoral neck and to the greater trochanter.

Anteroposterior view of knee joint showing (Fig. 10.23):

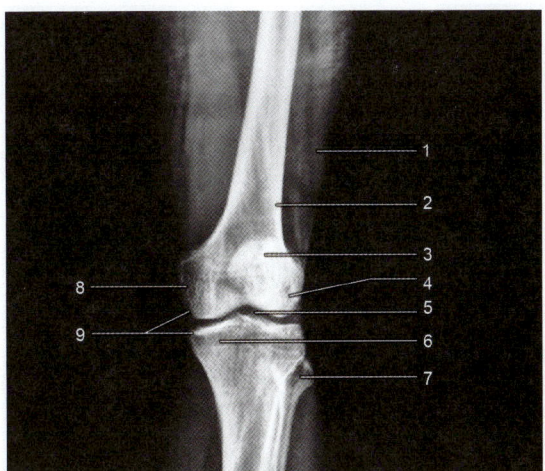

Fig. 10.23: Anteroposterior view of knee showing: 1. Soft tissue shadow, 2. Lower end of femur, 3. Outline of patella, 4. Lateral condyle of femur, 5. Knee joint space, 6. Lateral and medial condyles of tibia, 7. Head of fibula, 8. Medial condyle of femur, and 9. Articular end of femur and tibia

- *Articular ends of femur and tibia*: They are marked by thin white lines of cortical bone.
- Head and styloid process of fibula are seen considerably below the knee joint space on the lateral side and are superimposed by tibia.
- Knee joint space is normally 0.5 cm gap due to radiolucency of the articular cartilages and the two menisci.
- Intercondylar eminence of tibia presents a spinous appearance in a middle of upper surface of tibia.
- Intercondylar notch of femur is variable and superimposed by patella.
- Patella is a superimposed shadow on the lower end of femur and appears as a circular shadow with the lower edge lying 1.25 cm above the knee joint space (in fully extended position).

Lateral view of knee showing (Fig. 10.24):
- *Medial and lateral femoral condyles*: The anterior and posterior margins of two condyles are not superimposed due to the difference in their diameters.

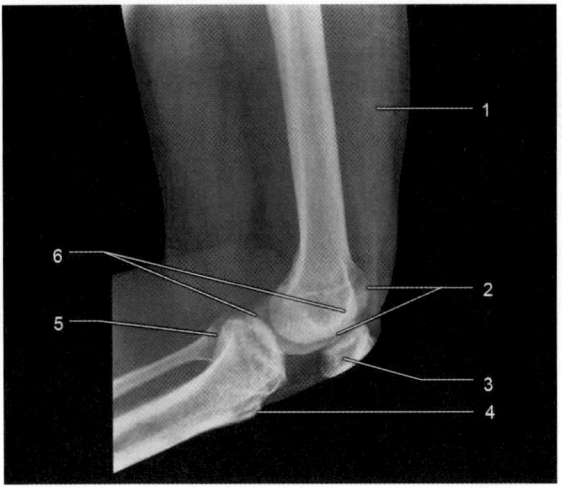

Fig. 10.24: Lateral view of knee joint showing: 1. Soft tissue shadow, 2. Lateral condyle of femur, 3. Patella, 4. Tibial tuberosity, 5. Head of fibula, and 6. Medial condyle of femur

- Intercondylar eminence of tibia is slightly overlapped by the femoral condyles.
- Knee joint space is not prominent by the overlapping of bones shadows.
- Patella is seen in front of the condyles of femur.

Anteroposterior view of ankle showing (Fig. 10.25):
- *Lower end of the tibia*: It is seen separated from upper surface of talus by the ankle joint space.
- Lower end of fibula is superimposed on tibia. The joint space is not visible in this view.
- Talus cast a four-sided shadow below the lower end of tibia and fibula.

Anteroposterior view of foot showing (Fig. 10.26):
- Calcaneum (3)
- Cuboid bone articulates directly with calcaneum on its proximal surface (5)

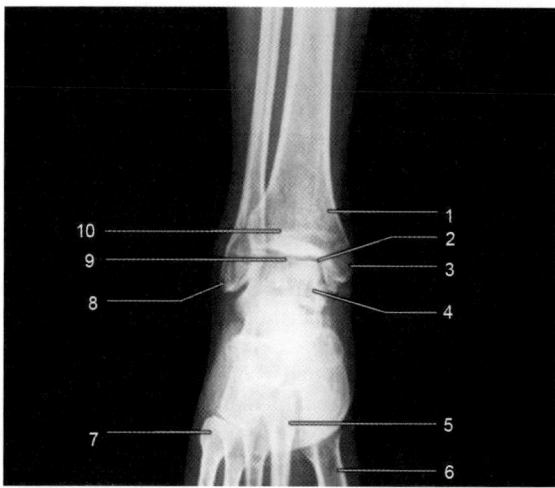

Fig. 10.25: Dorsoplantar or anteroposterior view of foot showing: 1. Lower end of tibia, 2. Ankle joint space (line), 3. Medial malleolus, 4. Talus, 5. Second metatarsal, 6. First metatarsal, 7. Styloid process of fifth metatarsal, 8. Lateral malleolus, 9. Trochlear articular surface of talus, and 10. Epiphyseal line

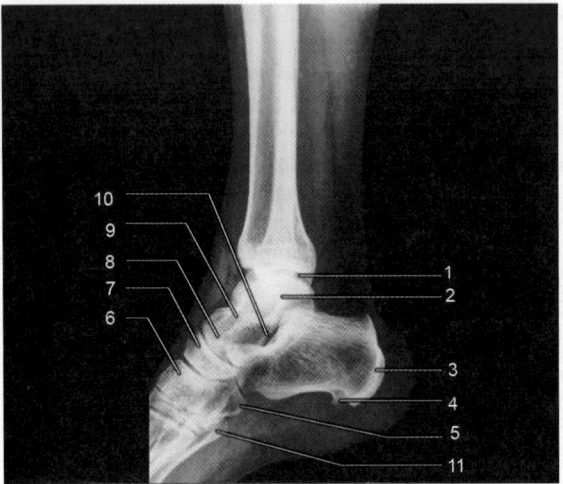

Fig. 10.26: Lateral view of foot showing: 1. Ankle joint space, 2. Lateral triangular-like articular surface of talus, 3. Calcaneum, 4. Calcaneal spur, 5. Cuboid, 6. Medial cuneiform, 7. Navicular, 8. Head of talus, 9. Neck of talus, 10. Trochlear articular area of talus, and 11. Tuberosity of fifth metatarsal (at base)

- Cuneiform bones medial, intermediate and lateral can be seen articulating with the navicular proximally.
- Intertarsal joint spaces are clearly visible.
- Navicular is an additional bone between the two rows of tarsal bones (7)
- Metatarsals are seen articulating with distal row of tarsal. The body of first metatarsal is heavy but the bodies of others are slender. The bases tend to overlap.
- Phalanges are seen separated by interphalangeal joints.
- *Sesamoid bones*: Prominent medial and lateral sesamoid bones are usually seen to overlap the head of first metatarsal bone.

Lateral view of ankle and foot showing (Fig. 10.27):
- *Calcaneum*: It is seen projecting backward. The pressure lamellae in the calcaneum is prominent.
- Cuboid shows its prominent projecting ridge on the plantar aspect.

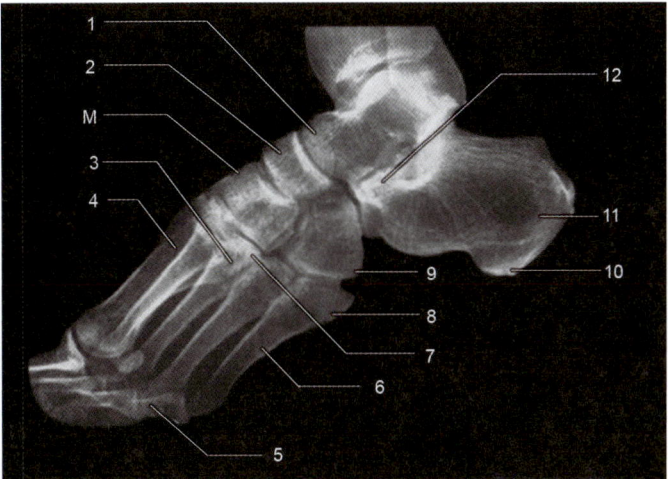

Fig. 10.27: Lateral view of foot showing: 1. Head of talus, 2. Navicular, 3. Base of second metatarsal, 4. First metatarsal, 5. Phalanx, 6. Fifth metatarsal, 7. Lateral cuneiform, 8. Styloid process of fifth metatarsal, 9. Cuboid, 10. Calcaneal tuberosity, 11. Calcaneum, and 12. Sinus tarsi. M: Medial cuneiform

- *Cuneiform*: These three bones are superimposed and their position can be decided by recognizing the articulation with the metatarsal.
- *Metatarsal*: The 1st, 2nd and 3rd tend to be partially superimposed. The 4th can be clearly demarcated. The 5th has a tubercle on its base.
- *Nevicular*: It is easily identified anterior to head of the talus.
- Talus is seen on the calcaneum and is itself lied over the lower end of tibia.
- Lower end of tibia is easily made out and the talotibial joint space is clearly visible.
- *Lower end of the fibula*: It is seen partially superimposed on tibia and talus. The shadow of lateral malleolus is lower and that of the medial malleolus.
- Sinus terri is visible like a semidark shadow above the calcaneum and below the neck of talus.

11

CHAPTER

Postgraduate Short Notes

CHAPTER OUTLINE

- Mutagenic Agents
- Role of Y Chromosome
- Mucous Membrane of Small Intestine
- Palmar Arterial Arch
- Ethmoid Air Sinus
- Endochondral Ossification
- Blood Supply of Breast
- Point Mutation
- Duchenne Muscular Dystrophy
- Embalming Techniques
- Renshaw Cells
- Apoptosis
- Endocrine Cells of Gut
- Coronary Circulation
  - Indication of Coronary Angiography
- Morphology and Maturation of T and B Lymphocyte
- Cervical Rib
- Immunohistochemistry
- Superior Colliculus and Its Connections
- Retina and its Structure
- Submandibular Salivary Gland
- Frey Syndrome (Auriculotemporal Syndrome or Gustatory Sweating)
- Pituitary
- Ossicles of Ear
- Movement of Ossicles
- Causes of Congenital Deafness
- Automatic Bladder
- Digital Synovial Sheath and Vinculae
- Role of Soft Palate in Swallowing and Phonation
- Acquired Immune Deficiency Syndrome
  - Subphrenic Space
- Stem Cell
- Reticular Formation of Brainstem
- Blood Circulation of Brain
- Subclavian Steal Syndrome
- Cleidocranial Dysostosis
- Papez Circuit
- Embryological Types of ASD
- Sphincters of Gut

MUTAGENIC AGENTS

Mutations are permanent changes in the genomic sequence. Substances causing mutation are called mutagens. Some of the mutagens are:
- Viruses
- Radiation
- *Transposons*: Deoxyribonucleic acid (DNA) sequences that can move themselves to new positions within the gene are known as transposons.
- Chemicals
- *Drugs*: Thalidomide

Mutations occur during meiosis or during DNA replication.

ROLE OF Y CHROMOSOME

Y chromosome is short and it is inherited from the father to the male offspring. It contains very few genes.

Y-linked disorders occur due to mutation on the Y chromosome. Since male offspring inherits the Y chromosome, every male offspring of the affected father will be affected by the disease. As female offspring inherit only X chromosome from their father they are never sufferers of the disease.

A few Y-linked diseases are:
- Male infertility
- Excessive hair on the pinna
- Retinitis pigmentosa
- Color blindness
- XYY syndrome.

MUCOUS MEMBRANE OF SMALL INTESTINE

Small intestine means duodenum, jejunum and ileum. The mucosal specifications of small intestine are (Figs 11.1 and 11.2):
- *Plica semilunaris*: The mucosa and submucosa form permanent folds which encloses the two-thirds of lumen. These increases mucosal absorptive surface. It is less prominent in ileum.
- *Villi*: These are finger- or leaf-like projections covering the mucosal surface. They consist of an epithelial lining and a core of lamina propria. A villus contains a central lacteal, blood capillaries and a strip of smooth muscle fibers from muscularis mucosa.

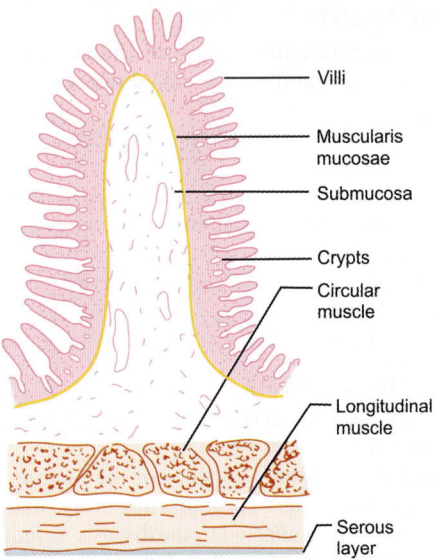

Fig. 11.1: Longitudinal section through a part of the small intestine seen at a very low magnification to show a circular mucosal fold (Schematic representation). Note the submucosa extending into the mucosal fold

- *Crypts of Lieberkühn (intestinal glands)*: These are simple tubular glands that extend through the entire thickness of mucosa.
- *Microvilli*: The apical surface of simple columnar epithelium is covered by microvilli. The microvilli increase the surface area by many times for better absorption.

Epithelium of villi consists of columnar cells and few goblet cells (unicellular mucous glands). The mucous secretion of the goblet cells lubricates the epithelium.

Epithelium of crypts are columnar in upper half and in the bottom there is less differentiated *stem cells*. They replenish the cells from the tip of the villi. At the base of the crypts there are also Paneth cells which secrete lysozyme that destroys bacteria in the gut. Apart from these, there are enteroendocrine cells which secrete secretin, cholecystokinin, motilin, etc.

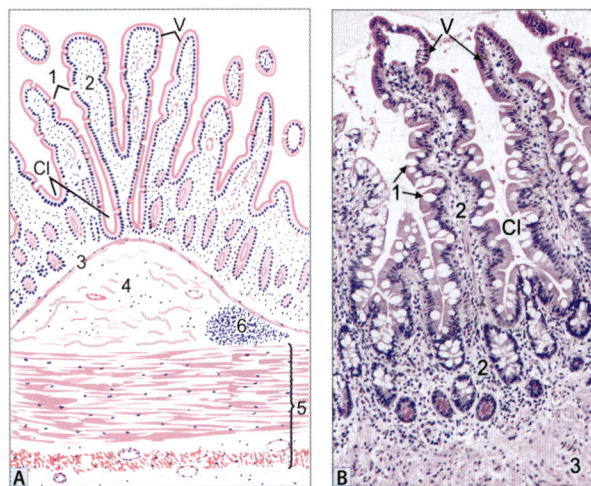

Figs 11.2A and B: Jejunum. A. As seen in drawing; B. Photomicrograph
Abbreviations: 1. Columnar epithelial lining with goblet cells. 2. Lamina propria; 3. Muscularis mucosa; 4. Submucosa; 5. Muscularis externa; 6. Lymph nodes; V, Villi; Cl, crypts of Lieberkuhn.
Courtesy: Ivan Damjanov. Atlas of Histopathology. Ist Edition. Jaypee Brothers.

Lamina propria fills up the spaces between crypts and consists of connective tissue, lymphocyte, macrophages, etc. In ileum large aggregated lymphatic nodule extends into submucosa and form *Peyer's patches.*

Muscularis mucosae is present and it has two layers of smooth muscles.

Clinical Anatomy of Mucous Membrane of Small Intestine

- *Gastritis:* This term is commonly employed for any clinical condition with upper abdominal discomfort where radiological abnormalities are absent.
- *Crohn's disease or regional enteritis:* It is an idiopathic chronic ulcerative bowel disease, characterized by transmural, non-caseating granulomatous inflammation affecting the terminal ileum.

- *Celiac sprue:* It is the most important cause of primary malasorption occuring in temperate climate. This disease produces significant loss of villi in the small intestine and there is diminished absorptive area. There are two form of celic sprue (i) Childhood form (ii) Adult form seen in adolescent and early childhood.

PALMAR ARTERIAL ARCH

- Terminal part of ulnar and radial artery form palmar arterial arches by anastomosis
- Two arches are present: (1) Superficial and (2) Deep

Superficial Palmar Arch

- This arterial arcade is situated beneath the palmar aponeurosis
- Lies in front of long flexor tendons, lumbrical muscles and palmar digital branch of median nerve
- Formed by superficial branch of ulnar artery joins with any one
  - Superficial branch of radial art
  - Arteria princeps pollicis
  - Arteria radialis indicis
- Major contribution of superficial palmar arch is by ulnar artery branch
- Convexity of arch is up to the distal border of outstretched thumb
- *Branches*: Four palmar digital artery.

Deep Palmar Arch

- Formed by terminal end of radial artery and deep branch of ulnar artery
- Major contribution by radial artery
- It lies deep to oblique head of adductor policies, long-flexar tendons and lumbrical muscles
- It crosses across the base of metacarpal bones
- Convexity lies at the level of proximal border of outstretched thumb, 1 cm proximal to superficial arch
- Branches
  - Three palmar metacarpal arteries
  - Three perforating arteries
  - Recurrent branches.

ETHMOID AIR SINUS
- This is an example of paranasal air sinus
- Situation between medial wall of orbit and lateral wall of nose
- Contained within labyrinth of ethmoid and completed by frontal maxillary and sphenoid bone
- *Number*: 3–11
- *Groups*:
    - *Anterior*: 3–7 numbers
    - *Middle*: 1–3 numbers
    - *Posterior*: 1–11 numbers
- *Opening*:
    - *Anterior*: Middle meatus of nose
    - *Middle*: Middle meatus of nose
    - *Posterior*: Superior meatus of nose
- *Blood supply*: Anterior and posterior ethmoidal artery, branch of ophthalmic artery
- *Lymph drainage*:
    - *Anterior and middle group:* Drains into submandibular node
    - *Posterior group:* Drain into retropharyngeal node.

ENDOCHONDRAL OSSIFICATION (FIG. 11.3)
- It is the cartilaginous ossification of bone
- Seen in most of bones of our body
- There is pre-existing hyaline cartilaginous model of the bone, surrounded by perichondrium
- Grows in length by interstitial method
- Grows in width by appositional method.

Cartilage cells arranged in rows of longitudinal columns (from above down words):
- Zone of proliferation by mitosis
- Zone of maturation
- Zone of hypertrophy
- Zone of calcification.

Mature cartilage cells form the matrix and secret alkaline phosphatase. This leads to calcification and calcination leads to death of cartilage cells due to lack of nutrition.
- Due to cell death, a gap is formed known as primary areolae.
- Perichondrium is vascularized and inner layer differentiates in osteoblastic layer.

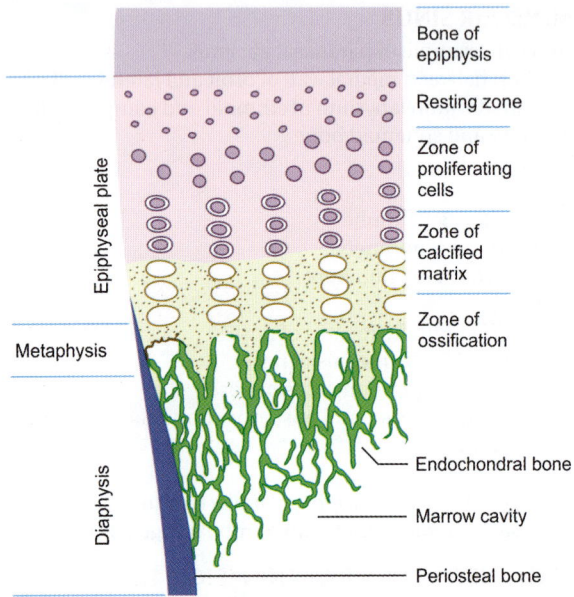

Fig. 11.3: Structure of an epiphyseal plate and endochondral ossification

Periosteal collar of new bone is formed by appositional growth.
- Osteogenic layer of periosteum forms periosteal bud. Through this blood vessel enter the model with osteoblast, osteoclast, and osteocytes.
- This enters into calcified matrix as primary center for ossification and perforation of bud persists as nutrient foramen.
- Osteoclast destroys calcified matrix and form a large space called secondary areolae.
- Secondary areolae filled by bone marrow and lined by osteoblast cells.
- Osteoclast divides and form new bone matrix and form cancellous bone.
- Osteoclast helps in resorption of bone spicules and formation of marrow cavity.
- Mineralization of bony matrix occurs

- Later other ossification centers arises for epiphysis called secondary ossification center and similar process described above repeated
- Epiphyseal cartilage persists as long as bone grows in length
- Remodeling and new bone formation occur lifelong.

BLOOD SUPPLY OF BREAST

Arterial Supply of Breast (Fig. 11.4)

It is Supplied by following arteries.
- *Lateral thoracic artery (branch of axillary artery 2nd part)*:
  - It provides lateral mammary artery
  - Supply lateral part of breast. It is the major supply of breast
- *Superior thoracic artery (small branch from axillary artery 1st part)*: Supplies upper part of breast.
- Perforating branches of 2nd, 3rd, and 4th internal mammary artery—provides medial mammary artery, supply medial part of the breast.

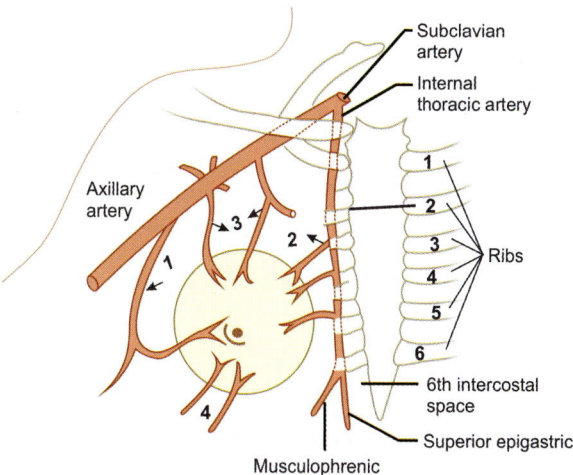

Fig. 11.4: Sources of arterial supply to the breast (1) Branches of lateral thoracic artery; (2) Branches of internal thoracic artery; (3) Branches of acromiothoracic and superior thoracic arteries; (4) Branches of 2nd, 3rd and 4th posterior intercostal arteries

- Lateral branches of 2nd, 3rd and 4th intercostal artery supply the gland from deep surface.

Venous Drainage

Vein forms circular venosus plexus beneath areola—form this veins radiales outward beneath skin—drains to axillary, internal thoracic and intercostal veins.

Clinical Anatomy

Through intercostal and azygos veins the blood communicates with internal vertebral venous plexus (Batson), intracranial sagittal and transverse sinus and this communicates with clavicle, humerus, vertebrae, so, carcinoma of breast may spread to bones.

POINT MUTATION

Replacement of single nucleotides with another nucleotide is known as point mutation or single base substitution.

It may produce an altered sequence of amino acid when protein is being synthesized. The newly formed protein may be ineffective.

CTGG A G
CTGG G G

One can arrange point mutation as:
- *Translation*: Replacement of a purine (adenine and guanine) with another purine or replacement pyrimidine (cytosine, thymine and uracil) with another pyrimidine.
- *Transversion*: Replacement of a purine with pyrimidine or vice versa.
- Translation mutations are more common than transversion mutations.

Point mutation can also divided into four types functionally. They are:
1. Missense mutation
2. Silent mutation
3. Conservative mutation
4. Nonconservative mutation

DUCHENNE MUSCULAR DYSTROPHY

- *Introduction*: This is an X-linked recessive disorder. Though both often carriers of the occurrence of Duchenne muscular dystrophy (DMD) 1 in 3,000 life births.
- *Genotype*: This disorder is caused by mutation the dystrophies gene located on the short arm of X chromosome.

- *Features*: Generally, symptom appears in male children before 5 years of age.
- The patient complains of:
    - Progressive proximal muscle weakness of legs and pelvis
    - Loss of muscle mass
    - Weakness spreading to the arms, neck and other areas
    - Use braces for walking
    - Difficulty in standing unaided or inability to ascend staircase
    - They may use a wheel chair
    - *Life span*: Their life span is less.
- Quality of Life: Poor
- Genetic Counseling.

Duchenne muscular dystrophy is an X-linked recessive disorder. Males of mutated gene is enough for producing the disease in males. Females are the carrier prenatal diagnosis can be performed for diagnosis of DMD. One can go for medical termination of pregnancy.

Commonly used techniques of embalming in anatomy department. Describe the role of formalin when used as embalming agent.

EMBALMING TECHNIQUES

The commonly used embalming techniques in anatomy department are formalin preservation. Previously the dead body preservation was done by Egyptian.

In India, a 6 cm long vertical incision is given on upper and medial side of thigh and femoral sheath is exposed. The sheath is excised and femoral artery is identified by tube like appearance. About 10–12 L of embalming fluid prepared by appropriate amount of formalin (10 L), glycerine (0.5 L) and alcohol (1 L) is put in the injector. The amount may be increased if the body is large. A nick is made in the femoral artery and the cannula of the injector machine is placed (Figs 11.5A and B) so that it points toward the head end. Five liters of fluid is pumped under 8 kg of pressure. The direction of cannula is reversed and the rest of the fluid is pumped in opposite direction. One should notice that froth is coming from mouth and nose and whole face will be swollen immediately. And this is the time when embalming is complete. The skin over the thigh is stitched. Salt may be mixed in embalming fluid. It will nicely preserve the muscle but there is chance of fungus formation in the body, if body remains outside for prolonged

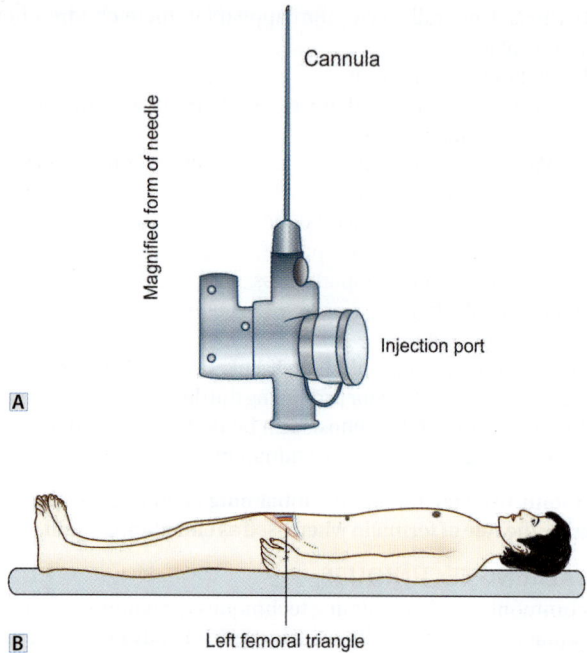

Figs 11.5A and B: Technique of embalming of body (dead). Injector—A machine by which embalming solution is introduced in the dead body

period. Local injections are given in palm, sole and dorsum of hand and foot as they are peripherally placed formalin may not go there, when formalin goes there, there is rounding of tips of fingers and toes.

RENSHAW CELLS

There are the interneurons of anterior gray column. The axon of Renshaw cell loops back to inhibit the corresponding alpha neurons and suppress the action of antagonistic muscle.

Clinical Anatomy

Tetanus toxin or strychnine suppress the action of Renshaw cells and produce convulsion.

APOPTOSIS

It is also known as programmed cell death. Here cell dies in tightly regulated suicide program. The cells plasma membrane remains intact but its structure is altered so that the cell ruptured immediately and cleared by phagocytosis before its content is leaked out.

Cause of Apoptosis

It can be physiologic or pathologic.

Physiologic Causes

- Programmed destruction of cells during embryogenesis.
- Hormone dependent involution of tissues (e.g. endometrium of uterus and prostate in adult)
- Death of cell supplies the useful purposes.

Pathological Causes

- Deoxyribonucleic damage due to hypoxia, radiation or cytotoxic drugs cause apoptosis.
- In case of neurodegenerative disorder due to accumulation of misfolded proteins.
- Cell death in viral infection like hepatitis.
- Pathological atrophy in parenchymal organ after duct obstruction.
- *Mechanism of apoptosis*: The process of apoptosis into an initiation phase, an execution phase (when the enzymes cause cell death).

Morphological and Biochemical Changes in Apoptosis

Morphological features of apoptosis include cell shrinkage, chromatic condensation and fragmentation and then these cell bodies are taken up by healthy cells or by macrophages.

ENDOCRINE CELLS OF GUT

The intestine contains some widely distributed cells called diffuse neuroendocrine system. Stimulation of these cells release secretary granules by exocytosis and the hormones exert paracrine or local or endocrine (blood-borne) effects.

Polypeptide secreting cells of digestive tract fall in two classes:

1. *Open type*: Here the apex of the cells present microvilli and in contact of the lumen of organ.
2. *Close type*: Here the cellular apices are covered by other epithelial cells.

In small intestine the endocrine cells of open type are more slender than the neighboring absorptive cells. The activity of digestive system is controlled by nervous system and modulated by a complex system of locally produced peptide hormone.

CORONARY CIRCULATION

Heart is supplied by two coronary arteries right and left.

Name	Beginning	Course	Branches	Area supplied
1. Right coronary artery (smaller than left coronary artery) (Fig. 11.6) P.G.E.	It arises from ascending aorta from the anterior aortic sinus	It passes downwards in between the root of pulmonary trunk and the right auricle, it winds round the inferior border, passes in the posterior part of atrioventricular groove and terminate by anastomosis with left coronary artery	• Marginal • Posterior inter-ventricular • Nodal (60% case)	It supplies all of the right ventricle, the variable part of diaphragmatic surface of left ventricle, post 1/3rd of inter-ventricular septum, the right atrium part of left atrium and nodal tissue
• Left coronary artery (Fig. 11.6) P.G.E.	It arises from ascending aorta from left posterior aortic sinus	It passes behind and then to the left of pulmonary artery. Between it and left auricle it divides into circumflex and anterior interventricular branch	• Anterior inter-ventricular (left anterior descending) • Left circumflex branch	It supplies most of left ventricle, small area of right ventricle, anterior 2/3rd of inter-ventricular septum, most of left atrium

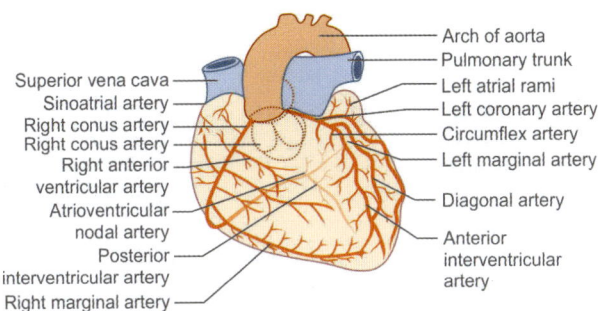

Fig. 11.6: Coronary arterial system

Clinical Anatomy

Angiography means the study of blood vessels by injection of contrast medium containing iodine in the vessel.

Indication of Coronary Angiography

To visually Vascularity appearance and narrowing of coronary artery.

Contraindication

- Bleeding tendencies.
- Cardiovascular disease like recent myocardial infarction.
- Hepatic failure.

Procedure

Local anesthetic at the site of puncture.

Puncture Site

1. Femoral artery
2. Axillary artery
3. Brachial artery.

By this procedure, we can detect the narrowing or dilatation of supplying artery. When there is narrowing of antery the cardiologist may insert stent to prevent myocardial infarction.

MORPHOLOGY AND MATURATION OF T AND B LYMPHOCYTE

The cell population of lymph node is made up of lymphocytes (Figs 11.7 and 11.8).

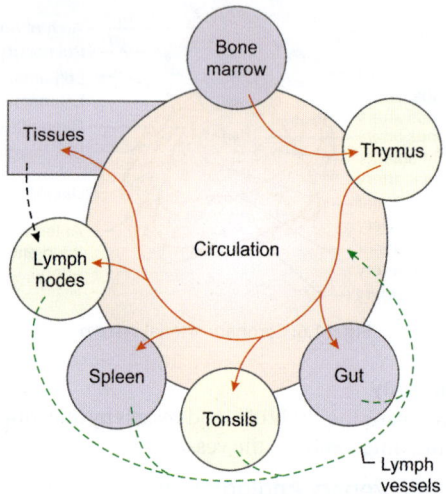

Fig. 11.7: Circulation of T-lymphycytes (schematic representation)

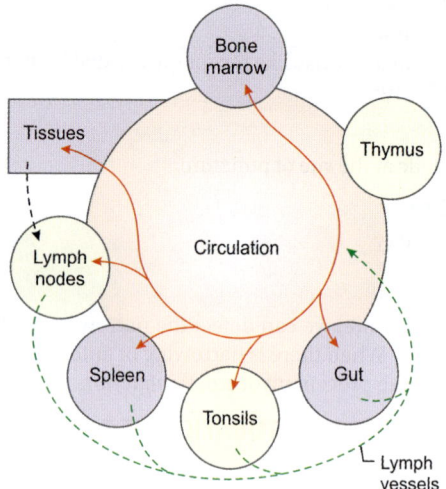

Fig. 11.8: Circulation of B-lymphocytes (schematic representation)

In the embryo the lymphocytes are derived from the mesenchymal cells derived from the wall of the yolk sac, in the liver and in the spleen. These cells then migrate to bone marrow. Lymphocytes from bone marrow then enter the blood. Depending upon their behavior they are classified as T lymphocyte and B lymphocyte.

Lymphocyte travels in the bloodstream to reach the thymus. Here they divide repeatedly and undergo certain changes and form T lymphocyte. Again they re-enter into blood circulation to reach the lymphoid tissue in the lymph nodes, spleen, tonsils and intestine. In lymph nodes T lymphocytes are found around lymphatic nodules. In the spleen it is found in the white pulp. About 85% of lymphocytes seen in blood are T lymphocyte.

B lymphocytes arise from stem cells of bone marrow. They enter the bloodstream but do not go through thymus. "B" means "bursa of Fabricius", a diverticulum of cloaca in birds. In birds B-lymphocytes are formed there and from here the name is derived.

In contrast to T lymphocytes that live in lymph nodes and spleen, B lymphocytes are seen in lymphatic nodules. The germinal centers are formed by dense aggregations of B lymphocytes, while the dark rims of lymphatic nodules are formed by dense aggregations of B lymphocytes. B lymphocytes like T lymphocytes also circulate between lymphoid tissues and bloodstream. Lymphocytes are important part of immune system of body which is important for defense mechanism.

CERVICAL RIB (FIG. 11.9)

- It is relatively common anomaly.
- Present in 1–2% of people.
- The costal elements of C7 cervical vertebra in front of foramen transversarium become abnormally enlarged and form sometimes a complete rib.
- In 60% cases the incidence is bilateral.
- The extra rib or a fibrous connection extending from its tip to first rib may elevate and place pressure on the structures that emerges from superior thoracic aperture—the subclavian artery or inferior trunk of brachial plexus and may cause thoracic outlet syndrome.

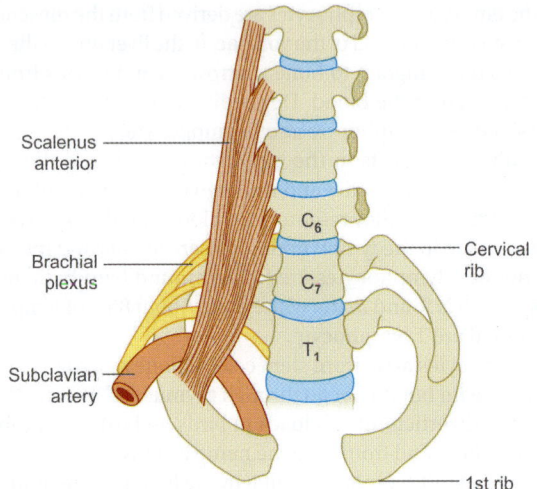

Fig. 11.9: Bilateral cervical ribs. On the right side the brachial plexus is shown. Cervical rib stretching its lowest trunk

IMMUNOHISTOCHEMISTRY

It denotes the process of selecting imaging antigens (e.g. protein) in the cells of a tissue section by taking the principle of antibodies binding specifically to antigens in biological tissues. Immunohistochemistry takes its name from the roots "immuno" in reference to antibodies used in the procedures, and "histo" meaning "tissue". The procedure was first implemented by Albert Coons in 1941.

Immunohistochemical staining is widely used in diagnosis of abnormal cells such as those found in cancerous tumors. Immunohistochemistry is also widely used in basic research to understand the distribution and localization of biomarkers and differentially expressed protein in different parts of biological tissue.

It is widely used in surgical pathology, neurosciences, salivary gland and head and neck carcinomas. Many clinical laboratories in tertiary hospitals will have 200 antibodies used as diagnostic and prognostic biomarkers.

Examples of biomarkers include:
- *Cytokeratins*: It is used for identification of carcinoma and sarcomas.
- *Alfa fetoproteins*: For yolk sac tumors and hepatocellular carcinomas.
- *CD15 and CD30*: It is used for Hodgkin disease.
- *CD10*: For renal cell carcinoma and acute lymphoblastic leukemia.
- *Prostate-specific antigen (PSA)*: For prostate cancer.
- *CD20*: It is used for identification of B cell lymphomas.
- *CD3*: It is used for diagnosis of T cell lymphomas.
- Immunohistochemistry can be used to asses which tumor is likely respond to therapy.

SUPERIOR COLLICULUS AND ITS CONNECTIONS

The superior colliculi are two pairs of elevated masses. They are the reflex center. Each superior colliculus is connected to the lateral geniculate body by superior brachium. The superior colliculum presents a laminar architecture, composed of layers of gray and white matter.

Afferent Connections
- From retina via retinotectal fibers
- From spinal cord via spinotectal tract
- From temporal and occipital cortex by corticotectal fibers
- From inferior colliculi.

Efferent Connections
- The tectospinal fibers decussate and relay in opposite side of spinal cord.
- The tectothalamic fibers end in the pulvinar of thalamus and tectocortical fibers reach the occipital cortex.
- The tectobulbar fibers connect it to cranial nerve nuclei, reticular formation and cerebellum.

Functions
- The superior colliculus is the reflex center for the movements of the eyes and head in response to visual stimuli.
- It is also involved in the control of vertical and horizontal gaze.

RETINA AND ITS STRUCTURE (FIG. 11.10)

Retina is the inner photosensitive complex layer of eyeball. It has the photoreceptor rods and cones.

The eye develops as an evagination of diencephalon known as optic vesicle. This vesicle forms a two layered optic cup later on. The outer layer develops into the pigment layer of choroid and the inner layer gives rise to rods and cones.

The photosensitive part of retina has nine layers.
1. *Layer of rods and cones*:
   - *Rods are cylindrical*. The outer part contains molecules of rhodopsin (visual purple). They are sensitive to dim light.
   - Cones are flask shaped. Their inner segment contains iodopsin that is sensitive to bright light. The cones are also responsible for color vision.
2. The next layer is the external limiting membrane. It is not a membrane but junctional complexes between Müller cells and photoreceptor cells.
3. *Outer molecular layer* consists of cell bodies of rods and cones.
4. *Outer plexiform layer* consists of axons of rods and cones forming synapses with bipolar cells.

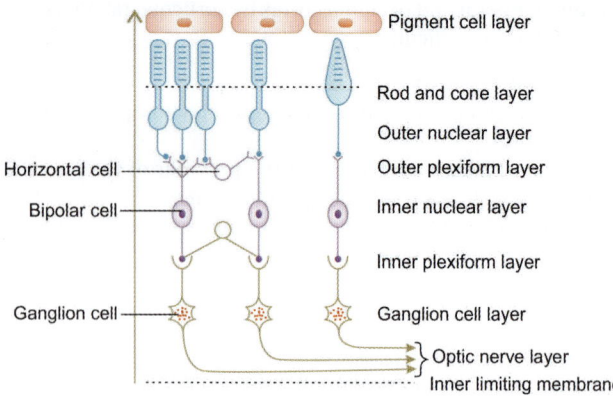

Fig. 11.10: Layers of retina

5. *Inner nuclear layer* contains nuclei of bipolar cells and nuclei of supporting Muller cells.
6. *Inner plexiform layer* consists of synapses between bipolar axons and dendrites of ganglion cells.
7. *Nerve fiber layer*: It is composed of unmyelinated axons of ganglionic cells. It runs in a parallel direction to reach the optic disc.
8. *Internal limiting membrane:* It is formed by the expanded ends of Müller cells and their basement membranes.

Clinical Anatomy

The pigment layer of retina is more firmly attached to the choroid than the nervous layer. This pigment layer may be detached from the nervous layer known as retinal detachment. It usually occurs in myopics.

SUBMANDIBULAR SALIVARY GLAND

It is a mixed type of compound racemose gland which pours viscous secretion into the floor of the oral cavity (Figs 11.11 and 11.12).

Parts: It consists of two parts:
1. A larger superficial part which is located below the mylohyoid muscle and almost fills the digastric triangle.

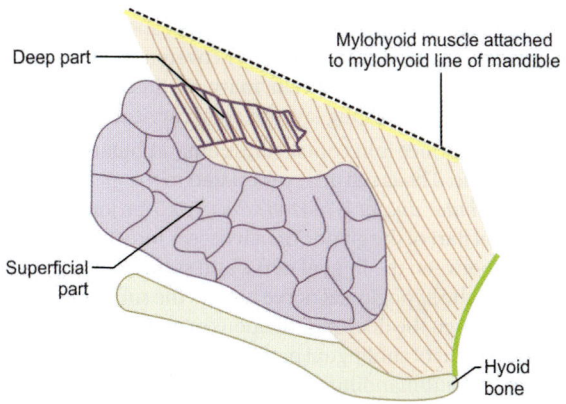

Fig. 11.11: Continuity of two parts of submandibular gland around the posterior margin of mylohyoid muscle

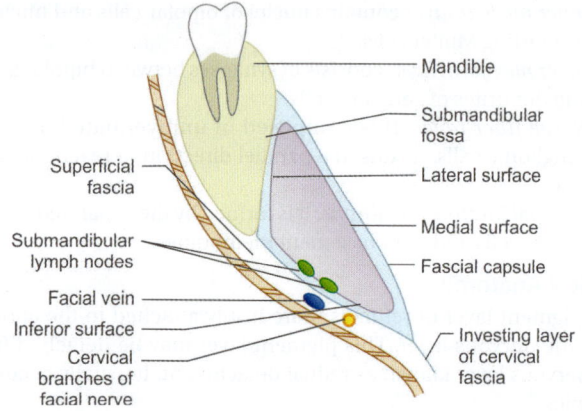

Fig. 11.12: Fascial capsule and surfaces of submandibular salivary gland

2. *Deep part*: Smaller, which is located above the mylohyoid muscle.

   The two parts are continuous with each other around the free posterior border of mylohyoid muscle.
   - *Facial capsule*: The gland is covered by investing layer of deep cervical fascia. The submandibular lymph nodes are almost embedded in the gland within the fascial capsule.
   - *Relations*: The superficial surface is covered by skin, superficial fascia with platysma, facial vein, marginal and cervical branch of facial nerve and investing layer of deep cervical fascia.

   The lateral surface is in contact on submandibular fossa on inner side of mandible. The facial artery is related to the gland twice.
   - *Submandibular duct or Wharton's duct*: It is 5 cm long. Begins from superficial part of the gland. Then it passes into the deep part. It is situated between the lingual nerve and submandibular ganglion above and the hypoglossal nerve below. The submandibular duct passes through the deep part. It opens over the floor of the mouth on the summit of sublingual papilla by the side of the frenulum of tongue. The submandibular duct has got triple relation with the lingual nerve that is lateral, inferior and medial aspect of the duct.

Clinical Anatomy
- About 80% salivary calculi occur in the submandibular salivary duct and 80% of them is radiopaque. Calculi are more common as the gland secrets more viscous fluid containing calcium.
- *Bimanual palpation of the gland*: The site of the gland may be assessed by placing two hands- (1) left hand at the floor of the mouth outside and (2) right hand should be placed within mouth by the side of the sublingual papilla.

FREY SYNDROME (AURICULOTEMPORAL SYNDROME OR GUSTATORY SWEATING)
- It is due to injury to auriculotemporal nerve, where the postganglionic parasympathetic fiber from otic ganglion becomes united to sympathetic nerves from the superior cervical ganglion (pseudosynapsis). Sweating and hyperesthesia occur in the area of skin supplied by the nerve skin of the auricle above the external auditory meatus and temple.
- It occurs in 10% of cases.
- *Causes*: Surgery or accidental injuries to the parotid.
- *Clinical features*: Flushing, sweating, pain and hyperesthesia over the skin supplied by auriculotemporal nerve, when there is mastication of food.

PITUITARY (FIG. 11.13)
- It is an endocrine gland. Situated within the pituitary fossa (sella turcica).
- It is oval in shape and weight is 0.5 g.
- Its transverse diameter is greater than anteroposterior diameter.
- It is attached by a stalk to the median eminence to tuber cinerium which is a part of hypothalamus.
- Pituitary is known as band master of endocrine orchestra because some of the hormone secreted by it controls the other endocrine gland activity.
- Pituitary gland consists of two lobes: (1) adenohypophysis and (2) neurohypophysis. The adenohypophysis is subdivided by a cleft into three parts:
  1. *Pars distalis*: The main anterior part containing chromophobe and chromophil cells.

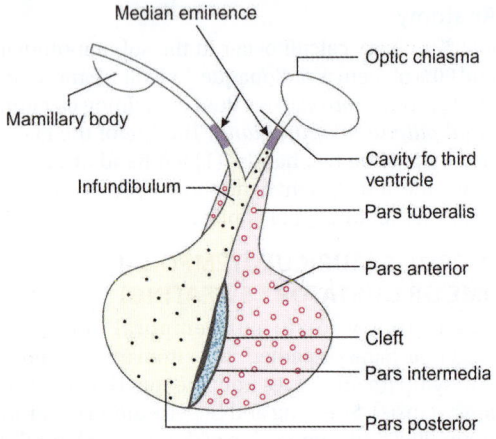

Fig. 11.13: Schemes to show sagittal section of the subdivisions of the hypophysis cerebri

2. *Pars tuberalis*: The cranial part of the distalis that surrounds the infundibulum.
3. Pars intermedium.
- The neurohypophysis is divided into two parts: (1) Pars nervosa—part that lies posterior to pars intermedia. It contains unmyelinated nerve fibers and (2) pituicytes.
- The endocrine system of pituitary gland is under direct control of hypothalamus.

Functions

- *Produces growth hormones*: Induces growth of linear by its stimulatory action on epiphyseal cartilage of long bones.
- Produces thyroid stimulatory hormone.
- Produces gonadotropin.
- Produces corticotropin.
- Produces lactogenic hormone.
- Produces antidiuretic hormone.
- Produces vasopressin.

Clinical Anatomy

- Tumors of pituitary are usually benign in type and cause excessive secretion of hormones (ACTH and GH). Tumor of adrenal cortex stimulates the corticotroph—produce large quantity of corticosteroid leading to Cushing's syndrome.
- Tumor of somatotrophs produces excess growth hormone causing gigantism in child and acromegaly in adults.
- Some tumor of pituitary produces no hormone but grow out sella turcica. It may compress the optic chiasmo-above, and produces bitemporal hemianopia.
- Deficiency of ADH due to lesion of hypothalamus may lead to a condition called diabetes insipidus (polyuria).

Pineal Gland (Fig. 11.14)

- *Introduction*: It is a small conical gland, projecting backward and downward between the two superior colliculi. It is situated below the splenium of corpus callosum. It is separated from splenium by tela choroidea of third ventricle.
- *Parts*: It has body and a stalk. Body is conical in shape, small. Stalk or peduncle is separated by a pineal recess of third ventricle. The superior lamina contains Habenular commissure and inferior lamina contains posterior commissure.

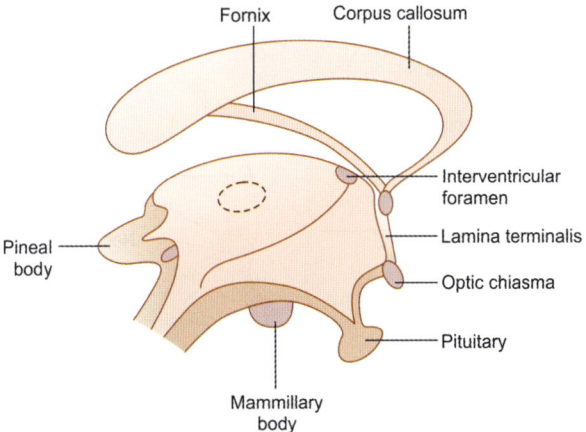

Fig. 11.14: Pineal and pituitary gland in respect to 3rd ventricle

- *Functions*: The function of pineal gland is that it plays an important role in development of gonads by influencing the output of gonadotropin—particularly in the period immediately before the sexual maturity.

  Melatonin and serotonin have been extracted from pineal body which are either directly or indirectly related to the sexual maturity. Effects of light, stress, temperature variation feeling, etc. on reproduction may be. Melatonin is secreted more during night.
- *Clinical anatomy*: Tumor of pineal gland is often associated with precocious puberty.

Gross anatomy, articulation and movement of ossicles of middle ear. Enumerate the causes of congenital deafness.

OSSICLES OF EAR (FIG. 11.15)

There are three ear ossicles: (1) malleus, (2) incus, and (3) stapes.
1. *Malleus* derived its name like its resemblance to mallet meaning "hammer". It is the smallest long bone in the body. It has head,

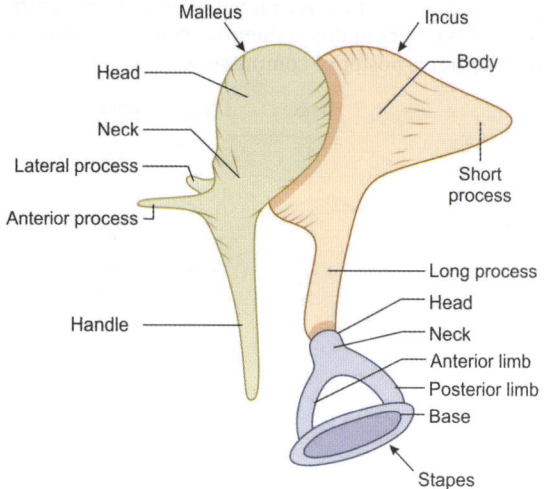

Fig. 11.15: Ossicles of the ear as seen from the medial side

handle and neck. Neck is a constriction between head and handle. The anterior and lateral processes arise just below the neck. The head lies in epitympanic recess and articulates with body of incus. Incudomalleal joint is a saddle shaped synovial joint. The neck gives attachment to the tensor tympani tendon. The lateral process gives attachment to the anterior and posterior malleolar folds.

2. *Incus* looks like premolar tooth but its name derived from anvil. It has body and two processes, long and short. The short process is attached to fossa of incudis in the posterior wall of middle ear. The long process goes down and its lower end articulates with head of stapes to form incudostapedial joint, which is ball and socket type of synovial joint.
3. *Stapes*: Resembles a stirrup. It is the smallest bone in the body. It has head, neck and two limbs of unequal length. These two limbs are joined with an oval plate called base or foot plate. The neck receives insertion of stapedius muscle. The foot plate is attached to the margin of fenestrum vestibuli by annular ligament.

MOVEMENT OF OSSICLES

When sound wave falls on the ear drum there is movement of the ossicles in a chain-like pattern. This movement ultimately vibrates the foot plate of stapes to the oval window and thus the sound wave passes from external ear to the internal ear up to organ of Corti.

CAUSES OF CONGENITAL DEAFNESS

Hereditary Group

Bad embryo: Defective development of cochlea, middle ear including otosclerosis and external ear.

Pregnancy Group

If mother suffers from
- Rubella
- Rh incompatibility
- Other infections
- Drugs
- Toxemia
- Threatened abortion
- Major surgeries under general anesthesia.

Birth Group
- Prolonged and difficult labor
- Premature birth
- Anoxia
- Convulsions
- Cerebral palsy
- Jaundice.

JUNCTIONAL COMPLEXES

Cells interact and communicate themselves by means of "junctional complexes". They are the following:

Tight Junction (Occluding Junctions)

It seals adjacent cells together and create a continuous barrier. It restricts the paracellular (between cells) movement of ions and other molecules. The junctions are formed from multiple transmembrane proteins including occludin, zonulin, claudin, etc. This area is a high resistant barrier and maintains the cellular polarity. Tight junctions are dynamic junctions that can dissociate and reform as required to facilitate epithelial proliferation or inflammatory cell migration.

Desmosomes (Anchoring Junction)

The cells are attached mechanically by means of belt and their intracellular cytoskeleton to other cell. Desmosomes are of following types:
- *Spot desmosomes (macula adherens)*: They are small revet like adhesion between cells.
- *Hemidesmosomes*: It is revet like adhesion between cells and transmembrane connector protein are called integrin.
- *Desmosomes* are formed by homotypic association of transmembrane glycoprotein called cadherin. In belt desmosomes the cadherins are associated with intracellular intermediate actin microfilaments, which can influence cell shape and motility.
- *Focal adhesion complexes*: These are large macromolecular complexes that localize to hemidesmosome and include proteins. This protein can generate intracellular signs when cells are under mechanical forces (e.g. endothelium in bloodstream or cardiac myocyte in a failing heart.

Gap Junctions (Communicating Junction)

It transfers the passage of chemical or electric signals between cells. The permeability of gap junctions is reduced by acidic pH or increased intracellular calcium. Gap junction plays an important role in cell to cell communication, e.g. in cardiac myocyte cell to cell calcium fluxes through gap junctions allow the myocardium to behave like a functional syncytium.

AUTOMATIC BLADDER

Sacral micturition center is situated at S2, S3, and S4 level.
This center is associated with two reflexes and are as follows:
1. *Bladder distension*: Stretch receptors are stimulated—impulse relay in lateral horn cell of S2, S3, S4, via pelvic splanchnic nerve. Detrusor contraction, dilatation of bladder neck and urine comes to urethra.
2. *Dilatation of proximal urethra*: Pelvic splanchnic nerve to spinal cord—lower motor neuron of anterior horn cell—inhibition—sphincter urethra is relaxed and urine pass through distal urethra.

After transactions of spinal cord above the level of S2, (above sacral micturition center) all reflexes are suppressed due to spinal shock. It leads to atonic, over distended bladder with overflow incontinence. After 2 weeks when spinal shock is over then micturition reflex returns without higher center control. In this case bladder capacity reduced, wall become hypertrophoid with residual urine. This is called automatic bladder.

DIGITAL SYNOVIAL SHEATH AND VINCULAE

- Flexor tendons of hand are situated within fibro-osseous tunnel in digits.
- To prevent fiction during movement the tendons are invested a tubular synovial sheath and called digital synovial sheath.
- It is closed at both ends.
- Has parietal and visceral layer.
- Parietal layer lines the wall of osseofibrous tunnel visceral layer lines the tendons.
- Continuity of two layers forms mesotendon posteriorly. Mesotendon gives passage to nerves and blood vessels.

- Due to frequent movement most of the portion of mesotendon disappears—only few area remains infect and forms vinculae.
- Types and number:
  - *Vinculae longa*: Three falciform fold
  - *Vinculae brevia*: Two triangular

Vinculae longa: Two attached with flexor with flexor digitorum superficialis tendon and one attached with flexor digitorum profundus tendon.

They are attached of proximal end of proximal phalanx and distal end of proximal phalanx, respectively.

Vinculae brevia: One attached with profundus tendon to distal interphalangeal and one attached with superficialis tendon to proximal interphalangeal.

- Digital synovial sheath of little finger is continuous with ulnar bursa, so spread of infection is high and that of thumb is continuous with radial bursa, but in other digits they are separated.

ROLE OF SOFT PALATE IN SWALLOWING AND PHONATION

Soft palate helps in 2nd stage of deglutition or pharyngeal stage of swallowing. This stage is involuntary stage. The bolus of food may pass to their direction from pharynx (1) regurgitation to mouth, (2) to nasopharynx and (3) to larynx to get esophagus.

The regurgitation to mouth is prevented by closing oropharyngeal isthmus by contraction of palatoglossus and pulling the root of tongue toward soft palate.

The passage to nasopharynx is prevented by closing pharyngeal isthmus by contraction of levator veli palatini and tensor veli palatini which leads to approximation of soft palate to Passavant's ridge.

This soft palate prevents wrong passage of food from pharynx.

Soft palate helps in resonance and articulation of speech. Changing the position the resonance of sound is changed and thus quality of sound is maintained by soft palate.

Articulations are formed by lip, teeth, palate and tongue. They are valves to stop the phonated exhaled air completely or through a narrow space for passage soft palate is slowed articulator for phonation.

ACQUIRED IMMUNE DEFICIENCY SYNDROME

This syndrome is caused by human immunodeficiency virus which is a group of retrovirus HIV-1 and HIV-2. This virus specially decreases CD4 cells leading to immunodeficiency. As a result, the individual is susceptible to infections by opportunistic microorganism and specific tumors. The incubation period is from 2 months to 4 years.

The main mode of transmission of HIVs are: (1) sexual contact (homosexual or heterosexual), (2) transplacental, (3) exposure to infected blood or tissue fluid and (4) through breast milk.

Mother-to-Child Transmission

The vertical transmission to neonates is about 30% through seropositive mother. Women with acquired immune deficiency syndrome (AIDS) are discouraged to become pregnant.

Pathogenesis

The virus predominantly affects the T lymphocyte. There is significant immunodeficiency (cell mediated) of the affected individual. As a result the individual suffers from a variety of infections and tumors.

Clinical Presentation

Initial presentation of an infected patient is fever, malaise, headache, sore throat, lymphadenopathy and maculopapular rash. Primary illness is followed by an asymptomatic period. Then there is progression of disease may lead to multiple infections with candida, tuberculosis, etc. Patients may present with neoplasms such as cervical carcinoma, lymphomas, etc. There may be weight loss and diarrhea.

SUBPHRENIC SPACE

The *subphrenic spaces* are potential spaces below the diaphragm produced by the peritoneal folds around the liver. The spaces are all intraperitoneal with the exception of small extraperitoneal compartment between the diaphragm and the bare area of liver.

Right Anterior Subphrenic Space

- Boundary
- *Superiorly*: Upper coronary ligament
- *Inferiorly*: General peritoneal cavity

- *Anterolaterally*: Diaphragm and anterior abdominal wall
- *Posteriorly*: Right lobe of liver
- *Medially*: Falciform ligament
- Right anterior subphrenic space is continuous with right posterior subphrenic space allowing infection to spread from one space to the other.

Left Anterior Subphrenic Space
- Boundary
- *Superiorly*: Left triangular ligament
- *Inferiorly*: General peritoneal cavity
- *Medially*: Falciform ligament
- *Laterally*: The space extends as far as spleen
- *Anterolaterally*: Diaphragm and anterior abdominal wall
- *Posteriorly*: Left lobe of liver.

Right posterior subphrenic space: Pouch of Rutherford-Morrison
- Boundary
- *Superiorly*: Lower coronary ligament
- *Inferiorly*: General peritoneal cavity
- *Laterally*: Lateral abdominal wall
- *Medially*: Lesser sac and foramen of Winslow
- *Anteriorly*: Inferoposterior surface of liver
- *Posteriorly*: Right kidney and hepatic flexure of colon.

Left Posterior Subphrenic Space: Lesser Sac
- Space lies between diaphragm, liver and stomach.
- Lateral boundary is inferior vena cava with abdominal portion of esophagus medially
- Anteroposteriorly the space extends from caudate lobe of liver to the right crus of diaphragm and the thoracic aorta.

Importance
- Subphrenic abscess is more common on the right side like appendicitis/perforation/liver abscess/cholecystitis.
- Postoperatively it develops commonly after gastritis, biliary/colonic surgeries and emergency surgeries.

Clinical Features
- Fever with chill and rigor
- Pain in right hypochondrium, epigastrium and lower thorax
- Hi-cough and tachycardia
- Bacteria causing subphrenic abscess—*Escherichia coli*, *Klebsiella*, Streptococci, etc.
- *Investigations*: Ultrasonography (USG) of abdomen.

Treatment
- *Antibiotic*: Ampicillin, gentamicin and metronidazole
- *Percutaneous drainage*: Ultrasound-guided aspiration is useful
- Open drainage is advisable when symptoms persists.

STEM CELL

Stem cells are characterized by their self-renewal capacity and their asymmetric replication. From one cell different types of cells develop. Asymmetric replication is a special property of stem cells. It means in every cell division one of the cells retain its self-renewal capacity while the other enter into differentiation pathway, and is converted into nondividing cells.

Stem cells are first identified as pluripotent cells in embryos and these are called embryonic. So stem cells are present in adult in many tissues to maintain the homeostasis of the body. Embryonic stem cells may be used to correct the damage cells like liver after necrosis of hepatocytes, heart (myocardium) after infarction.

Stem cell concept of healing—regenerative medicine. Nowadays stem cells are used for healing of tissues. Stem cells can differentiate into 220 types of cells, e.g. red cells, myocytes, neurons, etc.

Stem cells are in the following directions:
- *Bone marrow stem cells*: Hematopoietic stem cells taken from umbilical cord blood have been used for treatment of various forms of blood cancer and other blood disorder.
- *Neuron stem cells*: They are capable of generating neurons, astrocytes and oligodendrocytes. It may be possible to use these cells in neurodegenerative diseases like Parkinsonism, Alzheimer's disease and spinal cord injuries.
- *Skeletal muscle stem cells*: When introduced in damaged muscle it will regenerate.

- *Islet cell stem cells*: Clinical trials are in process of adult mesenchymal stem cells for islet cells in type 1 diabetes.
- *Cardiac stem cells* have the property to repair heart after myocardial infarction.
- Adult eye stem cells: The cornea of the eye contains stem cells in the region of limbus. These are useful in corneal opacities and damage of conjunctiva.
- *Skin stem cells*: In the skin the stem cells are located in the region of hair follicles and sebaceous gland. These stem cells can repair damaged epidermis.

RETICULAR FORMATION OF BRAINSTEM

- *Introduction*: It is defined as diffuse network of neurons and nerve fibers in the tegmentum of midbrain, dorsal part of pons and retroolivary region of medulla oblongata.
- *Extension*: Superiorly it extends up to diencephalon and inferiorly in the spinal cord. All ascending and descending tract of reticular formation is polysynaptic (Fig. 11.16).

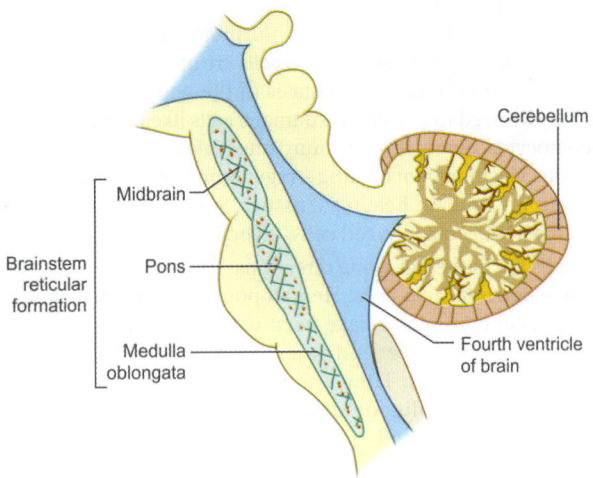

Fig. 11.16: Brainstem reticular formation extends throughout central tegmental core

- *Arrangement* of neurons of reticular formation in brainstem. They are arranged in three layers.
    1. *Median column* containing serotonergic raphe nuclei in the midline. Stimulation of raphe nuclei inhibits pain transmission from the posterior horn of spinal cord.
    2. The paramedian column contains ventral nucleus in pons and medulla. It controls the muscle tone.
    3. *The lateral column* contains neurons of small size (parvocellular nuclei). The word "parvus" means "small". These are situated in pons and medulla and locus coeruleus of fourth ventricle. The polysynaptic neuronal pathways are both ascending and descending and may be crossed or uncrossed. So unilateral stimulation of reticular formation produces bilateral and wide responses (Fig. 11.17).
    4. *Functional division of reticular formation*:
        - *Ascending reticular activating system*: It is responsible for state of alertness of mind. It is particularly formed by lateral column of reticular nuclei. It receives inputs

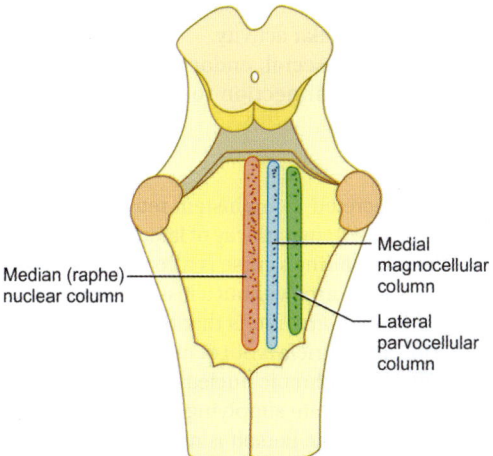

Fig. 11.17: Primary subdivision of brainstem reticular nuclei

either directly or through collaterals from various sensory pathways. It gives output to thalamus from where it goes to cerebral cortex and limbic system. When ascending reticular activating system (ARAS) is stimulated cerebral cortex is alert. Epinephrine and smelling salt stimulate ARAS activity. Some drugs like barbiturates, anesthetics suppress the ARAS results in drowsiness and sleep.
- *Descending reticular system*: This consists of descending pathway influenced by cerebral cortex, cerebellum, substantia nigra and red nucleus. It ends in autonomic center in brainstem and to anterior horn cell of spinal cord. The descending fibers ending in autonomic system in brainstem control the vital centers in the medulla. Thus, the respiratory center maintains automatic breathing during sleep.

5. *Function of reticular formation*:
   - Maintenance of alertness and wakeful state.
   - Essential for arousal from sleep.
   - Controls of cardiac and respiratory centers in medulla.
   - Modulation of pain sensation.
   - Central muscular activity.
   - It regulates visceral, endocrine and emotional activity through its connection to hypothalamus and limbic system.

Clinical Anatomy

- The serotonin secreted by brainstem reticular formation exerts inhibitory effect on pain pathway of lateral spinothalamic tract.
- *Ondine's disease*: Ondine's curse is a condition in which there is loss of automatic control without a loss of voluntary control. The reason for this phenomenon is that the respiratory function at the floor of fourth ventricle is out of function but pyramidal tracts are intact. Therefore phrenic nucleus is controlled by pyramidal tract during waking state supplying the intercostal muscle. But in the sleeping state the person is not able to breath due to lack of automatic breathing. So, patient must be put into artificial support during sleep.

BLOOD CIRCULATION OF BRAIN
Arterial Supply
The two vertebral and two internal carotid arteries supply the whole brain. The superolateral surface of cerebral hemisphere is mainly supplied by middle cerebral artery, Branch of internal carotid except upper 2.5 cm of superolateral surface and hole of paracentral lobule. The later part is supplied by anterior cerebral artery. The medial surface of hemisphere is mainly supplied by anterior cerebral (branch of internal carotid). The part along the parietooccipital sulcus up to the occipital bone is supplied by posterior cerebral artery, which also supplies the inferior surface of the cerebral hemisphere. The corpus striatum and internal capsule are supplied by central branches of anterior and middle cerebral arteries. The arterial circle of Willis is formed by the posterior cerebral, posterior communicating, anterior cerebral and anterior communicating artery. The circle of Willis equalizes the pressure of either side and also helps in establishing collateral circulation immediately (Fig. 11.18).

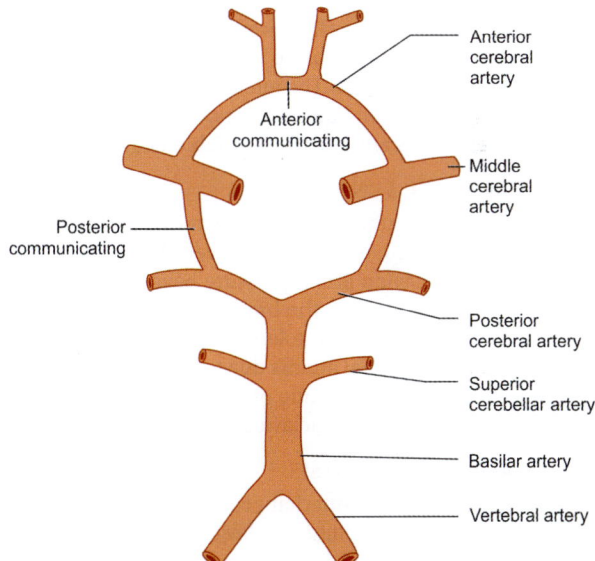

Fig. 11.18: Circle of Willis situated in interpeduncular fossa

Venous Drainage of the Brain

The veins draining in the brain are very thin-walled because their walls are devoid of muscle. They are also without valves. Functionally-they have to drain toward the direction of gravity. These veins drain their blood into dural venous sinuses. Before draining they pierce the arachnoid maters and inner layer of the dural mater. The brainstem and cerebellum are drain by unnamed veins into the dural venous sinuses of the posterior cranial fossa.

Table 11.1: Classification of cerebral veins

External cerebral veins	Internal cerebral veins
Superior cerebral veins	Thalamostriate vein
Superficial middle cerebral veins	Septal veins
Inferior cerebral veins	Choroidal vein
Anterior cerebral veins	Internal cerebral vein proper
Deep middle cerebral vein	Great cerebral vein

The cerebral veins are classified as external and internal cerebral veins. The external cerebral veins lie in subarachnoid space on the surface of cerebral hemisphere. The internal cerebral veins drain the internal part of cerebrum and ultimately pour their blood into great cerebral veins. The veins are described in Table 11.1.

SUBCLAVIAN STEAL SYNDROME

This condition is due to atherosclerotic narrowing of the subclavian artery proximal to the site of origin of the vertebral artery. There is reduction in the subclavian artery pressure beyond the stenosis. It results in retrograde flow from the brain stem down the vertebral artery up to the arm (so blood is stolen from brain). Exercises in the upper arm produces syncopal attacks due to ischemia of brain stem. Visual disturbance of the same side of affected arm. There may be supraclavicular bruit in the supraclavicular space.

CLEIDOCRANIAL DYSOSTOSIS

This is autosomal dominant inheritant condition, mainly affects the membrane bone, chiefly affecting the clavicle and the skull.

The patient is somewhat short with a large head and drooping shoulders. As the clavicles are partially absent the two shoulders of the patient can be brought in front of the chest. X-rays shows non-development of outer half of each clavicle. Wormian bones (sutural bones) may be present in the skull.

PAPEZ CIRCUIT

It is a circular pathway that inter connects certain important structure in limbic system. It contains the following structures, the hippocampus projecting via the fornix to mammillary nucleus. The mammillary nucleus projecting through mammillothalamic tract to the anterior nucleus of thalamus which project through cingulated gyrus and the cingulated gyrus projecting via the cingulum back to hippocampus.

It plays an important role and recent memory and the control of emotional behavior.

EMBRYOLOGICAL TYPES OF ASD

There are three types of ASD resulting in left to right shunts. 1. The ostium secondum defect is one of the most congenital heart defect. 2. The ostium primum defect is due to either faliure of septum primum to reach the endocardial cushion or due to defect in the endocardial cushion itself, so there is persistence of foramen primum. 3. Patent foramen ovale is due to failure of the septum primum and septum secondum fusion at birth. This is extremely rare. In ASD there is increase load on right side of the heart. Gradually, there is enlargement of right atrium, right ventricle and the pulmonary trunk. The disease manifest as fatigue and breathlessness on exertion. In the third or forth decade of life and thereafter.

Clinical anatomy: It is corrected by surgery.

SPHINCTERS OF GUT

Gut extends from lower end of pharynx (C6 level) to ano-cutaneous junction. It has several sphincters and valves to make the passage of food unidirectional.

1. **At starting of esophagus:**
   - At C6 level.
   - Formed by cricopharyngeus part of inferior constrictor.

- When thyropharyngeous constricts the cricopharyngeous relaxes and vice-versa, thus acts as effective sphincter.
- Due to miscoordination it may lead to Zenker's diverticulum.

2. **Cardioesophageal junction:**
   - No anatomical valve exists.
   - But physiological valve exists which prevents gastro-esophageal reflux.

3. **Pyloric end of stomach:**
   - Definite sphincter is seen.
   - Formed by thickening of circular muscle fibers of gut and deep layer and longitudinal muscle fiber.
   - The circular muscle fibers form the sphincter component and longitudinal muscle fiber dilator component.

4. **Sphincter of Oddi:** Interior of 2nd part of duodenum shows this sphincter which is formed by 3 sets of sphincters—sphincter choledochus, Sphincter pancreaticus and Sphincter of Oddi proper. They maintain the bile flow and pancreatic secretion to the 2nd part of a duodenum.

5. **Ileocecal orifice:**
   - It is guarded by a valve.
   - It has horizontal upper lip and crescentic lower lip.
   - It is formed by reduplication of mucosa, thickening of circular muscle layer and internal longitudinal muscle layer.
   - It maintains the flow of content from ileum to cecum and prevents regurgitation.

6. **Appendicular orifice:** The opening is guarded by the valve of Garlach.

7. **Rectum:**
   - Interior of rectum shows Houston valves; Horizontally directed and semilunar in shape.
   - Situated along concavities of lateral curve of rectum.
   - Formed by reduplication of mucosa, submucosa and thickening of muscle layer.
   - 1st valve lies at recto-sigmoid junction (righ/left)
   - 2nd valve present at 2.5 cm above 3rd valve (left side)
   - 3rd valve at opposite S3 (right side)

- 4th valve at 2.5 cm below 3rd valve (left side)
- When 3rd valve encircles whole rectum it is called Nelaton's sphincter.
- Function: support the weight of feces.

8. **Anal sphincter:**
    - Formed by sphincter ani internus and externus.
    - Sphincter ani internus: involuntary. Thickening of circular muscle fiber lies. In upper 2/3rd of anal canal.
    - Sphincter ani externus: Voluntary. Encircle whole length of anal canal. 3 parts—Subcutaneous, superficial and deep.
    - They keep the anus closed and make of continence of stool.

These are the valves of gut and their physiological action.

Index

Page numbers followed by *b* refer to box, *f* refer to figure, and *t* refer to table.

A

Abdomen 126, 362
    anatomy of 176
    radiograph of 364*f*
    surface marking of 177*f*
Abdominal testis 172
Abdominal wall
    anterior 169
    lower part of anterior 130
    posterior 109
Aberrant epiphysis 7
Abscess
    horseshoe-shaped 153
    ischioanal 175
    ischiorectal 175
Acetabular labrum 104
Acetabulum 372, 372*f*
Achalasia 27
Achondroplasia 6
Acne 282
Acquired immune deficiency syndrome 407
Acromioclavicular joint 14, 354*f*
Acromion 354*f*
Acromiothoracic arteries, branches of 385*f*
Addison's disease 277
Adductor muscles, paralysis of 110
Adductor tubercle 123, 124*f*
Adenine 297
Adrenal medulla 277
Air sinuses 234*f*
Albinism 294, 303
Alimentary system 328*f*
    development of 328
Allantoenteric diverticulum 307, 307*f*
Allelic gene 292, 292*f*, 293
Allograft 297
Alzheimer's disease 409
Amniocentesis 297
Amniogenic cells 312
Amnion 311
Amniotic cavity 311
Anal canal 175, 338
    distal part of 136, 137
Anal sphincter 417
Aneurysm, arterial 209
Angina pectoris 208
Angiography 352
Anhidrosis 27
Ankle 376
    anteroposterior view of 375
    joint space 375*f*, 376*f*
    perforating vein 100
Antibiotic 409
Aorta 359
    coarctation of 196, 204
    ends, ascending 86
    left dorsal 196
Aortic arch 326*f*
    arteries 326*f*
    derivatives 325
    left-fourth 196, 327
Aortic knuckle 327

Aortic sac
    left horn of 327
    left side of 195
Aphasia 261
Aponeurosis 213
    bicipital 66
Apoptosis 389
    cause of 389
    pathological causes in 389
    physiologic causes in 389
Appendicular orifice 416
Appendix 337, 337f
    base of 177
    microanatomy of 268
Aqueous humor 243
    composition 243
    formation 243
    function 243
    situation 243
Arachnoid granulations 244
    function 244
Arch of aorta 195, 195f, 207f
    begins 86
    ends 86
Areolar tissue, loose 214
Argyll Robertson pupil 256, 261
Arterial system 28
Arteriole 28
Arteriosclerosis 247
Artery 28, 32t, 58
    anesthetic 252
    brachial 66, 90, 89f
    development 139
    fastroepiploic 151
    intercostal 182f
    large size 28
    left anterior descending 206
    perforating 103
Arthroscopy 16
Articular cartilage 4
    degeneration of 4
Articulation, types of 258
Astrocytes 24

Atavistic epiphysis 6
Atherosclerosis 209
Atrial septal defect 203, 323, 323f
Atrium, right 187
Auditory meatus, external 253, 369f
Auditory radiation fiber 241
Auriculotemporal syndrome 399
Automatic bladder 405
Autonomic nervous system 24
Avascular necrosis 173
Axial sulcus 236
Axillary artery 58, 59f, 89f
    left 89
Axillary nerve 46, 47, 54
    anterior division 54
    posterior division 54
Axillary vein 73
Axonotmesis 27
Azygos lobe
    lower 185
    upper 185
Azygos vein 190, 190f
    lobe of 185
    situation 190

B

Bacteria 319
Banti's disease 137
Barium
    enema 364f
    meal 365
Barr body 291, 291f
Basal nuclei 241f
Basilic vein 73
Basivertebral foramen 164
Battledore placenta 308
Benedict's syndrome 249
Berry aneurysm 246f
Biceps brachii 20, 73
    muscle 40, 41f
    tendon of 66
Bicornuate uterus 162, 162f, 317
Bifid tongue 335

Bile duct, common 133, 133f
Bladder 367
    distension 405
Blastocyst 304
    formation of 304f
Blind spot 258
Blood
    borne effects 389
    brain barrier 238
    clots 259
    communication of 137f
    pressure, high 27
    supply 134
    transfusion of 80
    vessels 31, 271
    withdrawal of 80
B-lymphocytes, circulation of 392f
Bone 2, 39
    cells 2
    clinical anatomy of 8
    destroyer 2
    forming cells 2
    function of 2
    greenstick fracture of 16
    marrow stem cells 409
    tissue 4
Bony callus 8
Bowman's membrane 220, 221
Brachial artery, compression of 76
Brachial plexus 44, 45f, 46, 55t
    branches 44
    median nerve of 49t
    ulnar nerve of 51t
Brachialis 66
Brachii 42
Brachiocephalic veins, lower part of right 187
Brachioradialis 66
Brain 211, 235
    blood
        circulation of 413
        supply of 249

    venous drainage of 414
Brainstem reticular
    formation 410, 410f
    nuclei, primary subdivision of 411f
Branchial arch 332, 333t
    derivatives of 332, 332f
Branchial fistula 344
    course of 345f
Breast
    arterial supply of 385
    blood supply of 385
    cancer 75
    carcinoma 76
    sources of 385f
Bronchi 250
Bronchopulmonary segments 188, 189f, 189t
Bronchoscopy 190
Bronchus 187
    right 203
Brunner's gland 279
Bucket handle tear 13f
Buerger's disease 27, 83
Bulbus cordis 324

C

Calcaneal spur 376f
Calcaneal tuberosity 377f
Calcaneum 376f
Calcarine sulcus 236
Calices minor 146
Calot's triangle 134
Calyces, minor 366f
Canal boundaries, inguinal 129b
Canal, inguinal 128, 128f, 129, 129f
Cancer breast 75
Cancer stomach 170
Capsular ligament 111
Capsule, internal 241, 241f
Cardiac
    catheterization 73

impression 187
myocyte cell 405
orifice 176
Cardioesophageal junction 416
Cardiothoracic surgery 193
Carotid artery, common 262
Carpal tunnel
	syndrome 78
	transverse section of 71*f*
Cartilage 2, 2*t*
	cells, mature 383
	hypertrophic 14
	injuries 13
	types of 2, 3*f*
Cauda equina 236*f*
Caval system 32
Cecum 172, 337, 337*f*
Celiac
	artery, origin of 176
	sprue 382
	trunk 150, 151*f*
		origin of 86
Cells
	arrangement of 223*f*
	mature 2
Central nervous system 22
Central sulcus 236
Central tendon 205
Cephalhematoma 214
Cephalic vein 66, 93*f*
Cerebellar peduncle, superior 248*f*
Cerebellum
	histology of 281
	section of 281*f*
Cerebral
	artery, posterior 256
	peduncle 242, 248
	veins
		anterior 414
		classification of 414*t*
		external 414
		inferior 414
		internal 414
		superficial middle 414
		superior 414
Cerebrospinal fluid 244
Cervical
	ganglia 24
	pleura 183
	ribs 393
		bilateral 394*f*
		stretching 394*f*
	spine 370, 372
		seventh 262
Chest
	discomfort, complaining of 174
	X-ray of 359
Chimera 297
Cholecystectomy drain 166
Chorion 306, 306*f*
Choroidal vein 414
Chromophil cells 399
Chromosomal morphology 295
Chromosome 284
	classification of 285, 286*f*, 286*t*
	end of 284
	parts of 284*b*, 284*f*
	ring 295, 296*f*
	type of disorder of 293
Ciliary body 238
Circle of Willis 245, 246*f*, 249, 413, 413*f*
Circumvallate placenta 308
Clavicle 354
	fracture of 81*f*
Clavipectoral fascia 58, 62, 63, 63*f*
	incision of 64*f*
Claw hand 77
Cleft palate, types of 331*f*
Cleidocranial dysostosis 414
Club foot 123
Codominant genes 286
Cohn's syndrome 277
Collateral sulcus 236

Colles fascia 156
Colliculus, superior 395
Columnar epithelial lining 318
Communicating junction 405
Compact bone 357f
Compound epiphysis 80
Compression syndrome, type of 78
Congenital deafness, cause of 403
Conjunctival sac 215
Connective tissue 213
Conoid tubercle 354, 355f
Consanguinity 298
Coracoid process 39, 354f
    ligament at 39f
Cornea 220, 220f
    surfaces of 221
Corneal epithelium 220
Corona radiata 303
    fibers 241
Coronal suture 369f
Coronary
    angiography, indication of 391
    arterial system 391f
    artery
        left 192, 192t, 206, 390
        right 192, 192t, 193, 390
    bypass 209, 209f
    circulation 192, 193f, 390
    disease 203
    sinus 199, 199f
Coronoid fossae 356f
Corpus callosum 239, 240f
    parts of 240f
    splenium of 240
Corpus striatum 248
Cortex 355f
Corticonuclear fiber 260
Costal pleura 183
Costodiaphragmatic recess 184, 184f
Cramp 20
Cranial nerves, pairs of 22
Cremasteric reflex 163

Cricoarytenoid muscle, posterior 216
Cricoid cartilage 85
    anterior arch of 262
    border of 274
    larynx 260
Cri-du-chat syndrome 295, 296f
Crohn's disease 381
Cruciate anastomosis 102
Cryosurgery 210
Crypts of Lieberkühn 380
Cubital fossa 65, 245
    incision of 66f
    right 65f
Cubital tunnel syndrome 78
Cubital vein, median 66, 92f
Cubitus valgus 78
Cuneiform, lateral 377f
Cushing's syndrome 401
Cytokeratins 395

D

Daughter cell 288
Deep fascia 97f
Deep inguinal lymph nodes 116
Deep middle cerebral vein 414
Deep palmar arch 91f, 382
Deep perineal
    pouch 157
    spaces 157f
Deep peroneal nerve 108, 108f
    course 109
    origin 108
Deep-cervical fascia, part of 226
Deltoid ligament 112
    nature 112
    parts 112
    superficial part of 112f
Deltoid muscle 40
Dental caries 260
Denticulate suture 213
Deoxyribonucleic acid 284
Dermatome 281

Dermomyotome 314
Descemet's membrane 221
Desmosomes 404
Diabetes
    insipidus 401
    mellitus, development of 170
Diaphragm, right dome of 360*f*
Diaphragmatic pleura 184
Diaphysis, epiphyseal end of 3
Digastric muscle 252
    bellies of 252
Digital synovial sheath 405
Dislocation 14
Distal talofibular joint 103
Dizygotic twin 317, 317*t*
Dorsal digital expansion 58
Dorsal venous
    arch 93*f*
    network 100*f*
Down's syndrome 287, 287*f*, 293, 296
Duchenne muscular dystrophy 386
Duodenal ulcer 168
Duodenojejunal flexure 178, 363
Duodenum 268*f*, 336, 363
    histology of 267
    part of 168
    resembles, part of 171
    second part of 138, 138*f*, 139
    third parts of 138*f*
Dupuytren's contracture 77

E

Ear
    front of 214
    middle 262
    ossicles of 402
Ectopia vesicae 343
Ectopic pregnancy 313
Ectopic testis 148, 149*f*, 166
Ectopic thyroid 256
Elastic cartilage 2

Elbow joint 355, 356*f*, 357*f*
    anastomosis around 61, 61*f*
Elephantiasis 36*f*
Embalming of body, technique of 388*f*
Embryoblast derivatives 307
Embryology 300
Empyema 210
Endochondral ossification 383, 384*f*
Endocrine cells 389
Endoderm 308
Endothelium 221
Endothoracic fascia 183
Enteric fever 136
Ependymal cells 24
Epicondyles 356
Epicranial aponeurosis 213
Epigastric vessels, inferior 173
Epilepsy, chronic 240
Epiphyseal
    injury 14
    plate, structure of 384*f*
Epiphysis
    around knee joint 118
    law of union of 4
    types of 6, 6*f*
Epiploic foramen 142
Erb's palsy 47*f*
Erb's point 47*f*
Esophageal
    stricture 170
    varices 137
    wall, upper 274*f*
Esophagus 274, 336
    barium swallow X-ray of 361
    begins 85
    constrictions of 200
    histology of 274
    lower end of 136, 137
    starting of 415
Ethmoid air sinus 233, 369, 383

Euchromatin 298
Exomphalos 317
Extrahepatic biliary apparatus 134, 135*f*
Extrapyramidal system 248
Extremity, inferior 94, 372
Eye
    optic disc in 258
    stem cells 410
Eyeball 235, 238

F

Face, development of 329, 330*f*
Facial
    artery 252
        tortuous 254
    canal 253
    capsule 398
    nerve 252, 254
        injury 254
        intrapetrous part of 254
        palsy 253
        supranuclear lesion of 260
Falciform margin, sharp 97
Fallopian tube 153, 154*f*
    histology of 278
False ligaments 163
Fascia of Colles 161
Fascia of Scarpa 156
Fascia, superficial 213
Femoral artery, medial circumflex 103
Femoral cutaneous nerve, lateral 96
Femoral hernia 96, 116, 166, 173
Femoral pulse 83
Femoral triangle 95, 95*f*
Femur
    articular ends of 374
    head of 372*f*, 373
    lateral condyle of 373*f*, 374*f*
    lower end of 373*f*
    medial condyle of 373*f*, 374*f*
    neck of 372*f*, 373
Fertilized ovum 313*f*
    segmentation of 304*f*
Fibers
    shape of 17
    types of 216
Fibrous pericardium 197
Fibula
    head of 373*f*, 374*f*
    lower end of 377
Fibular collateral ligament 112
Fifth metatarsal, styloid process of 375*f*, 377*f*
Filum terminale 235
    ends 87
    externum 235
    internum 235
    parts 235
Fissure 231
Fit 240
Flexor pollicis longus 19
Flexor retinaculum 71
Focal adhesion complexes 404
Foot 376
    anteroposterior view of 375
Foramen
    boundaries of 143*f*
    cecum 258
Forearm
    interosseous membrane of 72*f*
    supinators of 41, 42*t*
Fossa
    exposure of 66
    interpeduncular 413*f*
    ischioanal 152, 153*f*
    ischiorectal 152
Fourth lumbar spine, tip of 178
Fracture
    comminuted 8
    compound 8

simple 8
stages in union of 10f
types of 8t, 9f
union of 8
Frey syndrome 399
Frontal air sinus 207f, 234, 368f, 370f
Fundic gas shadow 363f
Fusiform muscle 20

G

Galea aponeurosis 213
Gallbladder 169
    fundus of 176
    neck of 138
    pain 171
Gap junctions 405
Gastric 151
    triangle 131
Gastritis 381
Gastrosplenic ligament 160
Gastrulation 307
Gene 298
    recessive 298
Genetics, terms in 297
Genicular artery, superior lateral 102
Genitalia
    development of 344
    external 372f
Genome 298
Genu valgum, bilateral 5f
Genu varum, bilateral 5f
Gland
    bimanual palpation of 399
    intestinal 380
Glans penis 344
Glenoid cavity 354f, 355f
Glenoid fossa concavity of 75
Glenoid labrum 12
Glial cells 24
Glossopharyngeal nerve 218, 254
Gluteus medius 111
Goblet cells 318
Gonads, descent of 347
Great cerebral vein 414
Great saphenous vein 97, 98f
    formation 97
Great vessels, transposition of 203
Greater sciatic foramen 114, 114f
Greater splanchnic nerve 26
Greater trochanter 373
Greater tube 355f
Greenstick fracture 8
Growth hormones, produces 400
Gubernaculums 347
Gustatory cells 223
Gustatory sweating 399
Gut, sphincters of 415

H

Hand, sensory supply of 48f
Haversian system 5
Head 211
    and neck 263f, 367
        surface anatomy of 262
    blood supply of
    injuries, type of 257
Heart 208, 208f, 359
    anomalies of 323f
    apex of 206
    artery supply to 192
    attack 210
    development of 319
    failure 209
    left border of 208
    normal 323f
    right border of 206
    tube
        right and left 319f
        subdivisions of 320f
    venous drainage of 199
Heel dancing 122
Hemianopia
    bitemporal 255
    contralateral homonymous 256

Hemiazygos vein 191
    inferior 191
Hemidesmosomes 404
Hemivertebra 314
Hemorrhoids 167
Hepatic lobule, classical 273
Hernia
    congenital 317
    direct 130*f*
        inguinal 173
    inguinal 168
Herpes zoster 182
Hesselbach's triangle 130, 130*f*
Heterochromatin 298
Hilton's law 12
Hip, congenital dislocation of 117
Hip joint 111, 117, 166, 172, 372*f*
    anteroposterior view of 372
    dislocation of 118
    pathology of 118
    space 373
Hirschsprung's disease 27
Horn tear
    anterior 13*f*
    posterior 13*f*
Horner's syndrome 27, 205, 239, 259
Human leukocyte antigen 298
    complex 298
Human placenta 348
Humerus 75
    anatomical neck of 354
    epicondyles of 357*f*
    head of 354*f*
    lesser tubercle of 6
    surgical neck of 39
Hyaline cartilage 2, 250, 267
Hyoid bone 85, 260
    greater cornu of 262
Hyparterial bronchus 187
Hyperacusis 253, 254
Hyperplasia 168
Hypertension 27
    portal 167

Hypogastric nerve, branch of 174
Hypoglossal nerve 224, 224*f*, 224*t*
Hypophysis cerebri, subdivisions of 400*f*
Hysterosalpingogram 367

I

Ileocecal orifice 87, 159, 159*f*, 416
Ileum 279, 279*t*, 336, 364
    distal part of 364
Iliac crest 372*f*
Ilioinguinal nerve 174
Iliotibial tract 101, 101*f*
    attachments 101
Incision 68*f*
Incus 403
Infection 205
Inferior vena cava 187, 190
Infraorbital foramen 263
Inguinal canal
    obliquity of 130
    protection of 130
Inguinal lymph node
    distribution of 115*f*
    superficial 95, 116
Inguinoscrotal phase 348
Interatrial septum, development of 321, 322*f*
Intercostal vein, left superior 194
Intercostalis internus muscles 182
Intermuscular septum, anterior 106
Internal thoracic artery, branches of 385*f*
Interosseous
    membrane 103, 104*f*
    nerve, posterior 55, 56*f*, 76
Interventricular septum 321*f*, 324
    arterial supply of 193*f*
    blood supply of 193
    development of 323, 324*f*
Intestine 365
    small 381
Intracapsular fracture 117

Iris 238
 muscle of 239
Ischial spine 114
Islet cell stem 410
Isochromosome 295, 296*f*

J

Jaundice 171
Jejunum 279, 279*t*, 336, 364, 381*f*
Jerky rapid eye movement 294
Joint 13, 16
 atlanto-occipital 258
 blood supply of 11
 clinical anatomy of 13
 injuries, common 13
 intercarpal 56
 motion
  physiology of 12
  range of 12
 replacement 15
 stabilizing factor of 12
 xiphisternal 206
Junctional complexes 404

K

Karyotyping chromosome 285, 285*f*
Kidney 340
 coronal section of 146, 147*f*
 horseshoe-shaped 167, 340, 342*f*, 348
 stages of development of 324*f*
Klinefelter's syndrome 288, 290, 290*f*, 291, 297
Klumpke's paralysis 47
Knee joint 116, 166, 172, 374*f*
 anteroposterior view of 373
 extra-articular ligament of 111
 locking of 105
 menisci of 12
 space 373*f*
 unlocking of 105
Krukenberg's tumor 80
Kupffer cells 271, 273

L

Lacrimal apparatus 215, 215*f*
Lacrimal artery 216
Lacrimal canaliculi 216
Lacrimal ducts 215
Lacrimal gland 215, 253
Lacrimal sac 216
Lacunar ligament 166
Lamina propria 381
Large intestine, barium enema of 364
Laryngeal nerve 260
Larynx 228*f*
 ends 85
 intrinsic muscles of 216*f*
 watershed line of 252
Lateral thoracic artery, branches of 385*f*
Leg syndrome, anterior compartment of 121
Lens, suspensory ligament of 238
Lenticulostriate arteries 242
Leprosy 83
Levator ani 158
Lienophrenic ligament 160, 161
Lienorenal ligament 160
Ligamentum arteriosum 327
Ligamentum patellae 118
Limb
 lower 103, 104*f*
  longer 284
 short upper 284
Limiting sulcus 236
Lingual thyroid 255
Little's area of epistaxis 219
Liver 142*f*, 273*f*, 338
 bare area of 132, 132*f*
 pancreas, stages of development of 339*f*
Long bone, growing end of 4
Lumbar vertebra, caries spine of 122
Lumber vertebrae 367
Lumbrical canals 74*f*

Lumbrical muscle 81
Lunate sulcus 236
Lung 188*f*, 361
    azygos lobe of 185
    histology of 266
    left 186*f*, 187, 187*t*, 187*t*, 189, 189*f*
    lobes of 188*t*
    lower border of both 207*f*
    mediastinal surface of 185, 187*t*
    right 186*f*, 187, 187*t*, 189, 189*f*
    root of 187
    sectional view of 267*f*
    shadow of 355*f*, 359
Lymph capillary, formation of 33*f*
Lymph node 275*f*
    inguinal 115
    structure of 275
Lymphadenitis 36
Lymphangitis 36
Lymphatic duct, right 34
Lymphatic system 33
Lymphatic tissue
    aggregations of 136
    small masses of 34
Lymphedema 36, 36*f*
Lymphoid tissue 218
Lymphomas 37
Lyon's hypothesis 297

M

MacKenrodt's ligament 155
Macroglossia 335
Macula adherens 404
Macular sparing 256
Magnetic resonance imaging 352
Malleolus, lateral 375*f*
Malleus 402
Mammillary nucleus 415
Mandible, ramus of 368*f*
Maternal blood 310
Maternal hormones 319
Maxillary air sinus 368*f*, 370*f*
Maxillary sinus 233
McBurney's point 169, 177
Meckel's diverticulum 312, 313*f*, 340
Medial cuneiform 376*f*
Medial cutaneous nerve of
    arm 46
    forearm 46
Medial longitudinal arch 115, 115*f*
Medial malleolus, tip of 123
Median nerve
    lateral root of 46
    medial root of 46
Mediastinal pleura 183, 194
Mediastinum
    divisions of 194*f*
    superior 194
Medulla 275
Medullary cavity 355*f*
Meiosis cell division 288
Meiotic division starts 301
Membranous urethra 148
Meniscal tear, types of 13*f*
Mesenteric artery, origin of superior 176
Mesenteric vessels, superior 144
Mesodermal plate 316*f*
Metacarpals 359
    epiphysis of 81
Metaphysis 3
Microglia 24
Midbrain 247
    transverse section of 247*f*, 248*f*
Mitosis, repeated 301
Molecular layer, outer 396
Mongolism 287
Monozygotic twin 317, 317*t*
Morison, hepatorenal pouch of 140, 141*f*, 166
Morula 304
Mother-to-child transmission 407
Mouse-like appearance tissue 16
Mucosal cilia, loss of 263

Mucous membrane 278
    clinical anatomy of 381
    of small intestine 379
Müllerian duct 317
    fusses 317
    nonfusion of 317
Multiaxial shoulder joint 92
Muscle 19, 40, 42, 81, 254
    atrophy 20
    cardiac 18f
    coccygeus 158f
    fibers, direction of 21f
    injury 20
    interosseous 19
    intimus 182
    parallel 20
    strain 20
    tissue 16
    tone 19
    types of 17t
        parallel 20, 21f
Muscular layer 279
Muscular surface 229
Muscular system 16
Muscularis externa 268
Muscularis mucosa 268
Musculocutaneous nerve 46, 55, 55t
Mutagenic agents 379
Mutagens 379
Myelin sheath 27
Mylohyoid muscle 397f
Myocardial infarction 210
Myocytes 409

N

Nasal cavity 231, 370f
    parts of 232
Nasal conchae 232
Nasal regurgitation of fluid 259
Nasal septum 263, 368f
    blood supply of 220f
    major contribution 232

Nasion 262
Nasolacrimal duct 216, 233
Nasopharyngeal tonsil 219
Navicular bone, tubercle of 123
Neck 211, 371f
    anatomical 355f
    of fibula, fracture of 107, 120
    vein, enlargement of 205
Nerve 44, 46, 332
    block, intercostal 204
    entrapment of upper limb 82
    fiber 23
        layer 397
    in facial canal 253
    injury, median 75
    interosseous 82
    least splanchnic 26
    median 47, 48f, 82
    palsy, median 49f
    supply 17, 40, 41, 58, 105, 184, 214, 221, 227
        of joint 12
        of urinary bladder 163
    to pronator teres 66
    to subclavius 46
Nervous system 22
Nervous tissue, histology of 22
Neural crest cells 237
Neural tube, development of 305f
Neuroglia 24
Neuron 409
    stem cells 409
    structure of 23f
Neuropathy 27
Neuropores
    anterior 305f
    posterior 305f
Neuropraxia 27
Neurotmesis 27
Ninth costal cartilage, tip of 176
Nondisjunction 288
Non-Hodgkin's lymphomas 37

Index

Nose
    causes 250
    lateral wall of 232*f*
    pricking of 219
Notochord 305
Nuclei, position of 17
Nystagmus 294

O

Obstruction, intestinal 172
Obturator foramen 372*f*
Obturator nerve 109, 110, 110*f*
    origin 109
Occipital bone 258
Oculocutaneous albinism 294
Olecranon 357*f*
    fossae 356*f*
Olfaction, loss of 250
Oligodendrocytes 24
Omentum, lesser 145, 146*f*
Omphalocele 317
Ondine's disease 412
Oocyte, secondary 301
Oogenesis 301, 303*f*
Optic disc, papilledema of 259
Optic nerve 250, 258
    fibers 258
Orbicularis oculi 260
Orbital cavity 370*f*
Orbital fissure 230
    inferior 230, 231
    superior 230
Ossicles, movement of 403
Ossification 7, 7*f*
Osteoarthritis 4
Osteoblast 2
Osteoclast 2
Osteocyte 2
Otitis media 264
Ovarian diseases, pain in 116, 172
Ovarian fossa 150*f*
    of lateral pelvic wall 149
Oxygen from air 221

P

Palate, development of 329, 331*f*
Palatine tonsil 217, 217*f*
Palatoglossal arch 217
Palatopharyngeal arch 217
Palmar arch, superficial 90, 382
Palmar arterial arch 382
Palmar spaces 70*f*
Palmaris brevis 58
Palmaris longus 71
Palpebral artery
    lateral 216
    middle 216
Palpebral part, removal of 253
Pancreas, annular 340
Pancreatic tissue, accessory 340
Papez circuit 415
Papillae 222*f*
Paracentral lobule 237
Paramedian heart tubes 319
Paranasal air sinuses 232*f*, 233, 235*f*, 370*f*
Parasternal lymph node 80
Parathyroids, superior 258
Paravertebral veins 32
Parietal pleura 182
Parona, space of 69, 69*f*, 73
Parotid abscess 253
Parotid duct 207*f*, 227
Parotid gland 226
    deep part of 226*f*
    enlargement 257
    histology of 270
    inflammation of 261
    periphery of 226*f*
Parotidomasseteric fascia 226
Pars distalis 399
Pars tuberalis 400
Patella 374*f*
    outline of 373*f*

Patent ductus arteriosus 196
Peau d'orange 75
Pectoral nerve, lateral 46
Pectoral region, muscle of 42*t*
Pectoralis major muscles 42
Pectoralis minor 77
Pelvic
    diaphragm 158
        parts of 158
    kidney 340
    mesocolon 143
        attachment of 144*f*
    wall, lateral 150*f*
Pelvis 109
Pennate muscle 19
    types of 19*f*
Percutaneous drainage 409
Pericardial cavity 197, 198*f*, 320
Pericardial effusion 205
Pericardial sinus, oblique 198, 198*f*
Perineal body 346
Perineal pouch, superficial 156
Perineal tear 165
Peripheral arterial pulse 30*f*
Peripheral heart 121
Peripheral nerve 258
Peripheral nervous system 22
Peritoneal cavity 179*f*
Peritonitis 172, 179*f*
Peritonsillar abscess 218
Peroneal muscle atrophy 125
Peroneal nerve, superficial 106, 107*f*
Persistent interventricular foramen 324
Persistent truncus arteriosus 323*f*
Peyer's patches 136, 279
Phalanges 359
Phalanx 377*f*
    modified 81
Pharyngeal arches 332
Pharyngeal pouches, fate of 335*t*
Pharynx ends 85

Phenylketonuria 299
Philadelphia chromosome 294, 295, 296*f*
Phimosis 162
Phrenic nerves 184
Pimples 282
Pineal gland 401, 401*f*
Piriformis
    muscle 114
    syndrome 114
Pituitary
    fossa 369*f*
    gland 399, 401*f*
    tumor 255, 401
Placenta
    large 308
    previa 308, 310, 313*f*
        types of 310
    succenturiata rare 308
    types of 308, 309*f*
Placental barrier 310, 310*f*
Plane suture 213
Plantar calcaneonavicular ligament 113, 121
Pleiotropy 293
Pleura 183*f*
Pleural reflection 184*f*
Plexiform layer, outer 396
Plica semilunaris 379
Point mutation 386
Polycystic kidney 340, 342*f*
Polyuria 401
Popliteal ligament, oblique 112
Popliteus muscle 104, 105*f*
    course 104
    origin 104
Porta hepatis 141, 142*f*
Portosystemic anastomosis 135
Pregnancy group 403
Presbycusis 264
Pressure epiphysis 6
Pretectal nucleus, lesion of 261

Index

Pretracheal fascia 260
Primordial germ cells 301
Profunda femoris
    artery 102
    branches of 102
    vessels 96
Pronator syndrome 78
Pronator teres 66
Proprioceptive senses 221
Protein 303, 394
Proximal bulbar septum 324
Proximal segment of bone, avascular necrosis of 77
Proximal urethra, dilatation of 405
Puberty 282
Pubocervical ligaments 156
Pudendal canal 151, 152*f*
Pulmonary
    arch 327
    artery 187
    pleura 267
    trunk, bifurcation of 86
    vein 187
Pus, discharge of 251
Pyelogram 365
    ascending 365
    descending 365, 366*f*
Pyloric antrum 363*f*
Pyloric canal 363*f*
Pyriform fossa 251

Q

Quadratus lumborum 20

R

Radial artery 59, 60*f*
    in forearm 90
Radial blood vessels 66
Radial nerve 46, 52, 53*f*, 82
    in back of arm 91
    in cubital fossa will 79
    of brachial plexus 52*t*
    palsy 53*f*
Radial pulse 83
Radiography, contrast 362
Radioulnar joint 56
    superior 70
Radius, styloid process of 358*f*, 359
Raynaud's disease 27
Rectal fistulae, types of 346*f*
Rectovesical fistula 345
Rectum 338, 416
Rectus
    abdominis 20
    femoris 118
    sheath 127
        formation of 127*f*
Red cells 409
Renal fascia 139, 140*f*
Renal sinus 146
Renshaw cells 388
Respiratory epithelium 266
Respiratory part 266
Reticular formation, function of 411, 412
Reticular system, descending 412
Reticuloendothelial system 271
Retina 239, 251, 396
Retrosternal thyroid 256
Rheumatoid arthritis 15
Rhomboid fossa 244, 244*f*
Ribs, arching of 204
Rickets in children 5*f*
Right ventricle, small part of 187
Rods and cones, layer of 396
Roof of middle ear, fracture of 264
Rotator cuff
    muscle 42, 43*t*
    of shoulder 44*f*
Rugae 363*f*
Rutherford-Morrison, pouch of 408
Ryle's tube 200

S

Salivary gland 270
    parotid 270*f*

Saphenous opening 96
    measurement 96
Scalp 213
    bleed, wounds of 257
    dangerous layer of 255, 261
    injury 256
    laceration 257
Scapula
    caracoid process of 6, 39*f*
    lateral border of 354*f*
Schwann cells 27
Scleracorneal
    junction 238
    limbus 221
Sclerotome 314
Scrotum, swelling of 171
Sella turcica 399
Semiflexed hip and knee 124*f*
Septal veins 414
Septate uterus 317
Septum
    intermedium 203, 321, 324
    primum 203, 321
    secundum 203, 321
    transversum 316
Serous pericardium 197
Serratus anterior 77
Sertoli cells 301
Sex chromatin 291, 291*f*
Sex chromosome 291, 292*f*
Sex difference 173
Shenton's lines 373
Shoulder
    dislocation of 14*f*
    girdle, movement of 77
    joint 14, 16, 74, 79, 354*f*, 355, 355*f*, 356
        anteroposterior view of 354
    region, right 169
Sibso's fascia 183
Sinus venosus, fusion of 319*f*
Sinusoids 28, 28*t*

Skeletal muscle 18*f*
    stem cells 409
Skin 213, 271, 272*f*
    stem cells 410
Skull 369
Small intestine
    part of 380*f*
    proximal part of 364
Snuffbox, anatomical 57, 57*f*
Soft palate
    paralysis of 259
    role of 406
Somatotrophs, tumor of 401
Spasm 20
Spermatocytosis 301
Spermatogenesis 301, 302*f*
Spermatozoa, maturation of 303
Sphenoidal air sinus 234, 369*f*
Sphincter of Oddi 416
Sphincter pupillae 239
Spina bifida 314
    occulta 346
Spinal cord 22, 260
    commencement of 85
    histology of 280, 280*f*
    injuries 409
Spinal nerves 24
Spine 371*f*
    of scapula, root of 85
Splanchnic branches 25*f*
Splanchnic nerve, lesser 26
Splanchnic nerves 26
Spleen 340
    ligaments of 160, 160*f*
    section of 277*f*
Spot desmosomes 404
Sprain 13
Spring ligament 113, 121
Squamous epithelium, simple 266
Squamous suture 213
Stem cell 409
    cardiac 410

Sternal angle 181
Sternum anterior 181*f*
Stomach 336
    barium meal X-ray of 362, 363*f*
    bed 131
    carcinoma of 174
    fundus of 174, 360*f*
    greater curvature of 363*f*
    lesser curvature of 173, 363*f*
    part of 174
    pyloric
        end of 416
        orifice of 176
    pylorus of 87
    X-ray of 365
Stratum basale 272
Stratum corneum 272
Stratum granulosum 272
Stratum lucidum 272
Stratum spinosum 272
Stroma 221
Subclavian steal syndrome 414
Subcutaneous tissue 271
Submandibular duct 398
Submandibular gland, parts of 397*f*
Submandibular salivary gland 397, 398*f*
Subphrenic abscess 408
Subphrenic space 407, 408
Subscapular nerve
    lower 46
    upper 46
Substantia nigra 248
Substantia propria 221
Suckling milk 252
Sudden death, artery of 206
Sulcus 236
    lateral 236
    types of 236, 236*t*
Superfemale syndrome 291
Superior thoracic arteries, branches of 385*f*
Supinator 66
    muscle 73, 76
Supracondylar ridge 357*f*
Suprapatellar bursa 111
Suprarenal gland 29, 169, 276, 276*f*,
Suprascapular nerve 46
Sutural joint 212
    types 212
Sutures, types of 212*f*
Sympathetic trunk 24
    thoracic part of 25*f*
Symphysis pubis 127, 372*f*
Synovial fluid 12
Synovial joints 11, 16

T

T and B lymphocyte
    maturation of 391
    morphology of 391
Talipes equinovarus 123
Talocalcaneonavicular joint, ligament of 113
Talus 375*f*
    articular surface of 376*f*
    avascular necrosis of 119*f*
    fracture of 119
    head of 376*f*, 377*f*
    neck of 376*f*
Tapetum 239
Tarsal tunnel syndrome 125
Taste buds 222
Tectum 248
Tegmentum 249
Temporal bone
    mandibular fossa of 223
    petrous part of 368*f*, 369*f*
Temporalis muscle 223, 223*t*
Temporomandibular joint 14, 225, 225*f*
    movement of 225, 225*t*
Testis descent 347
Tetanus toxin 388

Tetralogy of Fallot 196, 197*f*, 323*f*, 324
    defects 196
Thalamostriate vein 414
Thalidomide 319
Third ventricle 242, 242*f*
Thoracic aorta, descending 86
Thoracic duct 34*f*, 201, 201*f*
Thoracic nerve, long 79
Thoracoabdominal diaphragm 205
Thoracodorsal nerve 46
Thorax 180
    median section of 194*f*
    surface anatomy of 206
Throat infection 251, 262
Thyroglossal duct 258
Thyroid
    cartilage 85, 260
    eminence 262
    fine-needle aspiration cytology of 230*f*
    gland 228, 228*f*, 259, 260
        isthmus of 262
    tissue 255
Tibia
    articular ends of 374
    lateral and medial condyles of 373*f*
    lower end of 375*f*
Tibial collateral ligament 111
Tibial nerve entrapment 125
Tibial tuberosity 374*f*
Tibialis anterior 19, 122
Tip-toe dancing 122
Tissue
    sensitive 353
    shadow, soft 373*f*
    soft 32*f*, 374*f*
Tongue
    development of 334, 334*f*
    muscles 254
    safety muscles of 250
    soft tissue of 368*f*
    tie 335
Tonsillar
    fossa 259
    ring 219*f*
    venous plexus 218
Tonsillectomy, performing 259
Tonsillitis 218, 258
    pain 262
Total knee replacement 15*f*
Trachea 228*f*, 250
    begins 85
    bifurcation of 86, 206
Tracheoesophageal fistula 204
Tracheostomy 210
Traction epiphysis 6
Transabdominal phase 347
Transitional epithelium 266
Translocation, example of 293
Transsphenoidal hypophysectomy 263
Transverse colon 338
Transverse pericardial sinus 197, 198*f*
Trendelenburg test 111
Trendelenburg's sign, positive 119
Truncus arteriosus 195
Tubes, fusion of 319*f*
Tumor, intracranial 259
Tunica vaginalis 171
Turner's syndrome 288, 289*f*
Twining 315*f*
Typhoid 136

U

Ulna, styloid process of 359
Ulnar artery 66
    in forearm 90
Ulnar nerve 46, 50, 50*f*, 71, 72, 82
    hickening of 83
    in forearm 91
    palsy 50*f*

Ulnar paradox 72
Ulnar vessels 71
Umbilical cord 311, 311*f*
Umbilical hernia, physiological 316, 316*f*
Umbilical opening 312*f*
Umbilical region 136, 138
Upper limb
    interosseous membrane of 72
    surface anatomy of 88
Urachal fistula 343
Ureter
    histology of 269
    pelvis of 366*f*, 367
    transverse section of 270*f*
Ureteric colic
    pain in 165
    upper 165
Urinary and congenital anomalies bladder 343*f*
Urinary bladder 342, 366*f*
    base of 147, 148*f*
Urinary incontinence 165
Urogenital
    sinus 346
    triangle 157*f*
Uterine tube, section of 278*f*
Uterosacral ligaments 156
Uterus
    anomalies of 318*f*
    cavity of 153
    ligamentous supports of 155*f*
    removal of 166
    round ligaments of 155
    true ligaments of 155
Uveal tract, part of 238

V

Valveless veins 165
Valves 99
Valvular disease 209
Varicocele occurs 164

Vascular surface 229
Vaso-occlusive disease 27, 83
Vastus intermedius 118
Vastus lateralis 118
Vastus medialis 118
    muscle 102
Vein 32, 32*t*, 66, 137, 221
    cardiac 199, 199*f*
    perforating 100
    portal 135, 136*f*
    superficial 66
Velamentous insertions of cords 308
Vena cava, superior 187, 190, 194
Venous
    drainage 386
    system, portal 32
Ventricle 324
Ventricular septal defect 197, 289, 323
Ventricular septum proper 323
Vermiform appendix 269*f*
    blood supply of 161
Vesicourethral canal 343
Villi 379
Vinculae brevia 406
Vinculae longa 406
Viral infection 182
Virchow's lymph gland 174
Virus 319
Vitamin
    A 319
    D deficiency 5
        affects 5
    D resistant rickets 299
Voice, hoarseness of 259
Volkmann's ischemic contracture 78
Voluntary muscle, classification of 20, 21*f*

W

Waldeyer's ring 218, 219*f*
Weber syndrome 249

Wedge-and-groove suture 213
Wharton's duct 398
Wrist
    and hand, posteroanterior view of 358f
    drop 53f
    joint 359

X

X chromosome inactivation 291, 291f
X syndrome, triple 288

Y

Y chromosome, role of 379
Young bone 8
Young vascular tissue 8

Z

Zona fasciculata 276, 277
Zona glomerulosa 276, 277
Zona pellucida 303, 305
Zona reticularis 276, 277
Zygomatic arch 226, 251
Zygote, gene of 318